Orofacial Disorders

João N.A.R. Ferreira • James Fricton
Nelson Rhodus
Editors

Orofacial Disorders

Current Therapies in Orofacial Pain and Oral Medicine

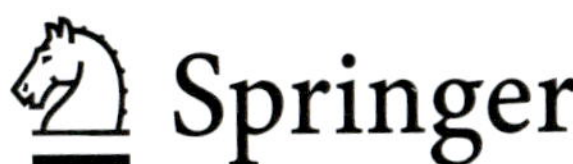

Editors
João N.A.R. Ferreira
Faculty of Dentistry
National University of Singapore
Singapore

Nelson Rhodus
Diagnostic and Surgical Sciences
University of Minnesota
Minneapolis, MN, USA

James Fricton
Diagnostic and Surgical Sciences
University of Minnesota
Edina, MN, USA

ISBN 978-3-319-84670-5 ISBN 978-3-319-51508-3 (eBook)
DOI 10.1007/978-3-319-51508-3

Softcover reprint of the hardcover 1st edition 2017

Printed on acid-free paper

This Springer imprint is published by Springer Nature
The registered company is Springer International Publishing AG
The registered company address is: Gewerbestrasse 11, 6330 Cham, Switzerland

To our families,
this book is affectionately dedicated

Preface

Orofacial disorders are common in the general population causing chewing dysfunction, dental pain, intraoral pain, facial pain, jaw pain, earaches, and/or headache. Orofacial disorders including oral cancer and lesions, oral candidiasis, salivary gland dysfunctions, temporomandibular disorders, occlusal dysfunction and dysesthesia, orofacial pain disorders, oral neurosensory disturbances, malodor, orofacial dystonias and dyskinesias, burning mouth syndrome, oral parafunctions, sleep apnea and snoring disturbances, and others are very common in all dental and medical practices with a collective prevalence of over 40% of the population. Management of these disorders differs from traditional dental practice because the dentist spends significant clinic time providing medically based evaluation and treatment for these patients. Services are usually reimbursed by time for consultation and procedures through the patient's medical insurance plans similar to physicians.

This guide is a quick reference for practicing clinicians. Its purpose is to provide a concise evidence-based clinical summary of diagnosis, etiology, and management of the most common orofacial disorders. Each chapter includes succinct bullet points, tables, and illustrations that summarize important points in understanding each orofacial disorder. In addition, interdisciplinary and multidisciplinary orofacial pain management recommendations are presented to improve effectiveness while providing patient care. Integrative therapies for pain management such as biofeedback and hypnotherapy are also presented. The last section/chapter offers a comprehensive strategy on how to conduct a structured history taking and physical exam for orofacial disorders. The guide includes the following sections: Pearls of Wisdom, Introduction and Diagnostic Subtypes, Clinical Presentation, Etiology, Epidemiology, Pathophysiology and Mechanisms, Diagnosis and Diagnostic Criteria, Rationale for Treatment, Treatment Options, Treatment Goals and Sequencing of Care, and References.

We hope this guide is helpful to your daily care of patients with these disorders.

Sincerely,

João N.A.R. Ferreira — Singapore, Singapore
James Fricton — Edina, MN, USA
Nelson Rhodus — Minneapolis, MN, USA

In Memoriam

To Dr. Sol Silverman, Dr. Jonathan Ship, and Dr. Steven Graff-Radford our compassionate colleagues and enthusiastic educators.

Contents

Part I Oral Cancer and Premalignant Lesions

1 **Leukoplakia** 3
Isaäc van der Waal

2 **Oral Cancer** 15
Douglas E. Peterson and Nelson L. Rhodus

3 **Orofacial Pain in Cancer** 21
Gary D. Klasser and Joel Epstein

Part II Oral Mucosal Diseases

4 **Herpes Simplex** 35
Andres Pinto

5 **Oral Vesiculobullous Diseases** 41
Francina Lozada-Nur and Chelsia Sim

6 **Oral Candidiasis** 53
Scott S. De Rossi and Katharine Ciarrocca

Part III Oral Diseases of the Senses

7 **Chemosensory Disorders** 63
Joseph A. D'Ambrosio

8 **Oral Malodor** 71
Patricia Lenton

Part IV Salivary Gland Dysfunctions

9 **Salivary Gland Dysfunction and Xerostomia** 89
Mahvash Navazesh

10 **Gene Therapy for Radiation-Induced Salivary Hypofunction** 95
Bruce J. Baum

11 **Salivary Hypofunction in Aging Adults** 105
Catherine Hong and João N.A.R. Ferreira

Part V Oral Parafunctions and Sleep Disorders

12 **Oral Parafunctional Behaviors** 115
Alan G. Glaros and James Fricton

13 **Obstructive Sleep Apnea and Snoring** 127
Antonio G. Romero and João N.A.R. Ferreira

Part VI Temporomandibular Disorders and Occlusal Dysfunction

14 **Temporomandibular Joint Disorders** 145
Jeffrey P. Okeson, Cristina Perez, and James R. Fricton

15 **Temporomandibular Muscle Disorders** 159
Edward F. Wright

16 **Orofacial Dystonias and Dyskinesias** 171
Gary M. Heir and José L. de la Hoz

17 **Occlusal Dysesthesia and Dysfunction** 189
Somsak Mitrirattanakul, Tan Hee Hon, and João N.A.R. Ferreira

Part VII Orofacial Pain Disorders

18 **Non-odontogenic "Tooth" Pain** 197
Flavia P. Kapos and Donald R. Nixdorf

19 **Trigeminal Neuropathic Pain and Orofacial Neuralgias**............ 213
David A. Sirois and Teekayu P. Jorns

20 **Burning Mouth Syndrome** 223
Miriam Grushka and Nan Su

Part VIII Headaches

21 **Chronic Daily Headache**.. 235
Roger K. Cady and Kathleen Farmer

22 **Migraine**.. 245
Steven B. Graff-Radford

23 **Cluster and Facial Headache**................................... 257
Robert G. Kaniecki

24 **Migraine Variants** 269
Robert L. Merrill

Part IX Health Care Approaches in Orofacial and Widespread Pains

25 Interdisciplinary and Multidisciplinary Approaches to Orofacial Pain Care 283
Shawn McMahon

26 Transformative Care for Orofacial Disorders 301
James R. Fricton

27 Integrative Approaches to Orofacial Pain: Role of Biofeedback and Hypnosis 317
Gabriel Tan, Alan Glaros, Richard Sherman, and Chin Yi Wong

Part X A Comprehensive Approach to Orofacial Disorders

28 History Taking and Physical Examination for Orofacial Disorders 327
David Ojeda Díaz and Thomas P. Sollecito

Part I

Oral Cancer and Premalignant Lesions

Leukoplakia

1

Isaäc van der Waal

Pearls of Wisdom

- Oral leukoplakia is the most common premalignant lesion or disorder of the oral mucosa.
- The expert clinician is occasionally surprised by the presence of epithelial dysplasia or even invasive squamous cell carcinoma in a leukoplakia lesion, irrespective of its clinical presentation.
- The annual malignant transformation rate amounts approximately 1–2%. Of the many predictors of future cancer development, including a vast number of genetic and molecular biomarkers, the presence and degree of epithelial dysplasia is still the most important one.
- Dysplastic leukoplakias in non-smokers carry a higher risk of cancer development.
- Malignant transformation may also occur in non-dysplastic leukoplakias.
- Spontaneous regression is rather rare. In small lesions, e.g., less than 2–3 cm, the taking of an excisional biopsy is recommended.
- Leukoplakias persisting for more than 3 months should be biopsied at least once, and, if left untreated, a biopsy should be performed thereafter if clinical changes occur.
- Symptomatic leukoplakias should always be biopsied as soon as possible.
- In case of larger or multiple lesions, surgical removal may be limited to the clinically most suspicious area, if any, and may be combined with CO_2 laser evaporation.

I. van der Waal, DDS, PhD
VU University Medical Centre/ACTA, Department of Oral and Maxillofacial Surgery/Pathology, P.O. Box 7057, 1007 MB Amsterdam, The Netherlands
e-mail: i.vanderwaal@hotmail.com

J.N.A.R. Ferreira et al. (eds.), *Orofacial Disorders*,
DOI 10.1007/978-3-319-51508-3_1

- Because of the lack of prospective randomized trials, it is questionable whether removal of leukoplakias does truly eliminate or reduce the risk of future development of oral cancer.
- All patients with leukoplakias, being actively treated or not, should be followed up with intervals of 3–6 months, depending on the histopathological findings.

1.1 Introduction

Leukoplakia is primarily a clinical term for a predominantly white lesion that cannot be wiped off and that cannot be characterized as any other definable white lesion of the oral mucosa. It is the most common premalignant lesion of the oral mucosa.

A premalignant or potentially malignant lesion is a lesion that carries a significantly increased risk of transforming into cancer. Some prefer to refer to leukoplakia as a disorder instead of a lesion since cancer development may not only occur in or adjacent to the leukoplakic area but also elsewhere in the oral cavity or the head-and-neck region.

1.2 Clinical Presentation

- Oral leukoplakias are clinically classified into homogeneous and nonhomogeneous leukoplakias.
- Homogeneous leukoplakias are consistently white and flat and usually do not cause symptoms (Fig. 1.1).
- Nonhomogeneous leukoplakias comprise lesions with a mixture of white and red changes (erythroleukoplakias) and nodular or speckled leukoplakias

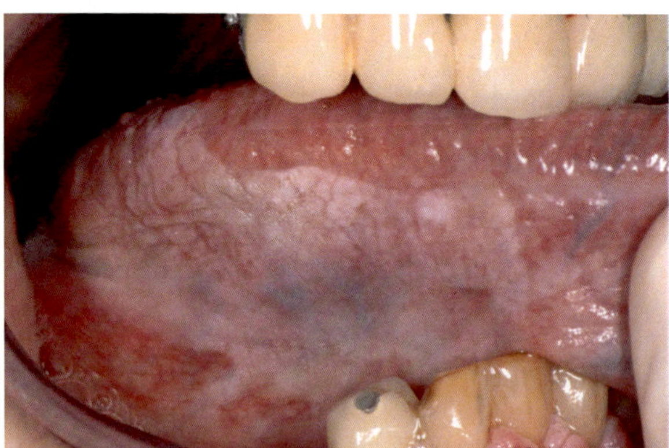

Fig. 1.1 Homogeneous (flat and thin) leukoplakia

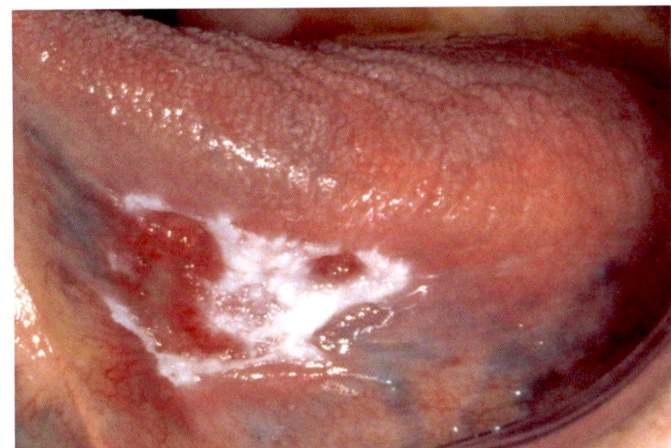

Fig. 1.2 Nonhomogeneous (erythematous) leukoplakia ("erythroleukoplakia")

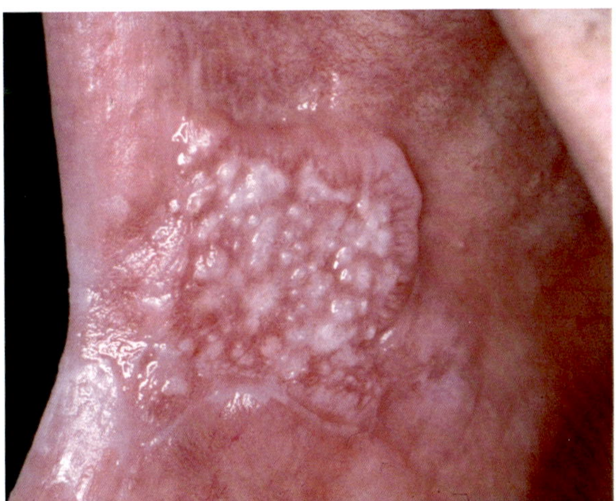

Fig. 1.3 Nonhomogeneous (nodular) leukoplakia

(Figs. 1.2 and 1.3); these nonhomogeneous leukoplakias usually cause some discomfort. Another type of nonhomogeneous leukoplakia is the verrucous leukoplakia in which there is a somewhat exophytic, verrucous texture (Fig. 1.4). Verrucous leukoplakias are usually asymptomatic. A rare subtype of verrucous leukoplakia is proliferative verrucous leukoplakia (PVL), characterized by widespread occurrence and resistance to treatment. Recurrences of PVL are, indeed, common and malignant transformation may be inevitable in many if not all patients [1].

- When redness is the predominant color of a lesion that cannot be recognized as any other definable red lesion or disorder of the oral mucosa, the term erythroplakia is applied (Fig. 1.5). Erythroplakias are usually symptomatic with a localized burning pain. Erythroplakias are less common than leukoplakias, but the risk of malignant transformation is much higher than in leukoplakias.

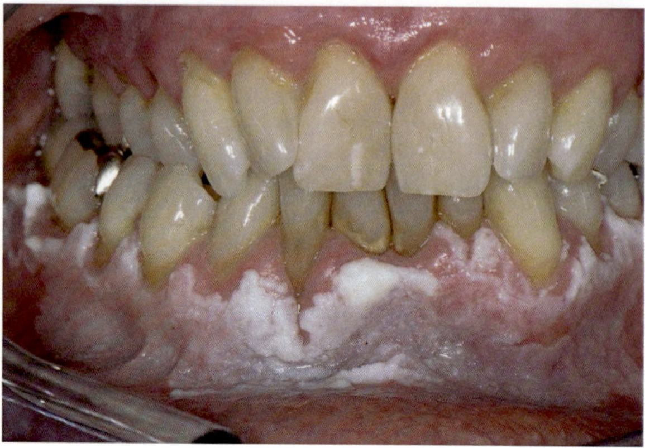

Fig. 1.4 Nonhomogeneous (verrucous) leukoplakia

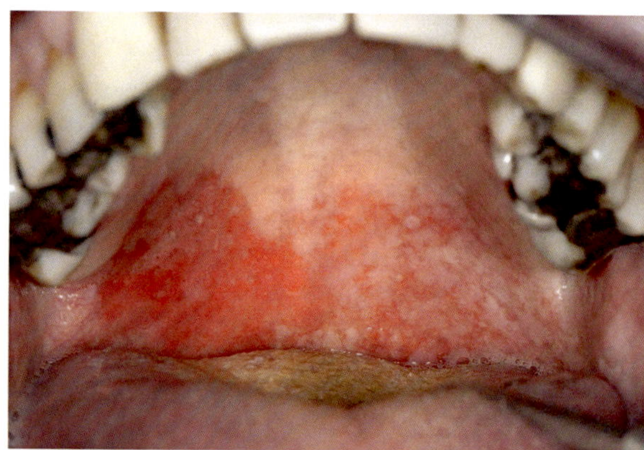

Fig. 1.5 Erythroplakia of the palate

1.3 Etiology and Epidemiology

- Oral leukoplakias occur much more often in smokers than in non-smokers.
- Other possible etiologies for oral leukoplakia include *Candida albicans* and certain human papillomaviruses.
- Limited information is available on the epidemiology of oral leukoplakia. The reported prevalence rates vary between 1.0% and 2.7% [2].
- Most affected patients are in the fourth decade of life or above.
- The male-female ratio varies in different parts of the world. In the Western world, there is no distinct gender predilection.

1.4 Pathophysiology and Mechanisms

- In patients who smoke, the epithelial changes that result in the development of leukoplakia are thought to be brought about by the carcinogens of tobacco products.
- In non-smokers with oral leukoplakia, the pathophysiology is currently unknown.
- The possible role of *Candida albicans* in the development or the malignant transformation of leukoplakia is poorly understood.
- Suggested determinants contributing to malignant potential include advanced age, female gender, size exceeding 200 mm^2, nonhomogeneous clinical type, and higher grades of epithelial dysplasia [3]. In many of the reported studies, location on the tongue is another risk factor.
- Apparently, dysplastic leukoplakias in non-smokers carry a higher risk of cancer development than in smokers [4].
- Of the numerous suggested genetic and molecular biomarkers that may be predictive of future malignant transformation, loss of heterozygosity at 9p and mutated p53 in biopsies of oral leukoplakias are at present the most promising ones [5, 6].

1.5 Diagnosis and Diagnostic Criteria

- The diagnosis of oral leukoplakia is in most cases primarily based on clinical aspects.
- White lesions that may be caused by friction, such as vigorously toothbrushing, may be diagnosed as frictional lesions but only so if the lesions have disappeared after changing the brushing habits. Otherwise, the term leukoplakia should be applied.
- Occasionally, it may be difficult to distinguish leukoplakia from other white lesions and disorders (Table 1.1); this particularly applies to the plaque type or erosive, erythematous type of lichen planus.
- Whitish or reddish changes of the oral mucosa may also be the result of direct contact with large dental restorations, particularly amalgam, being referred to as "contact lesions."
- For diagnostic purposes there is hardly a role for exfoliative cytology, brush cytology, or vital staining, such as by toluidine blue, except in case of erythroleukoplakia or erythroplakia. Nevertheless, the use of toluidine blue staining may aid in determining the site of the biopsy [7]. Preference is given to one or more incisional biopsies or, in case of a lesion less than a few centimeters in diameter, by an excisional biopsy.
- The biopsy should be taken at the site of induration, redness, or symptoms, if present. In multiple or large leukoplakias, the taking of multiple biopsies should be considered. The pathologist should be provided with proper clinical information, among others with regard to the site where the biopsy has been taken.

Table 1.1 Definable white lesions and disorders that may have a leukoplakic appearance

Lesion	Main diagnostic criteria
Alveolar ridge "keratosis"	Primarily a clinical diagnosis of a flat, white change of the mucosa of an edentulous part of the alveolar ridge; may overlap frictional lesion ("keratosis")
Aspirin burn	History of prolonged local application of aspirin tablets (paracetamol may cause similar changes)
Candidiasis, pseudomembranous, hyperplastic	Clinical aspect (pseudomembranous, often symmetrical pattern) Somewhat questionable entity; some refer to this lesion as candida-associated leukoplakia
Darier-White diseases	Associated with lesions of the skin and the nails; rather typical histopathology
Frictional "keratosis"	Disappearance of the lesion within an arbitrarily chosen period of 6–12 weeks after elimination of the suspected mechanical irritation (e.g., habit of vigorous toothbrushing); therefore, it is a retrospective diagnosis only
Geographic tongue	Primarily a clinical diagnosis; characterized by a wandering pattern in time
Glassblower lesion	Occurs only in glassblowers; disappears within a few weeks after cessation of glassblowing
Hairy leukoplakia	Clinical aspect (bilateral localization on the borders of the tongue); histopathology (including EBV immunohistochemical stain)
Lesion caused by a dental restoration (often amalgam)	Disappearance of the anatomically closely related (amalgam) restoration within an arbitrarily chosen period of 6–12 weeks after its replacement; therefore, it is a retrospective diagnosis only
Leukoedema	Clinical diagnosis (including symmetrical pattern) of a veil-like aspect of the buccal mucosa
Lichen planus, reticular type and erythematous type	Primarily a clinical diagnosis (including symmetrical pattern); histopathology is not diagnostic by its own
Linea alba	Clinical aspect (located on the line of occlusion in the cheek mucosa; almost always bilateral)
Lupus erythematosus	Primarily a clinical diagnosis (including symmetrical pattern); almost always cutaneous involvement as well. Histopathology is not diagnostic by its own
Morsicatio (habitual chewing or biting of the cheek, tongue, lips)	History of habitual chewing or biting; clinical aspects
Papilloma and allied lesions, e.g., condyloma acuminatum, multifocal epithelial hyperplasia, squamous papilloma, verruca vulgaris	Clinical aspect; medical history; HPV typing of a biopsy may be helpful
Skin graft, e.g., after a vestibuloplasty	History of a previous skin graft
Smokers' lesion	Disappearance of the lesion within an arbitrarily chosen period of 6–12 weeks after cessation of the tobacco habits; therefore, it is a retrospective diagnosis only
Smokers' palate ("stomatitis nicotinica")	Clinical aspect; history of smoking
Syphilis, secondary ("mucous patches")	Clinical aspect; demonstration of *T. pallidum*; serology
Verrucous hyperplasia and verrucous carcinoma	Clinicopathological entities
White sponge nevus	Family history; clinical aspect (often symmetrical pattern)

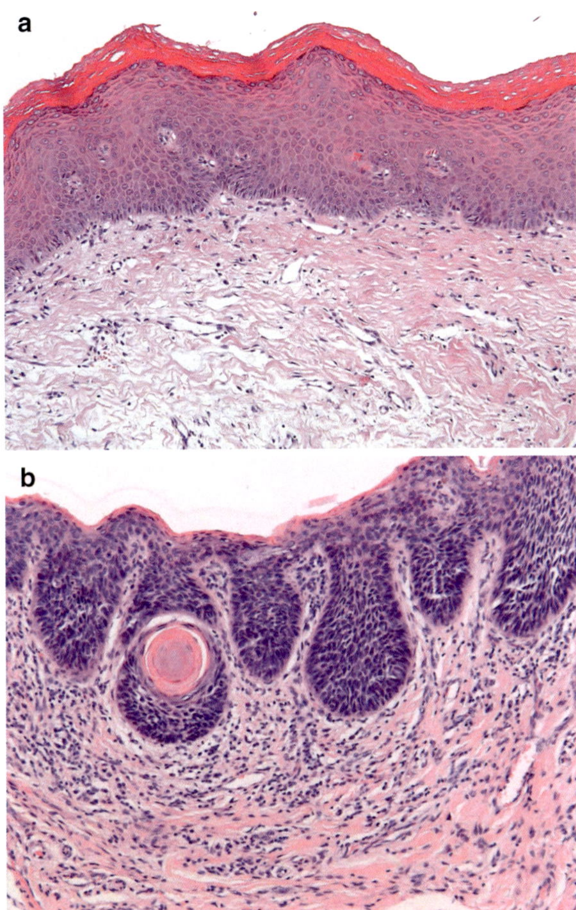

Fig. 1.6 Mild hyperkeratosis; no epithelial dysplasia (**a**); moderate epithelial dysplasia (**b**)

- The pathologist report should include a statement on the absence or presence of epithelial dysplasia and, if present, its degree. Usually three such grades are recognized, being mild, moderate, and severe (Fig. 1.6a, b). The difficulties encountered in establishing a reproducible way of dysplasia grading are well discussed in a study by Speight et al. [8].
- In rare cases, particularly in erythroplakias, carcinoma in situ or invasive squamous cell carcinoma is seen in a biopsy of a leukoplakic lesion. In such instances the diagnosis of leukoplakia is replaced by the histopathological diagnosis. In all other cases a final diagnosis of dysplastic or non-dysplastic leukoplakia remains.

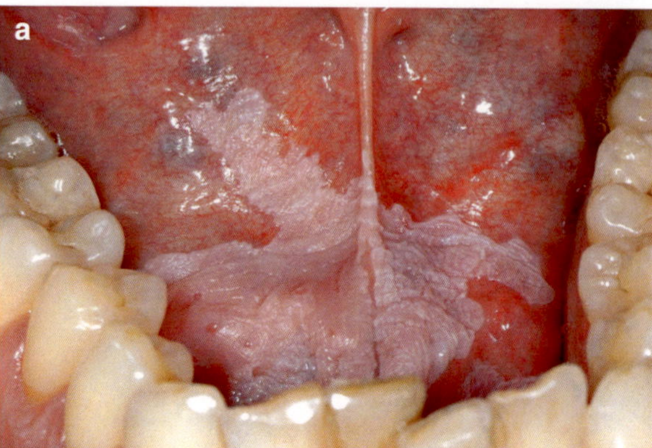

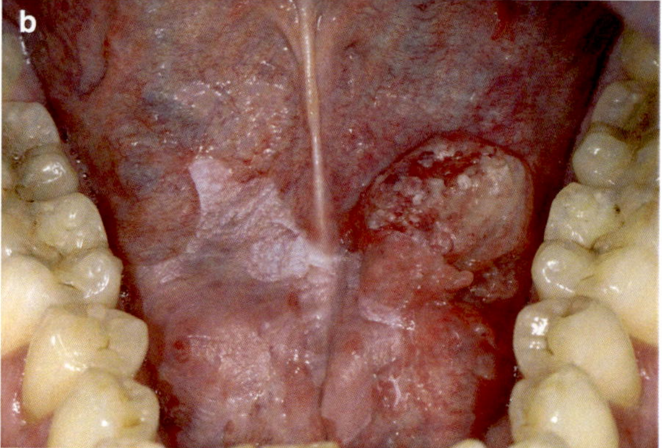

Fig. 1.7 Leukoplakia of the floor of the mouth; no treatment instituted (**a**); squamous cell carcinoma developing 4 years later (**b**)

1.6 Rationale for Treatment

Treatment is directed at removal of symptoms, if any, but above all at prevention of malignant transformation. Unfortunately, such removal may actually not entirely eliminate or reduce the risk of future development of oral cancer [9–11]. This also applies to all other surgical and nonsurgical treatment modalities.

If untreated, transformation into a squamous cell carcinoma occurs at an annual rate of approximately 1–2%. The absence or presence of epithelial dysplasia, and, if present, the degree of dysplasia as assessed by histopathological examination of a biopsy, is at present still the most reliable predictive factor of malignant transformation. Nevertheless, malignant transformation may occasionally occur in non-dysplastic leukoplakias, while some dysplastic leukoplakias may remain unchanged or regress (Fig. 1.7a, b) [12].

1.7 Treatment Options

- Spontaneous regression of oral leukoplakia is rare.
- Possible mechanical and chemical etiologic factors should be eliminated, particularly any tobacco habits, cheek and mucosal biting, sharp and irritating teeth, alcohol, and others.

- In lesions that are in close contact with large amalgam restorations, replacement of such restorations, e.g., by composite type of material or porcelain, should be considered; no reliable tests are available to predict the result of such replacement.
- Lesions smaller than a few centimeters may be excised or vaporized by CO_2 laser (but only after the taking of a biopsy), although recurrence rates may vary from 10% to 30%; in larger lesions or in case of multiple occurrences, the morbidity of treatment should be weighted against the relative low risk of malignant transformation.
- In widespread lesions, surgical intervention (including laser-based) may have to be limited to the clinically most suspicious part of the leukoplakia.

1.8 Treatment Goals and Sequencing of Care

A flowchart for the sequence of care of oral leukoplakia is showed in Table 1.2. Nevertheless, the following goals and recommendations should be taken into consideration while managing these lesions:

- Goals of treatment include a healthy mouth and a minimal risk of developing oral cancer.
- Initial treatment is aimed at cessation of tobacco habits, if any, excessive intake of alcohol, and reduction of oral habits such as cheek or mucosal biting.

Table 1.2 Flowchart with the sequence of care for the management of oral leukoplakia

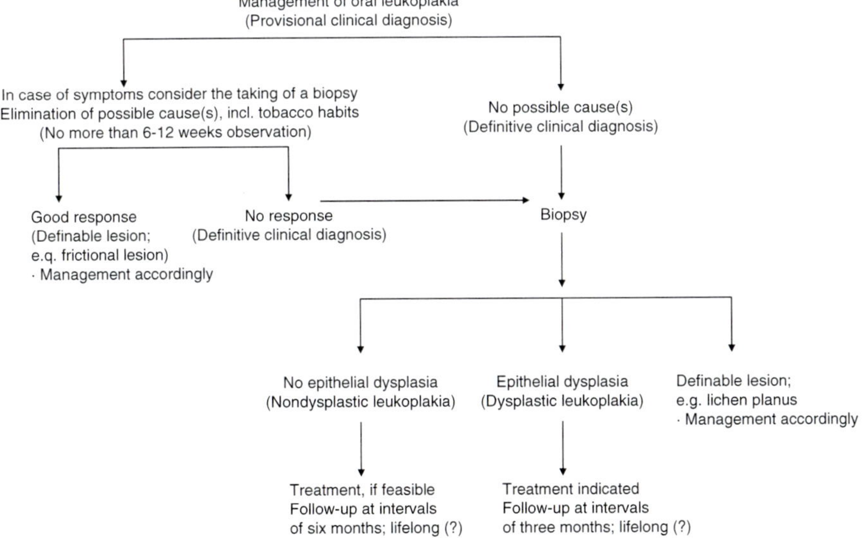

- Possible other etiologic factors should be eliminated, such as sharp edges of teeth or large amalgam restorations that are in close contact with the lesion. In symptomatic cases, it is a safe practice to first perform a biopsy.
- In the absence of etiologic factors or in persisting lesions of more than 3-month duration, performing one or more biopsies should be considered in an early stage in order to be informed about the presence and, if so, of the degree of epithelial dysplasia.
- Although removal of leukoplakia may actually not eliminate or reduce the risk of future development of oral cancer, a wait-and-see policy is for most patients, particularly in case of a small lesion, not an acceptable strategy. Such strategy may be more acceptable in non-dysplastic lesions that are too large for simple excision or (CO_2) laser treatment.
- In a few studies, wide surgical excision has resulted in a lower rate of recurrence and progression to malignancy in comparison to lesions that have been excised in a more conservative way [13, 14].
- Surgical removal is preferable above laser evaporation because of the availability of a surgical specimen that allows additional histopathological examination of the entire leukoplakic lesion.
- Cessation of smoking habits may reduce the risk of unfavorable events after surgical removal of leukoplakias in smokers [15].
- Intervals of follow-up in treated and untreated patients are largely dependent on the degree of epithelial dysplasia; in the absence of dysplasia, intervals of 6 months seem to be justified, while in case of untreated dysplastic lesions, intervals of 3 months are recommended.
- Follow-up visits are aimed at early detection of recurrences or, in untreated leukoplakias, at changes in size, color, or texture of the leukoplakia or the presence of symptoms.
- No strict rules can be provided for the length of follow-up; in patients in whom complete removal has been obtained of a non-dysplastic leukoplakia, follow-up may be completed after 3 years.

References

1. Parashar P. Proliferative verrucous leukoplakia: an elusive disorder. J Evid Based Dent Pract. 2014;(Suppl):147–53.
2. Petti S. Pooled estimate of world leukoplakia prevalence: a systematic review. Oral Oncol. 2003;39(8):770–80.
3. Warnakulasuriya S, Ariyawardana A. Malignant transformation of oral leukoplakia: a systemic review of observational studies. J Oral Pathol Med. 2015; doi: 10.1111/jop.12339. Epub ahead of print.
4. Ho MW, Risk JM, Woolgar JA, Field EA, Field JK, Steele JC, et al. The clinical determinants of malignant transformation in oral dysplasia. Oral Oncol. 2012;48(10):969–76.
5. William Jr WN. Oral premalignant lesions: any progress with systemic therapies? Curr Opin Oncol. 2012;24(3):205–2010.
6. Graveland AP, Bremmer JF, de Maaker M, Brink A, Cobussen P, Zwart M, et al. Molecular screening of oral precancer. Oral Oncol. 2013;49(12):1129–35.

7. Chainani-Wu N, Madden E, Cox D, Sroussi H, Epstein J, Silverman Jr S. Toluidine blue aids in detection of dysplasia and carcinoma in suspicious oral lesions. Oral Dis. 2015;21(7):879–85.
8. Speight PM, Abram TJ, Floriano PN, James BS, Vick J, Thornhill MH, et al. Interobserver agreement in dysplasia grading: toward an enhanced gold standard for clinical pathology trials. Oral Surg Oral Med Oral Pathol Oral Radiol. 2015;120(4):474–82.
9. Holmstrup P. Can we prevent malignancy by treating premalignant lesions? Editorial Oral Oncol. 2009;45(7):549–50.
10. Anderson A, Ishak N. Marked variation in malignant transformation rates of oral leukoplakia. Evid Based Dent. 2015;16(4):102–3.
11. Balasundaram I, Payne KF, Al-Hadad I, Alibhai M, Thomas S, Bhandari R. Is there any benefit in surgery for potentially malignant disorders of the oral cavity? J Oral Pathol Med. 2014;43(4):239–44.
12. Kuribayashi Y, Tsushima F, Morita K, Matsumoto K, Sakurai J, Uesugi A, et al. Long-term outcome of non-surgical treatment in patients with oral leukoplakia. Oral Oncol. 2015;51(11):1020–5.
13. Kuribayashi Y, Tsushima F, Sato M, Morita K, Omura K. Recurrence patterns of oral leukoplakia after curative surgical resection: important factors that predict the risk of recurrence and malignancy. J Oral Pathol Med. 2012;41(9):682–8.
14. Arnaoutakis D, Bishop J, Westra W, Califano JA. Recurrence patterns and management of oral cavity premalignant lesions. Oral Oncol. 2013;49(8):814–7.
15. Vladimirov BS, Schiødt M. The effect of quitting smoking on the risk of unfavorable events after surgical treatment of oral potentially malignant lesions. Int J Oral Maxillofac Surg. 2009;38(11):1188–93.

Oral Cancer

2

Douglas E. Peterson and Nelson L. Rhodus

Pearls of Wisdom

- Oral squamous cell carcinoma (SCC) is largely a preventable malignancy, if patients either never use tobacco or permanently discontinue its use.
- Systematic oral examinations by an experienced clinician are important for early detection and management.
- High durable cure rates (e.g., >90%) occur if the oral SCC is detected in Stage I.

2.1 Introduction

Oral and pharyngeal squamous cell carcinoma (SCC) is projected to the sixth most common malignancy [1]. Primary cause continues to be associated with tobacco use in most but not all cases. Currently, the most rapidly developed oropharyngeal cancer is caused by HPV [2, 3]. Thus, it is one of only a few human cancers that are largely preventable based on current understanding of carcinogenesis.

D.E. Peterson, DMD, PhD
Department of Oral Diagnosis, School of Dental Medicine, Pittsburgh, PA, USA

Oral Oncology Program, Neag Comprehensive Cancer Center, University of Connecticut Health Center, Farmington, CT, USA

N.L. Rhodus, DMD, MPH, FICD (✉)
Division of Oral Medicine, School of Dentistry, University of Minnesota, Minneapolis, MN, USA

Department of Otolaryngology, School of Medicine, University of Minnesota, Minneapolis, MN, USA
e-mail: rhodu001@umn.edu

J.N.A.R. Ferreira et al. (eds.), *Orofacial Disorders*,
DOI 10.1007/978-3-319-51508-3_2

Oral SCC typically both grows relatively slowly and doesn't metastasize in the early months of clinical presentation. Over time, untreated oral SCC can gradually lead to compromised oral function including speech, mastication, and/or use of dental prostheses. Early detection and treatment offers the highest incidence of long-term survival and minimizes the deleterious impact of the progressing tumor on oral symptoms and signs including pain.

2.2 Clinical Presentation

The most common sites for oral SCC include the posterior lateral tongue and floor of the mouth, lip, and oropharynx. Pain as a first complaint occurs in up to 66% of these patients, although lip pain is least frequent (27%) as an initial reason for seeking dental medical evaluation [3]. Importantly, patients are often unaware of the presence of oral SCC in its early clinical stages (Fig. 2.1). Thus, although pain is often an initial reason that causes patients to have evaluation, the pain itself may not occur until several months after clinical appearance of the lesion.

As oral SCC expands in size (Fig. 2.2), pain may develop secondary to trauma associated with the elevated mucosal surface. This is particularly common when the lesion involves the posterior lateral tongue (Fig. 2.3), a site easily traumatized during normal oral functions.

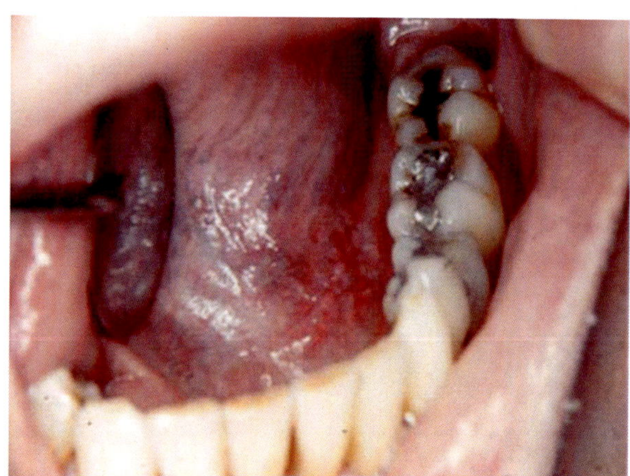

Fig. 2.1 Early squamous cell carcinoma of the left floor of mouth

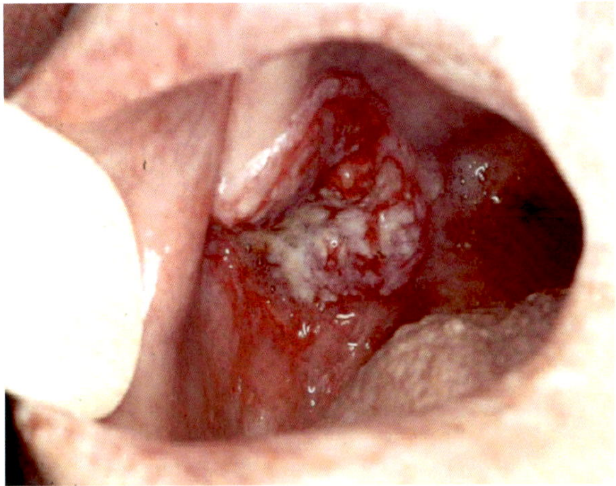

Fig. 2.2 Advanced squamous cell carcinoma of the posterior soft palate complex

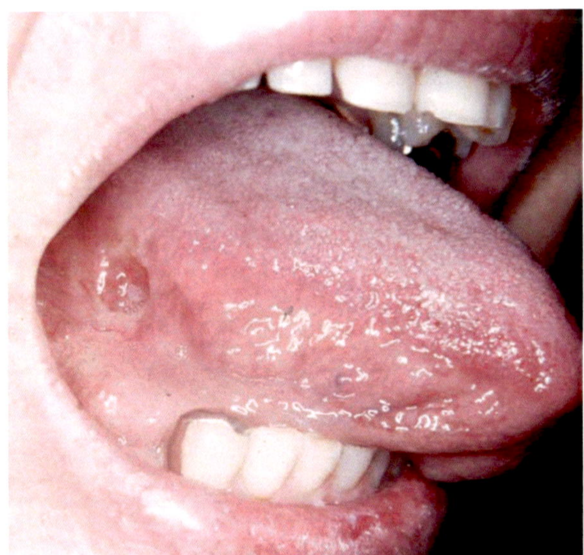

Fig. 2.3 Squamous cell carcinoma of the posterior lateral tongue (the most common location)

2.3 Etiology and Epidemiology

Etiology of oral SCC can best be viewed as a multifactorial process [2, 3]. Tobacco use, with or without alcohol abuse, has classically been identified linked with causation in >90% of these cancers. However, over the past two decades, there has been an emerging subset of patients who develop oral SCC without these obvious risk behaviors. Thus, other mechanisms including genetic alterations, mucosal immune surveillance, as well as other cofactors have been implicated as well.

Oral and pharyngeal cancers accounted for over 45,000 cases and more than 9,000 deaths in 2015 [1].

2.4 Pathophysiology and Mechanisms

The carcinogenesis model for oral SCC includes several components which can be viewed as strongly, possibly, or weakly associated with actual cancer risk [3].

Strongly associated components include:

- Tobacco use, with or without alcohol abuse
- Loss of p53 suppressor genes
- Activation of proto-oncogenes
- Diminished mucosal immune surveillance

Factors possibly linked to oral SCC carcinogenesis include [3]:

- Deficiencies in antioxidant vitamins and nutrients
- Viruses (herpesviruses, papilloma virus)

Other factors have been investigated relative to their role in carcinogenesis and have to date not been demonstrated to be important cofactors. These cofactors include:

- Deficiency or excess of dietary proteins, fats, or carbohydrates
- Denture trauma
- Dental radiographs
- Fluoridated water

2.5 Diagnosis and Diagnostic Criteria

The gold standard for diagnosis remains incisional or excisional biopsy followed by histopathologic confirmation [3]. Selection of the biopsy site as well as of the histopathology sections to be interpreted is critically important to maximizing detection of malignancy. This diagnostic strategy, coupled with additional clinical and radiographic assessment, is typically sufficient to both confirm the final diagnosis and to define the staging of the patient.

This approach needs to be considered in the context of screening and prevention, as well as the essential need for detailed inspection of the oral mucosa by a health professional well experienced in detecting subtle physical changes in the tissue. The requirement for experienced examiners is heightened by the fact that the oral cancer may be located on oral mucosal tissue that cannot be easily inspected without careful manipulation of the oral soft tissue. Since many oral SCCs are located on posterior lateral tongue, floor of mouth, and retromolar pad, detailed and systematic inspection of all oral mucosal tissues at risk is required.

Adjunctive diagnostic aids [3] include:

- *Toluidine blue oral rinse*: metachromatic dye that may enhance selection of biopsy site when broad field of suspicious tissue is present
- *Oral cytology and brush biopsy*: minimally invasive technique that can be useful in determining whether incisional or excisional biopsy may be required

Additional diagnostic strategies including imaging (computed tomography, magnetic resonance imaging) are also important regarding staging, once the diagnosis of oral cancer has been confirmed histopathologically.

2.6 Rationale for Treatment

Treatment rationale is directed to surgical removal, combined with cytotoxic therapy (radiation with or without chemotherapy) in more advanced cases [3]. Decisions as to which treatment strategy will be used are principally governed by the following considerations:

- Tumor histopathologic diagnosis
- Location of tumor in relation to normal oral hard and soft tissue
- Tumor stage of patient

2.7 Treatment Options

Stage I tumors are typically removed surgically, with >90% cure rates resulting. No additional therapy, including radiation therapy or chemotherapy, is generally indicated. Chronic morbidity resulting from the surgery is rare, given the relatively conservative surgical approach and the location of most tumors [3].

Surgical treatment of more advanced tumors is typically the primary therapeutic choice as well. If there is evidence of metastasis, radiation therapy with or without concomitant chemotherapy is indicated.

Treatment may thus be single modality or multimodality, depending on stage:

- Surgical removal is the primary therapy for Stage I and early Stage II (*confirm II*).
- Surgery followed by radiation is the primary therapy for advanced Stage II and Stage III.
- Surgical debulking, followed by radiation and concomitant high-dose chemotherapy, is frequently utilized for the most advanced stages.

2.8 Treatment Goals and Sequencing of Care

Durable cure is the ideal treatment goal. However, diagnosis of advanced tumors (e.g., Stage III or IV) results in higher mortality rates sooner, versus cancers that are diagnosed at an early clinical stage.

For all stages of oral cavity and pharyngeal cancers, approximately 85% of patients are alive 1 year following diagnosis [1]. Overall, the 5- and 10-year survival rates are 59% and 44%, respectively [1]. Furthermore, there is a population bias such that American black men have a disproportionately high 5-year mortality rate [1].

References

1. Siegel RL, Miller KD, Jemal A. Cancer statistics, 2016. CA Cancer J Clin. 2016;65:5–29.
2. Silverman Jr S. Epidemiology. In: Silverman Jr S, editor. Oral cancer. 5th ed. Hamilton: BC Decker; 2003. p. 1–6.
3. Rhodus NL, Kerr AR, Patel K. Oral cancer: leukoplakia and squamous cell carcinoma (Chapter 6). In: Sollectio TS, editor. Dental clinics of North America. Oral lesions. Saunders: Philadelphia; vol. 57, issue 3; 2014. p. 143–56. ISBN-978-0-323-28995-5.

Orofacial Pain in Cancer

3

Gary D. Klasser and Joel Epstein

Pearls of Wisdom

- Mild-to-moderate pain is present in the majority of HNC patients at the time of diagnosis.
- Orofacial pain due to HNC is the most common reason patients seek diagnosis.
- Pain arising in cancer patients usually have a multifactorial etiology and require a multidisciplinary management approach.
- The approach to treatment of pain from malignant origin and all cancer therapies that are pain focused must follow guidelines of WHO analgesic ladder, including topical therapy for oropharyngeal pain, and use of adjunctive medications and pain management strategies.

3.1 Introduction

Pain in cancer patients may develop due to the primary disease and/or be due to single or multimodal cancer therapy, all of which can damage epithelial and connective tissues (Table 3.1). Head and neck cancer (HNC) patients report pain

G.D. Klasser, DMD (✉)
Louisiana State University Health Sciences Center, School of Dentistry, Department of Diagnostic Sciences, 1100 Florida Avenue, Box 140, New Orleans, LA 70119, USA
e-mail: gklass@lsuhsc.edu

J. Epstein, DMD, MSD, FRCD(C), FDS RCS (Edin)
Samuel Oschin Comprehensive Cancer Institute, Cedars Sinai Health System, 8700 Beverly Drive, Los Angeles, CA 90048, USA

Division of Otolaryngology and Head and Neck Surgery, City of Hope, 1500 East Duarte Road, Duarte, CA 91010, USA

J.N.A.R. Ferreira et al. (eds.), *Orofacial Disorders*,
DOI 10.1007/978-3-319-51508-3_3

Table 3.1 Classification of orofacial pain in cancer patients

Orofacial pain due to cancer
Pain due to direct effects of tumor
Orofacial pain due to cancer management
Pain due to chemotherapy, targeted therapy, immunotherapy
Pain due radiotherapy
Pain due to surgery
Orofacial pain due to other etiology

symptoms that often include both nociceptive and neuropathic components. Noteworthy, is that orofacial pain due to HNC is the most common reason patients seek diagnosis.

3.2 Clinical Presentation and Diagnostic Subtypes

Mild-to-moderate pain is present in up to 85% of HNC patients at the time of diagnosis. In a study by Potter et al. [1], it was reported that pain was identified in 56% of patients with HNC at diagnosis, and they found mixed nociceptive and neuropathic pain in 93% of those with pain. Pain due to HNC therapy is a well-recognized adverse effect of treatment. It presents unique challenges due to the extensive innervation of the orofacial region. Additionally, oral intake, swallowing, speech, and other motor functions of the head, neck, and oropharynx are constant orofacial pain triggers.

Furthermore, the oral mucosa is susceptible to the effects of systemic chemotherapy and regional radiotherapy, often resulting in painful mucositis and neuropathy. Pain due to oropharyngeal mucositis is the most debilitating complaint impacting quality of life during cancer therapy in HNC patients and in those receiving hematopoietic cell transplant (HCT). Pain due to oropharyngeal mucositis impacts all aspects of oral function, including intake of food and medications, and frequently requires opioid analgesics for pain management. Mucositis may lead to admission to hospital, prolong hospital admissions, and admission to intensive care. This may negatively affect cancer treatment as it will delay, interrupt, or discontinue previously planned cancer therapies.

3.3 Etiology and Epidemiology

In a retrospective study of 1,412 patients with oral cancer, pain was identified as the first sign of cancer in 19%, and pain was commonly reported with tumor recurrence [2]. Others reported cancer-related pain in 52% of hospitalized patients, with pain directly related to tumor in 29% and to surgery in 50% [3, 4]. In large surveys of pain characteristics in cancer including HNC [5, 6], patients experienced pain associated with the tumor (87–92.5%) or cancer therapy (17–20.8%) or both. Mechanistically, as the tumor progresses, pain may progress; unfortunately, diagnosis remains common at advanced stage disease rather than at initial presentation, thereby reducing performance status, increasing anxiety and depressive symptoms, weakening quality of life, and rising morbidity and mortality.

Optimal pain management requires recognition of etiological/contributing factors (which may be multiple), an understanding of the neurobiology of pain, and addressing the components of the patient's pain. Successful management may require multidisciplinary approaches to care and must address the complex sensory and physiologic components, affective and cognitive dimensions, as well as behavioral and sociocultural issues.

Orofacial pain may be due to the following sources:

- Regional disease
- Metastatic cancer with the most common metastases to the head, neck, and oral cavity from breast, lung, gastrointestinal tract, and prostate cancers
- Oral involvement by systemic cancers (e.g., hematologic malignancies)
- Referral of pain from remote cancer most commonly from the lungs

Pain due to cancer may have multiple causes: may be due to mechanical factors and biochemical factors (Table 3.2). Leukemia, lymphoma, and multiple myeloma may cause head and neck manifestations with direct involvement of oral tissues or secondary infection due to immunosuppression and myelosuppression. Pain may present as temporomandibular disorders (TMD) as reported in a study of patients with nasopharyngeal cancer [7]. Orofacial neuropathic pain may occur with tumor involvement of cranial nerves, with intracranial tumors or as result of cancer therapy.

Table 3.2 Mechanisms of pain in oncology – mechanical and biochemical processes

Type of pain			Processes
Pain due to tumor			Mass, ulceration, invasion, pressure, ischemia, molecular sensitization, and stimulation
Pain due to treatment	Surgery	Acute	Incision, inflammation, ischemia, infection, discontinuity, inflammation, molecular sensitization, and stimulation
		Chronic	Neuropathy, ischemia, fibrosis, molecular sensitization, and stimulation
	Radiation therapy	Acute	Mucositis, infection, molecular sensitization, and stimulation
		Chronic	Neuropathy, atrophy, hyposalivation, ischemia, fibrosis, molecular sensitization, and stimulation
	Chemotherapy/targeted therapy, immunotherapy	Acute	Mucositis, infection, molecular sensitization, and stimulation
		Chronic	Neuropathy, fibrosis, molecular sensitization, and stimulation
Pain not related to cancer or cancer therapy			
Psychosocial factors			

3.4 Pathophysiology and Diagnosis: Importance on Understanding Mechanisms

3.4.1 Mechanisms of Orofacial Pain from Cancer

Progresses in the study of mechanisms of cancer-related pain are being made [8–18]. The malignant disease may cause pain due to several mechanisms:

- Tissue damage and release of inflammatory and pain mediators (Table 3.3).
- Traction, invasion, or compression of pain-sensitive structures including nerves, vessels, bone, and skin or mucosal ulceration.
- Malignancy associated with bone pain includes stretching or invasion of periosteum, nerve root infiltration, and compression and reactive muscle involvement.
- Ischemia due to obstruction of blood vessels may lead to necrosis and release of cellular products and cytokines.
- Malignant cells may lead to local release of numerous proteolytic enzymes, sensitizers, and mediators including prostaglandins [19, 20], growth factors, neurotransmitters, interleukins, endothelins, glutamate, calcitonin gene-related peptide, serotonin, norepinephrine, and prodynorphin. Additionally, there is an upregulation of expression of COX-2 [21].
- Some cancers including those of the oropharynx may elaborate circulating humoral factors, including cytokines, that cause central sensitization that may lead to persisting pain [19–21]. Uric acid production is increased in malignancies with rapid cell turnover, and with rapid cell kill due to treatment, a decrease in the threshold for the transient receptor potential vanilloid receptor (TRPV1 – the capsaicin receptor) and evoke response [22] via the acid-sensing ion channel (ASIC) receptor family may occur [23, 24].

3.4.2 Mechanisms Due to Nonsurgical Management of Cancer

Chemotherapy may cause neuropathy that may present in the head, neck, and oral cavity as treatments result in numerous changes to cellular structure and function, including loss of sensory terminals in the skin, and alterations of membrane

Table 3.3 Mechanisms of pain due to tumor

Tissue damaged	Mechanisms
Mucosa	Infiltration, ulceration, inflammation, secondary infection
Bone	Infiltration, microfractures, inflammation, hypoxia
Muscle	Hypoxia, inflammation, spasm, fibrosis
Vessel	Traction, compression, obstruction, inflammation
Neural	Local sensitization, inflammation, ectopic firing, compression, central sensitization, reduced descending inhibition

receptors, intracellular signaling, neurotransmission, excitability, and metabolism all of which can negatively influence neuronal and glial cell phenotypes [25]. Commonly used neurotoxic agents such as the taxanes (paclitaxel, docetaxel), vinca alkaloids (vincristine, vinblastine), platinum-based compounds (cisplatin, oxaliplatin), antimitotics (methotrexate, cytosine arabinoside, and fluorouracil), thalidomide, and bortezomib and targeted cancer therapies are responsible. Chemotherapeutic drugs usually affect sensory nerves (positive and negative symptoms), but motor (muscle weakness and atrophy) and autonomic nerves (hypotension, cardiac conduction irregularities, impotence, and bowel and bladder involvement) may also be affected [26]. Interestingly, both small diameter sensory fibers – unmyelinated C fibers and thinly myelinated A-delta fibers – and large myelinated A-beta fibers are affected by chemotherapeutic agents with the large fibers being preferentially injured by chemotherapeutic agents such as vinca alkaloids, taxanes, and platinum-based compounds. The timing of presentation of neuropathic symptoms after chemotherapy is quite variable after cancer therapy. Agents such as cisplatin manifest signs of neuropathy, which occur about 1 month after the therapy, while oxaliplatin may produce symptoms within 30–60 min after the infusion. Neuropathic pain associated with vinca alkaloids may begin several days after administration and may involve the trigeminal and glossopharyngeal nerve distributions.

Radiation therapy has also been associated with neuropathic pain. The severity of the neuropathic pain is related to radiation exposure, the dose of radiation, and vicinity to major nerves or nerve plexus. The mechanism of radiation-induced neuropathies is not well understood, but possible causes include radiation-induced tissue fibrosis and associated factors such as ischemia, oxidative stress, and inflammation [27]. Acute symptoms that may present with hypoesthesia and with triggered neuralgia-like pain occur during therapy but are uncommon. Radiation-induced neuropathy can present from 6 months to 20 years after receiving treatment. Radiation therapy also results in hypocellular, hypovascular, and hypoxic tissue leading to reduced capacity of bone to recover from injury leading to risk of osteonecrosis. The current prevalence rate of osteoradionecrosis is less than 4%. Pain, bad breath, taste alteration, and trismus are among the major symptoms associated with osteonecrosis. The onset varies and may appear decades following radiotherapy. Recently, reports of necrosis have been seen in patients on antiresorptive therapies (bisphosphonate or monoclonal antibody) and other drugs affecting vascular function (e.g., bevacizumab, sunitinib). Although no specific studies are available on the mechanisms of pain in osteonecrosis, it is possible that the ischemia, reduced pH, inflammatory mediator release, and secondary infection are associated with pain. Secondary bacterial infection and pathologic fracture in osteonecrosis may occur thereby compounding symptoms. Muscle fibrosis is another complication associated with radiation therapy (in addition to surgical intervention), and this may lead to change in function of the jaw, which coupled with stress, and anxiety/depression may result in TMD and pain or complicate pre-existing TMD. In addition, scar tissue formation may alter local anatomy and function, leading to pain and dysfunction.

Taste is also altered as an early response to radiation therapy and may present as a reduction in taste sensitivity (hypogeusia), an absence of taste sensation (ageusia), or a distortion of normal taste (dysgeusia) [28]. Taste impairment greatly impacts the quality of life of the patient, and coupled with other radiation therapy-related comorbidities such as mucositis, hyposalivation, dysphagia, and reduced food enjoyment, radiation therapy may affect the nutritional status and overall health of the patient [29, 30]. Ninety percent of all patients experience a loss of taste when the cumulative dose has reached 60 Gy. Direct radiation damage to the taste buds or innervating fibers is the proposed caused of taste loss in addition to the reduction in salivary flow. Histologically, taste buds show signs of degeneration and atrophy at 10 Gy (2 Gy per day), while at therapeutic levels, the architecture of the taste buds is almost completely destroyed. Taste loss is usually transient, gradually returning to normal or near normal levels within 1-year postradiation therapy; however, it also may be prolonged.

Oropharyngeal mucosal pain may be aggravated by hyposalivation and secondary mucosal infection (e.g., fungal, bacterial, viral). Pain may also arise in salivary glands due to sialadenitis during early phases of radiation therapy and in cases of secondary infection of the salivary glands associated with hyposalivation.

Oral graft versus host disease, a result of donor cells leading to immune-mediated inflammation and damage of recipient tissues of the host, may involve the mucosa that is associated with pain and may be associated with hyposalivation that may in turn lead to mucosal sensitivity, mucosal infection, mucosal ulceration, and risk of trauma as well as increased risk of salivary gland infection.

3.4.3 Mechanisms Due to Surgical Procedures for Cancer

Acute surgical pain is an easily understood complication of head and neck and oral pain in cancer patients, and residual neurosensory impairment following mandibular resection is common, although some recovery may occur over time (Table 3.3). Postsurgical neuropathy involving anesthesia and dysesthetic, allodynic, and hyperpathic pain which may become chronic occurs following surgery involving cervical procedures which are commonly part of HNC. In addition to tissue injury from resection of the tumor and radical neck dissection, local trauma due to endoscopy or intubation may result in oropharyngeal pain. Surveys of surgically treated cases of oral cancer show chronic pain are common despite treatment with different classes of analgesics and physical therapy [31, 32]. Shoulder complaints are a common site of pain in HNC patients, followed by the oral cavity, neck, and temporomandibular joint each accounting for approximately 5% of postoperative complaints. Orofacial and head and neck complaints are reported by approximately 50% of treated cancer patients, affecting their quality of life.

Table 3.4 Cancer therapy and oropharyngeal mucositis

Disease/therapy		% of patients
UADTCa	RT alone	>80% RT
	Chemo/RT	Up to 100%
Intensive chemotherapy with HCT rescue		Up to 75% with HSV prophylaxis
Solid cancers of GI/GU, breast with neutropenia inducing chemotherapy		Up to 50% of courses, ulcerative mucositis in up to 20% of courses

UADTCa upper aerodigestive cancer, *RT* radiation therapy, *Chemo* chemotherapy, *HCT* hematopoietic cell transplant, *GI/GU* gastrointestinal, genitourinary, *HSV* herpes simplex virus

3.4.4 Mechanisms Due to Secondary Effects from Radiotherapy and/or Chemotherapy (Mucositis)

Pain may arise as erythema develops during mucositis development and intensifies with formation of ulceration and/or pseudomembrane presentation (Table 3.4). Oral pain associated with mucositis in HNC patients and in HCT/leukemia patients commonly require opioids for pain management. In HNC patients treated with the combination of radiation and chemotherapy, an increase in pain may be seen at week 3 that may peak at week 5 with persistence due to mucositis with gradual remission occurring as mucositis resolves [33].

Mucositis and pain due to chemotherapy may arise within 7–10 days of treatment, with resolution in 1–3 weeks. In addition, mucosal pain may persist long after mucositis resolves and sensitivity persisting at 1-year follow-up is common and may be related to mucosal atrophy and neuropathy in the treatment volume. Targeted chemotherapy may cause neurotoxicity and may also cause mucosal ulceration with aphthous-like presentation and result in pain [34, 35]. Further, immunotherapies (immune check point inhibitors) may stimulate immune/inflammatory reactions leading to pain presenting in the oral mucosa and oropharynx as part of the gastrointestinal tract [36].

The direct stomatotoxic effect of chemoradiotherapy results in connective tissue and epithelial changes resulting in generation of free radicals, release of pro-inflammatory cytokines, and reduced epithelial renewal that may result in mucositis (Tables 3.3 and 3.5). Studies of potential nociceptive compounds in mucositis have been considered [37]. Cellular necrosis and apoptosis and secondary inflammation may enhance pain by nociceptor sensitization and direct stimulation of nociceptors. Inflammatory substances released from damaged tissue and from inflammatory cells directly stimulate or increase the excitability of nociceptors. Degranulation of mast cells and platelets and breakdown of tumor and normal cells may result in release of cellular contents including histamine and cytokines. Inflammatory mediators directly activate and sensitize primary afferent nociceptors [37]. Tumor acidity and inflammation also lead to lower pH that may activate proton-induced pain pathways. As mucositis progresses to ulcerative stages, secondary bacterial colonization may further stimulate cytokine release, which may enhance the inflammatory response and aggravate pain.

Table 3.5 Potential molecular sensitizers and mediators of pain in cancer

Neurotoxicity:
Radiotherapy, chemotherapy, targeted therapies
Cellular necrosis and apoptosis:
Cell contents enhance inflammation and nociception
Tumor acidity and inflammation lower pH, activate proton-induced pain
Inflammatory substances: damaged tissue and inflammatory cells
Cytokines/growth factors:
Tumor necrosis factor (TNF), interleukins (IL-1, IL-6), platelet-derived growth factor (PDGF), epidermal growth factor (EGF), transforming growth factor (TGF), vasoactive intestinal peptide (VIP), vascular endothelial growth factor (VEGF), nerve growth factor (NGF), endothelins
Sensory neurotransmitters:
Serotonin, noradrenaline, bradykinin, substance P, calcitonin gene-related peptide (CGRP), excitatory amino acids (e.g., glutamate, which activates N-methyl-D-aspartate receptors) and hydrogen ions (protons), reactive oxygen species
Inflammatory mediators:
Pro-inflammatory cytokines, histamine
Arachidonic acid metabolites: prostaglandins, leukotrienes
Adenosine, adenosine 5′-triphosphate, nitric oxide
Other:
Infection:
Microbial waste products, pH, increase inflammation, pro-inflammatory cytokines, inflammatory cell activity
COX-2 upregulation

3.4.5 Orofacial Pain Due to Other Etiologies

Pain unrelated to cancer or its therapy includes all types of pain due to pulpal or periodontal origin and musculoskeletal pain including TMD. Pain occurring in cancer patients is likely to be associated with heightened anxiety which impacts pain experience, presentation, and pain behavior. The psychological state influences all pains, and the longer a patient suffers, the greater the influence of these factors.

3.5 Rationale for Treatment

Pain prevention and management will be improved with further understanding of molecular and neurophysiologic mechanisms underlying the pain complaint [38–41]. Current management requires assessment of the components of the presenting pain, treating the primary disease and the components of pain, diagnosis, and treatment of contributing factors of pain.

3.6 Treatment Options, Goals, and Sequence of Care

The approach to treatment of pain from malignant origin and all therapies that are pain focused should follow guidelines of WHO analgesic ladder, including topical therapy for oropharyngeal pain (Table 3.6), and the use of adjunctive medications and pain management strategies (Table 3.7). Several factors may have potential for a targeted therapy:

- Serotonin
- Norepinephrine
- Substance P

Table 3.6 Current management of orofacial cancer pain

Diagnosis and treatment of primary disease:
Cancer therapy
Diagnosis and treatment of infections:
Herpesviruses, candida, dental and periodontal and salivary gland infection
Symptom management:
Topical agents: anesthetics, analgesics (cytokines, prostaglandins, etc.)
WHO ladder:
Topical anesthetics/analgesics
Analgesics (prostaglandins, COX2)
Nonsteroidal analgesics, acetaminophen
Mild opioid combination agents
Strong opioids and nonsteroidal analgesics, acetaminophen
Adjunctive centrally acting medications:
Anticonvulsants
Antidepressants
Tricyclics, gabapentinoids, serotonin norepinephrine reuptake inhibitors
Anxiolytics, sleep promoters
Muscle relaxants
Adjunctive techniques:
Physical therapy including orofacial appliances, acupuncture, low-level laser therapy (LLLT), psychological techniques
Assessment and management of hyposalivation
Address dentinal sensitivity

Table 3.7 Additional and complimentary pain management techniques in oncology

Palliative radiation therapy
Cold/moist heat applications
Low-level laser therapy
Hypnosis
Acupuncture
Psychological:
Cognitive/behavioral therapy
Distraction techniques
Relaxation/guided imagery techniques
Music therapy; drama therapy
Counseling

- Calcitonin gene-related peptide (CGRP)
- N-methyl-D-aspartate (NMDA)
- Prostaglandins
- COX-2
- Tumor necrosis factor alpha (TNFα)
- Nerve growth factor (NGF)
- Vascular endothelial growth factor (VEGF)
- Nerve growth factor inducible (NGFi)
- Altered tissue pH
- Interleukins
- Nociceptor sensitization and stimulation

These targeted therapies may provide hope for improvement in pain management. Multidisciplinary management, rational use of topical and systemic analgesics, adjuvant medications, and additional/adjunctive pain management techniques provide the optimal pain management due to tumor presence and to complications of cancer therapies.

References

1. Potter J, Higginson IJ, Scadding JW, Quigley C. Identifying neuropathic pain in patients with head and neck cancer: use of the Leeds Assessment of Neuropathic Symptoms and Signs Scale. J R Soc Med. 2003;96(8):379–83.
2. Cuffari L, Tesseroli de Siqueira JT, Nemr K, Rapaport A. Pain complaint as the first symptom of oral cancer: a descriptive study. Oral Surg Oral Med Oral Pathol Oral Radiol Endod. 2006;102(1):56–61.
3. Holtan A, Aass N, Nordoy T, Haugen DF, Kaasa S, Mohr W, et al. Prevalence of pain in hospitalised cancer patients in Norway: a national survey. Palliat Med. 2007;21(1):7–13.
4. Ripamonti C, Zecca E, Brunelli C, Groff L, Boffi R, Caraceni A, et al. Pain experienced by patients hospitalized at the National Cancer Institute of Milan: research project "towards a pain-free hospital". Tumori. 2000;86(5):412–8.
5. Caraceni A, Portenoy RK. An international survey of cancer pain characteristics and syndromes. IASP Task Force on Cancer Pain. International Association for the Study of Pain. Pain. 1999;82(3):263–74.
6. Grond S, Zech D, Diefenbach C, Radbruch L, Lehmann KA. Assessment of cancer pain: a prospective evaluation in 2266 cancer patients referred to a pain service. Pain. 1996;64(1):107–14.
7. Epstein JB, Jones CK. Presenting signs and symptoms of nasopharyngeal carcinoma. Oral Surg Oral Med Oral Pathol. 1993;75(1):32–6.
8. Mantyh PW. Bone cancer pain: from mechanism to therapy. Curr Opin Support Palliat Care. 2014;8(2):83–90.
9. Middlemiss T, Laird BJ, Fallon MT. Mechanisms of cancer-induced bone pain. Clin Oncol (R Coll Radiol). 2011;23(6):387–92.
10. Zhu XC, Zhang JL, Ge CT, Yu YY, Wang P, Yuan TF, et al. Advances in cancer pain from bone metastasis. Drug Des Dev Ther. 2015;9:4239–45.
11. Schmidt BL, Hamamoto DT, Simone DA, Wilcox GL. Mechanism of cancer pain. Mol Interv. 2010;10(3):164–78.
12. Basbaum AI, Bautista DM, Scherrer G, Julius D. Cellular and molecular mechanisms of pain. Cell. 2009;139(2):267–84.

13. Dubner R. The neurobiology of persistent pain and its clinical implications. Suppl Clin Neurophysiol. 2004;57:3–7.
14. Grace PM, Hutchinson MR, Maier SF, Watkins LR. Pathological pain and the neuroimmune interface. Nat Rev Immunol. 2014;14(4):217–31.
15. Okuse K. Pain signalling pathways: from cytokines to ion channels. Int J Biochem Cell Biol. 2007;39(3):490–6.
16. Oranger A, Carbone C, Izzo M, Grano M. Cellular mechanisms of multiple myeloma bone disease. Clin Dev Immunol. 2013;2013:289458.
17. Villa A, Sonis ST. Mucositis: pathobiology and management. Curr Opin Oncol. 2015;27(3):159–64.
18. Lippitz BE. Cytokine patterns in patients with cancer: a systematic review. Lancet Oncol. 2013;14(6):e218–28.
19. Daughaday WH, Deuel TF. Tumor secretion of growth factors. Endocrinol Metab Clin N Am. 1991;20(3):539–63.
20. Mantyh PW, Clohisy DR, Koltzenburg M, Hunt SP. Molecular mechanisms of cancer pain. Nat Rev Cancer. 2002;2(3):201–9.
21. Sanchez OH. Insights into novel biological mediators of clinical manifestations in cancer. AACN Clin Issues. 2004;15(1):112–8.
22. Tominaga M, Caterina MJ, Malmberg AB, Rosen TA, Gilbert H, Skinner K, et al. The cloned capsaicin receptor integrates multiple pain-producing stimuli. Neuron. 1998;21(3):531–43.
23. Julius D, Basbaum AI. Molecular mechanisms of nociception. Nature. 2001;413(6852):203–10.
24. Sutherland SP, Cook SP, McCleskey EW. Chemical mediators of pain due to tissue damage and ischemia. Prog Brain Res. 2000;129:21–38.
25. Boyette-Davis JA, Walters ET, Dougherty PM. Mechanisms involved in the development of chemotherapy-induced neuropathy. Pain Manag. 2015;5(4):285–96.
26. Dropcho EJ. Neurotoxicity of cancer chemotherapy. Semin Neurol. 2010;30(3):273–86.
27. Dropcho EJ. Neurotoxicity of radiation therapy. Neurol Clin. 2010;28(1):217–34.
28. Epstein JB, Barasch A. Taste disorders in cancer patients: pathogenesis, and approach to assessment and management. Oral Oncol. 2010;46(2):77–81.
29. Coa KI, Epstein JB, Ettinger D, Jatoi A, McManus K, Platek ME, et al. The impact of cancer treatment on the diets and food preferences of patients receiving outpatient treatment. Nutr Cancer. 2015;67(2):339–53.
30. Alvarez-Camacho M, Gonella S, Ghosh S, Kubrak C, Scrimger RA, Chu KP, et al. The impact of taste and smell alterations on quality of life in head and neck cancer patients. Qual Life Res. 2016;25(6):1495–504.
31. Gellrich NC, Schimming R, Schramm A, Schmalohr D, Bremerich A, Kugler J. Pain, function, and psychologic outcome before, during, and after intraoral tumor resection. J Oral Maxillofac Surg. 2002;60(7):772.
32. Weymuller EA, Yueh B, Deleyiannis FW, Kuntz AL, Alsarraf R, Coltrera MD. Quality of life in patients with head and neck cancer: lessons learned from 549 prospectively evaluated patients. Arch Otolaryngol Head Neck Surg. 2000;126(3):329–35.
33. Al-Ansari S, Zecha JA, Barasch A, de Lange J, Rozema FR, Raber-Durlacher JE. Oral mucositis induced by anticancer therapies. Curr Oral Health Rep. 2015;2(4):202–11.
34. Boers-Doets CB, Raber-Durlacher JE, Treister NS, Epstein JB, Arends AB, Wiersma DR, et al. Mammalian target of rapamycin inhibitor-associated stomatitis. Future Oncol. 2013;9(12):1883–92.
35. Watters AL, Epstein JB, Agulnik M. Oral complications of targeted cancer therapies: a narrative literature review. Oral Oncol. 2011;47(6):441–8.
36. Jackson LK, Johnson DB, Sosman JA, Murphy BA, Epstein JB. Oral health in oncology: impact of immunotherapy. Support Care Cancer. 2015;23(1):1–3.
37. Miaskowski C. Biology of mucosal pain. J Natl Cancer Inst Monogr. 2001;29:37–40.
38. Van Sebille YZ, Stansborough R, Wardill HR, Bateman E, Gibson RJ, Keefe DM. Management of mucositis during chemotherapy: from pathophysiology to pragmatic therapeutics. Curr Oncol Rep. 2015;17(11):50.

39. Mallick S, Benson R, Rath GK. Radiation induced oral mucositis: a review of current literature on prevention and management. Eur Arch Otorhinolaryngol. 2016;273(9):2285–93.
40. Vadalouca A, Raptis E, Moka E, Zis P, Sykioti P, Siafaka I. Pharmacological treatment of neuropathic cancer pain: a comprehensive review of the current literature. Pain Pract. 2012;12(3):219–51.
41. Hunt SP, Mantyh PW. The molecular dynamics of pain control. Nat Rev Neurosci. 2001;2(2):83–91.

Part II

Oral Mucosal Diseases

Herpes Simplex

4

Andres Pinto

Pearls of Wisdom

- A careful history of patients who complain of oral lesions will guide the astute clinician toward a correct differential diagnosis for herpes simplex.
- Particular attention should be placed to early prodromal symptoms of herpes simplex.
- Early treatment (within 24–48 h of the prodromal cycle) of suspicious herpes simplex lesions is suggested for the efficacy of systemic treatment.
- Most clinical trial data is derived from studies on HSV-2 or primary infection cases. Concrete evidence for recurrent herpes labialis or recurrent intraoral herpes is limited.

4.1 Introduction

The term herpes simplex refers to a subgroup of infectious mucocutaneous diseases that may affect the craniofacial complex [1]. As occurs with other viral diseases, herpes simplex infections usually follow up a prodromal stage of malaise, lymphadenopathy, itching, burning, or fever [2, 3]. Gastrointestinal symptoms may also be present. A majority of the population is exposed to this virus in infancy. However, few individuals manifest clinically oral or dermatologic lesions of primary infection [1, 4]. Herpes simplex viridae are divided into HSV-1 and HSV-2. Herpes simplex virus type 1 usually affects the skin or the mucosa above the waistline. This virus is also associated with meningeal inflammation. Herpes simplex virus type 2 is linked to anogenital lesions [5, 6].

A. Pinto, DMD, MPH, MSCE, FDS RCS (Edin)
Oral and Maxillofacial Medicine and Diagnostic Sciences, University Hospitals Case Medical Center and Case Western Reserve School of Dental Medicine, Cleveland, OH, USA
e-mail: andres.pinto@case.edu

J.N.A.R. Ferreira et al. (eds.), *Orofacial Disorders*,
DOI 10.1007/978-3-319-51508-3_4

4.2 Clinical Presentation

The clinical presentation of infection by both types of HSV is similar and characterized by vesicular eruptions followed by erosion of the epithelium. The mucosal lesions are characterized by irregular superficial ulcers with clear erythematous margins and coalescing distribution (Figs. 4.1 and 4.2). Primary infection with the virus in immune-competent patients usually occurs within the initial 6 years of life [2, 6]. It is possible that, depending on lifestyle and location, primary infection occurs in patients older than 30 years of age. Most primary infections are characterized by prodromal symptoms. The appearance of the mucosal lesions in HSV-1

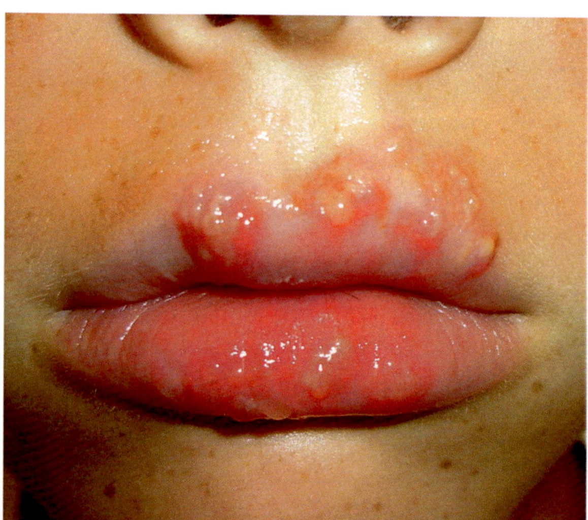

Fig. 4.1 Herpes simplex lesions in the upper and lower lips and perioral skin characterized by irregular superficial ulcers with clear erythematous margins and coalescing distribution

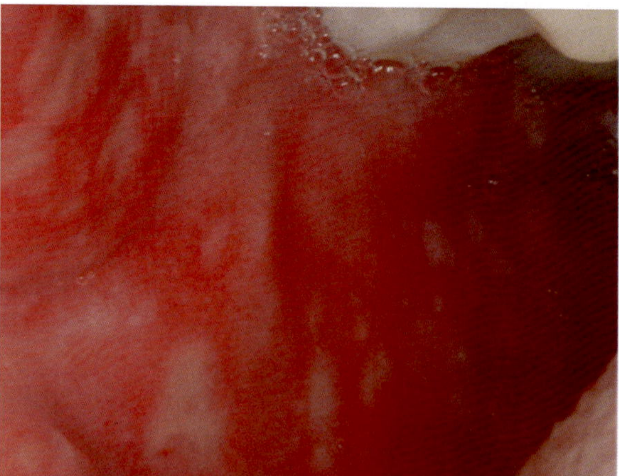

Fig. 4.2 Intraoral herpes simplex lesions in the oral mucosa vestibule

infection is termed primary gingivostomatitis [7]. The clinical appearance of the stomatitis is of severe generalized erosion that may impair oral intake. HSV is neurotrophic. Therefore, after primary infection, they remain within a latent stage in ganglionic and peripheral distributions of facial nerves. The recurrent presentation of disease can either occur on the lips, nasal cavity or skin, inside the mouth, or other distribution of the trigeminal nerve. Labial lesions are described as recurrent herpes labialis.

Typical sites of onset follow the dermatomal distribution of the cranial nerves. Standard intraoral sites are heavily keratinized tissues that include the hard palate and gingiva. Clinical lesions usually appear within 24–48 h of the occurrence of prodromal symptoms. The natural history of infections with HSV is usually of 8–10 days in immune-competent patients. The clinical presentation in immune-compromised individuals has a broad range of appearances. The ulcers may present in non-keratinized issue, may affect multiple dermatomes the same time, and may be extensive in size. Viral infections in immune-compromised patients are the second most common opportunistic infection. Therefore, HSV-related infections may prolong for more than 2 weeks in these individuals if untreated.

4.3 Etiology and Epidemiology

Exposure to herpes virus is almost universal and is dependent on geographic location, population group, and other lifestyle factors. Early onset in life is characteristic of primary infection, although primary infection after 60 years of age has been reported. Exposure to the virus does not directly imply the development of primary or recurrent clinical infection. Factors such as immune status, exposure to ultraviolet light, stress, and nutrition may impact the degree of expression of the virus in its mucosal sequelae. The prevalence of HSV infection in the United States has been tracked in the past decade. The National Health and Nutrition Examination Survey (NHANES) reported a decrease prevalence of HSV-2 infection in a stable HSV-1 infection rate in the 1999–2004 cohort. Within this time, the prevalence of HSV-2 infection (serologic) was reported to be 17%, with a 95% confidence interval of 15.8–18.3%. The prevalence of HSV-1 infection was reported to be 57%, with a 95% confidence interval of 55.9–59.5% [8].

4.4 Pathophysiology

Herpes simplex viridae are double-stranded DNA viral particles. The characteristic neurotropism of this group allows HSV to elude normal immune surveillance. Besides, proteins like ICP 0 increased resistance to inflammatory mediators such as interferon. The components of the virus are the core, the capsid, the tegument, and an outer envelope [9]. The DNA part is a 152 kg base string that can assume several structural appearances. The virus enters into host cells, replicates in epithelial cells, and causes cell lysis. After replication, the virus moves into the nerve ending and migrates to one of the several ganglia that include trigeminal, sphenopalatine, and geniculate ganglions and gains latency by entering neuronal cell nuclei [9].

4.5 Diagnosis

The diagnosis of acute infection is made by a combination of careful history and either polymerase chain reaction (PCR) testing, direct fluorescent antibody assay (DFA) testing, Tzanck smear, viral culture, or tissue biopsy [5, 10]. The most common diagnostic test is PCR given its high positive predictive value. When biopsies are performed, histologic findings include giant cells and viral inclusions. Serologic testing that may prove useful to differentiate primary versus recurrent infection are IgM and IgG antibody levels against the virus.

4.6 Rationale for Treatment

The rationale for treatment of herpes simplex infection is based on the limitation of the replication ability of the virus by interacting with its DNA processing [11]. Current treatments also aim to shorten the duration of mucosal/skin erosions and reduce pain [11].

4.7 Treatment Options

Therapeutic options include topical and systemic delivery of antiviral medications. Currently available evidence-based approaches for adults are described in Table 4.1. Novel approaches using topical medications as alternative therapy have proven efficacy in pilot clinical trials. The only FDA-approved topical formulations in the United States are 5% acyclovir and 1% penciclovir [3, 7, 11–13].

Table 4.1 Pharmacological options for herpes simplex treatment

Medication	Dose[a]	Precautions
Acyclovir	200 mg 5×/day for 10 days	Renal or hepatic impairment, dehydration, elderly patients
Valacyclovir	1000 mg 2×/day for 10 days	Advanced immune suppression, renal impairment
Famciclovir	250 mg 3×/day for 10 days	Renal impairment

[a]Some evidence of efficacy of single dose of 1,500 mg of valacyclovir or 2 gm twice a day of famcyclovir as abortive approach for recurrent herpes labialis

4.8 Treatment Goals

The primary treatment goals include limitation of acute discomfort and increasing the healing rate of lesions. Shortening of the natural history of the viral infection cycle, accompanied by the improvement in the quality of life, is among the important outcome measures used in clinical trials. Systemic therapy should be the initial line of treatment because it shortens the duration of viral infection dramatically and is complemented by FDA-approved topical formulations.

References

1. Stoopler ET, Alfaris S, Alomar D, Sollecito TP. Recurrent Intraoral Herpes. J Emerg Med. 2016. pii: S0736-4679(16)30128-7. doi: 10.1016/j.jemermed.2016.05.001. [Epub ahead of print].
2. Stoopler ET, Sollecito TP. Oral mucosal diseases: evaluation and management. Med Clin N Am. 2014;98(6):1323–52.
3. Radulescu M. The pharmacologic management of common lesions of the oral cavity. Dent Clin N Am. 2016;60(2):407–20.
4. Corstjens PL, Abrams WR, Malamud D. Saliva and viral infections. Periodontol 2000. 2016;70(1):93–110.
5. Miller RM. Diagnosis of herpes simplex virus in patients with erythema multiforme. JAMA. 2014;312(10):1060–1.
6. Balasubramaniam R, Kuperstein AS, Stoopler ET. Update on oral herpes virus infections. Dent Clin N Am. 2014;58(2):265–80.
7. Goldman RD. Acyclovir for herpetic gingivostomatitis in children. Can Fam Physician. 2016;62(5):403–4.
8. Xu F, Sternberg MR, Kottiri BJ, et al. Trends in herpes simplex virus type 1 and type 2 seroprevalence in the United States. JAMA. 2006;296(8):964–73.
9. Kolokotronis A, Doumas S. Herpes simplex virus infection, with particular reference to the progression and complications of primary herpetic gingivostomatitis. Clin Microbiol Infect. 2006;12(3):202–11.
10. Sarnoff DS. Treatment of recurrent herpes labialis. J Drugs Dermatol. 2014;13(9):1016–8.
11. Al-Ghazawi FM, Ramien ML, Brassard A, Shear NH, Beecker J. Management of pain associated with selected conditions in dermatology. Am J Clin Dermatol. 2016;17:463–74.
12. Zhao M, Zheng R, Jiang J, et al. Topical lipophilic epigallocatechin-3-gallate on herpes labialis: a phase II clinical trial of AverTeaX formula. Oral Surg Oral Med Oral Pathol Oral Radiol. 2015;120(6):717–24.
13. Chi CC, Wang SH, Delamere FM, et al. Interventions for prevention of herpes simplex labialis (cold sores on the lips). Cochrane Database Syst Rev. 2015;(8):CD010095.

Oral Vesiculobullous Diseases

5

Francina Lozada-Nur and Chelsia Sim

Pearls of Wisdom

- Match the level of complexity of the management program with the complexity of the patients and use a clinical team approach (dermatologist, PCP, oral hygienist) to facilitate success in complex patients.
- Ensuring that focus is on paradigms of self-care and education will enhance long-term outcomes and maintain positive relationships with the clinician.

5.1 Introduction

The diagnosis and management of *o*ral *v*esiculo-*e*rosive *d*iseases (OVEDs) are often quite complex due primarily to the fact that clinically they can mimic one another (e.g., oral lichen planus and lichenoid lesions or pemphigus vulgaris and oral erythema multiform). This frequently leads to an incorrect diagnosis and as a result ineffective selection and use of medications.

Improving clinicians' recognition and management of OVED is the aim of this chapter. To begin with, it is important to know that therapeutic approaches vary among patients and diseases. These therapies are not recipes, and they are ruled by disease severity and pattern and by the underlying medical condition of the patient.

F. Lozada-Nur, DDS, MS, MPH, BCOM
Division of Oral Medicine, Department of Oro-facial Science, University of California, San Francisco School of Dentistry San Francisco, San Francisco, CA 99143, USA

C. Sim, BDS, MS, BCOM (✉)
Department of Oral Maxillofacial Surgery, National Dental Center, Clinical Lecturer, Faculty of Dentistry, National University of Singapore, Singapore, Singapore
e-mail: sqxchel@gmail.com

J.N.A.R. Ferreira et al. (eds.), *Orofacial Disorders*,
DOI 10.1007/978-3-319-51508-3_5

Therefore, before starting any therapy, a clinician must first have at least a provisional diagnosis and/or a tissue biopsy (definitive diagnosis). This allows the clinician to know what she/he is treating and be able to select the most effective drug(s) and/or treatment protocol to treat that particular condition. Furthermore, having the correct diagnosis will add to patient understanding of what to expect and likely improve the outcome (prognosis).

Starting therapy without this safeguard increases the chance of therapeutic failure and the risk of drug adverse side effects, due to poor therapy choices, and worsens patient's frustrations. Thus, instead of helping patients, one may do just the opposite by disguising the original diagnosis.

Oral vesiculo-erosive diseases form a group of chronic inflammatory and/or autoimmune conditions which affect the oral mucous membrane, occasionally involving other mucous membranes (e.g., genital, esophagus, nasal, eye-conjunctiva), and/or skin. It is important to remember that the oral mucosa can be the first site of involvement and should alert the clinician to consider referral to the appropriate specialist to evaluate the involvement of other sites (e.g., dermatologist, ophthalmologist, ENT, gynecologist).

In this chapter, we will address the most common entities often seen by the oral medicine specialist: oral lichen planus (OLP), oral erythema multiforme (OEM), mucous membrane pemphigoid (MMP), and pemphigus vulgaris (PV).

5.2 Clinical Presentation

5.2.1 Common Symptomatology

1. Pain can be spontaneous or triggered by trauma while eating or from toothbrushing or tooth cleaning.
2. Discomfort and swelling, which is proportional to amount of inflammation, primarily on the buccal and gingival mucosa. Swelling is commonly reported by patients with OLP (especially among those with severe reticular and atrophic components), OEM, and PV.
3. If a patient reports having a burning sensation, a secondary yeast infection and/or burning mouth syndrome should be ruled out.
4. Spontaneous bleeding often reported in patients with MMP can be triggered by trauma (eating and tooth brushing) in all of them, when the gingival mucosa is involved.

5.2.2 Signs

1. *Possess consistent clinical patterns of disease distribution according to each condition:*

   Oral Lichen Planus: must have a bilateral and/or symmetrical clinical distribution. Otherwise, consider lichenoid disease either due to an allergic reaction or an early sign of dysplasia. Most commonly affected oral sites include buccal mucosa, lateral borders of the tongue, lower labial mucosa, and hard palate. However, any site can be involved except vermillion border of the lip. Classic clinical presentation includes bilateral or symmetric lacey-like white striaes with or without ulcers covered by pseudomembranes and erythematous changes. The lacey-like changes must always be present in OLP, given that it is a hallmark of the disease (Fig. 5.1) [1].

Oral Erythema Multiforme: as its name suggests, OEM is characterized by nonspecific erythematous changes. As shown by our studies, and to help clinicians in recognizing this condition, OEM has been divided into three clinical groups: intraoral alone, intraoral and lip, and intraoral and skin. Ulcers tend to be shallow and irregular with well-demarcated margins anywhere in the oral cavity with or without involving the vermilion border of the lip [2–4]. However, vermilion border of the lips is a hallmark of OEM (Fig. 5.2).

Mucous Membrane Pemphigoid: clinically characterized by desquamative gingivitis (a hallmark of MMP), shallow ulcers covered by pseudomembrane, and tense or sluggish looking bullae filled with blood, often on the gingival mucosa, soft palate, and buccal mucosa (Fig. 5.3). These bullae can be painful due to pressure caused by blood [5, 6].

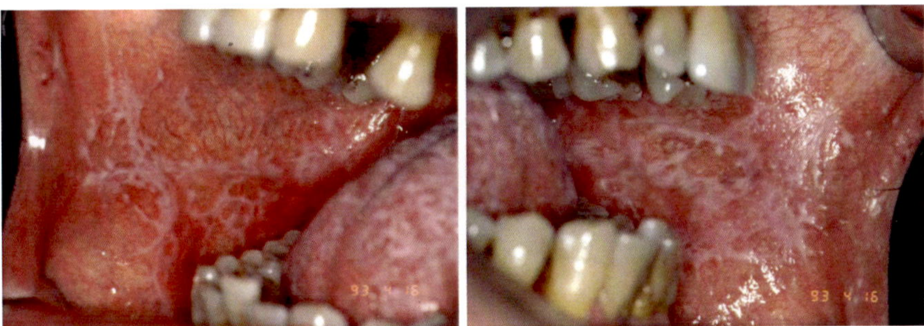

Fig. 5.1 Oral lichen planus (*OLP*) located bilaterally on buccal mucosa with typical diffuse, white reticular striations

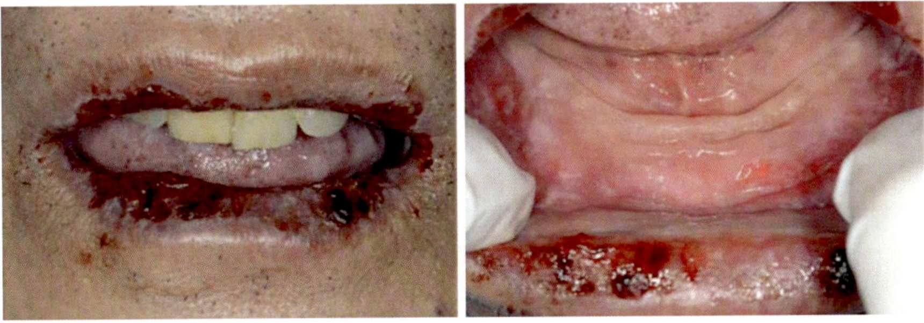

Fig. 5.2 Oral erythema multiforme (*OEM*) with a characteristic generalized crusting of the lips with multifocal ulcerations within the oral cavity

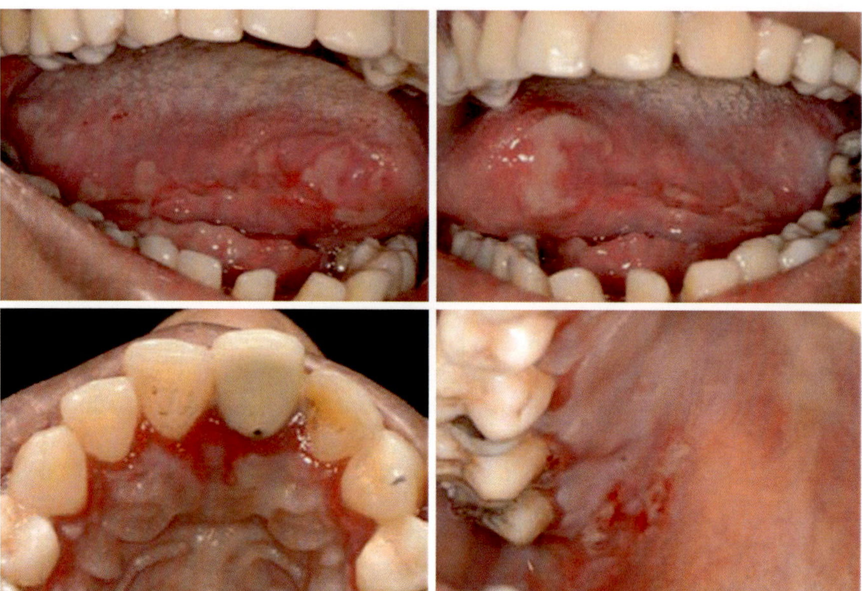

Fig. 5.3 Mucous membrane pemphigoid (*MMP*) showing generalized pseudomembrane-covered ulcers involving both keratinized and nonkeratinized mucosa. Gingival involvement is common

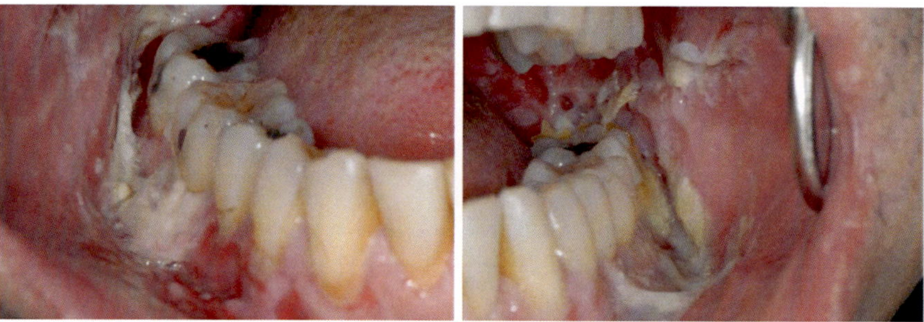

Fig. 5.4 Pemphigus vulgaris (*PV*). Generalized epithelial sloughing with extensive erosions on bilateral mandibular buccal sulcus and buccal mucosa

Pemphigus Vulgaris: clinically characterized by true and deep erosions and edema affecting the buccal mucosa, often with a bilateral distribution (Fig. 5.4). PV can affect any site of the oral cavity, and it is very painful when affecting the lateral tongue, soft palate, and esophageal area. By and large oral lesions precede skin, on average by 3–6 months. In severe cases, PV may affect the vermilion surface of the lip, which leads to a misdiagnosis of OEM. *Paraneoplastic pemphigus* (PNPV) is a different entity from PV and is indicative of an underlying malignancy, which clinically mimics oral erythema multiforme. However, it has a more aggressive clinical presentation and fails to respond to conventional treatment for OEM.

2. *Extraoral sites*, which shall be evaluated include:
   - *Ocular and nasal (MMP, PV)*
   - *Genital (OLP, MMP, PV)*
   - *Skin (OLP, OEM, MMP, PV)*
   - *Vermilion border of the lip (OEM, PV, PNPV)*
3. *Chronic clinical course (OLP, MMP, PV)*
4. *Chronic clinical course with a cyclic pattern of occurrence (OEM)*

5.3 Etiology and Epidemiology

The prevalence of OVED is unknown due to its rarity as well as clinical variability. Lack of population-based epidemiological studies makes it difficult to know the true incidence and prevalence of OVED. However, based on several observational studies performed in some tertiary centers, rough estimates are reported, depending on geographic distribution:

- OLP: Prevalence varies from 0.22% to 5% worldwide; incidence of up to 2.2%. OLP occurs in those between 30 and 80 years of age, with greater prevalence in females [1, 7, 8].
- MMP: Incidence varies from 1 in 12,000 to 1 in 20,000 of the adult population.
- PV: Incidence varies from 0.1 to 0.5 in 100,000 of the adult population, influenced by geographic location and ethnicity, higher rates in India, Southeast Europe, and the Middle East as well as among Jews especially the Ashkenazi Jews.
- OEM: Incidence and prevalence varies widely, from 1.1% to 3.7%, and tends to occur in young adults between 20 and 50 years of age, with no sexual predilection or race [2–4].

5.3.1 Etiological Considerations According to Each Condition

OLP: Etiology unknown.

- Potential triggering factors include local and systemic inducers of cell-mediated hypersensitivity (e.g., dental materials, flavoring agents), stress, and autoimmune response to epithelial antigens etc. [9].

  MMP: Genetic predisposition and environmental factors [6].

- Virus or drugs with structural similarity to endogenous antigens of the BMZ
- HLA-DQB1**0301 allele

  PV: Genetic predisposition with environmental factors.

- Drugs such as penicillamine, antibiotics, ACE inhibitors, and NSAIDs.
- Ultraviolet exposure.

- HLAD-R4 and DR14; HLA-DRB1 0402 is associated in Ashkenazi Jews, and DRB1 1401/04 and DQB1 0503 are associated in non-Jewish patients of European or Asian descent.

  OEM: Etiology unknown.

- Environmental factors
  - Drugs (e.g., antibiotics, anticonvulsants, antihypertensives, diuretics, sulfa drugs, nonsteroidal anti-inflammatory drugs, birth control pills)
  - Alcohol
  - Endocrine triggers
  - Local or systemic infections:
    - Viral: HSV, EBV, HCV, HIV
    - Bacterial: *Mycoplasma pneumoniae*, *Mycobacterium leprae*
    - Fungal: *Candida albicans*

5.4 Pathophysiology and Mechanisms

- OLP: Studies suggest that OLP is a T-cell-mediated autoimmune disease in which cytotoxic T cells react against epithelial keratinocytes [1, 10–12].
- MMP: Studies show that MMP is a type II, cytotoxic autoimmune disease with autoantibodies targeted at BP180, laminin 5 and 6, VII collagen, and beta 4 integrin.
- PV: Studies show that PV is a type II, cytotoxic autoimmune mucocutaneous disease with autoantibodies targeting to intercellular adhesion molecules, desmoglein 3 (dsg3) and desmoglein 1 (dsg1). PV with only oral involvement involves dsg3, while in both oral and skin involvement, dsg1 and dsg3 are targeted.
- OEM: Studies suggest that OEM is a result of a type IV, T-cell-mediated hypersensitivity reaction to triggering factors [13].

  Some of the comorbid conditions and complicating factors may include:

- Medication from underlying chronic medical conditions, specifically high blood pressure medication, cholesterol-lowering agents, antihyperglycemic agents, and antidepressants
- Oral candidiasis
- Psychological factors such as stress, anxiety, and depression

5.5 Diagnosis and Diagnostic Criteria

5.5.1 Clinical Diagnostic Criteria for OVED

- The presence of persistent shallow ulcers or erosions covered by yellowish-white fibrinous exudate with surrounding erythematous mucosa.

- Rarely seen are blood-filled bullae or blisters on attached and free mucous membrane.
- Desquamative gingivitis may be observed in OLP and MMP; in the former, usually white striations are present.
- For OLP, post-inflammatory hyperpigmentation of the involved oral mucosa may be observed especially in dark-skinned patients.

5.5.2 Laboratory Diagnostic Criteria for OVED

Routine histological examinations using hematoxylin and eosin (H&E) stains are to be performed, and at times, direct immunofluorescence and serologic tests are carried out to aid in diagnosing OVED. *Location of tissue obtained for histopathological examination is crucial in order for the test to be diagnostic*. For MMP and PV, peri-lesional tissue with intact mucosa should be submitted for H&E and direct immunofluorescence tests. Specimens for DIF are submitted in Michel's solution. Serologic tests such as indirect immunofluorescence or ELISA involve collection of patients' blood to detect circulating autoantibodies that bind to epithelial antigens.

5.6 Treatment

5.6.1 Rational for Treatment

Treatment is aimed at controlling sign and symptoms and to prevent disease progression.

5.6.2 Treatment Options

- Once diagnosis is established, patients should be referred to an oral hygienist to have a thorough oral prophylaxis and be instructed on proper oral hygiene/ home care.
- Treatment approach should be determined by disease severity and patient's medical history (Table 5.1).
- Disease limited to the mouth should be managed with high-potency topical steroids and/or intralesional injections (OLP, OEM, MMP) and good oral hygiene. Disease involving other mucous membrane and/or skin (OLP, MMP, and PV) should be treated with a combination of systemic and topical medication (Table 5.2) [16, 18].
- The most severely involved site should determine treatment course.
- Regular oral hygiene (3–4 months) is crucial, especially early on in the course of treatment when symptoms prevent the patient from optimal oral care.

Table 5.1 Biopsy, histological, and immunofluorescence findings according to each OVED condition

OVED	Location of tissue biopsy	Routine H&E	DIF	IIF
OLP	Lesional tissue[a] for H&E and DIF	Hyperparakeratosis, acanthosis with sawtooth rete ridges; atrophic epithelium or ulceration, depending on clinical features Cytoid bodies (civatte bodies) within surface epithelium Band-like chronic inflammatory infiltrates subjacent to surface epithelium, predominantly lymphocytes Basal liquefactive degeneration	Deposition of fibrinogen in a shaggy pattern along the basement membrane zone (BMZ) in the absence of IgG, IgM, IgA, and C3	NA
MMP	Peri-lesional tissue adjacent to erosions/bullae for H&E and DIF Blood for IIF	Separation of epithelium from underlying connective tissue with preservation of basal keratinocytes Scant chronic inflammatory infiltrate in lamina propria	Deposition of IgG ± C3 in the basement membrane zone in a smooth, continuous linear pattern At times, IgM, IgA, and fibrinogen can be present	Circulating IgG may be present in approximately 20% of cases No correlation between antibody titers and disease activity Less likely to detect autoantibodies in those with localized oral lesions than those with oral and skin involvement
PV	Peri-lesional tissue adjacent to erosions/bullae for H&E and DIF Blood for IIF	Intraepithelial cleavage with acantholysis (Tzanck cells) in the suprabasal region Retention of basal keratinocytes along the basement membrane zone, giving rise to "row of tombstones" Sparse inflammatory infiltrate in the lamina propria with eosinophils	Deposition of IgG at the epithelial intercellular spaces, giving a "chicken-wire" pattern. Staining with C3 may also be present	Circulating IgG targeted at intercellular molecules in active disease Antibody titers may or may not correlate with disease activity May not be useful for monitoring response to therapy

Table 5.1 (continued)

OVED	Location of tissue biopsy	Routine H&E	DIF	IIF
OEM	Peri-lesional tissue adjacent to erosions/bullae for H&E and DIF	Intraepithelial and intracellular edema Increase vascularity with perivascular inflammatory infiltrates in the lamina propria Numerous eosinophils seen	Only if needed to rule out MMP or PV	NA

H&E hematoxylin and eosin, *DIF* direct immunofluorescence, *IIF* indirect immunofluorescence, *Ig* immunoglobulin, *C3* complement 3

[a]Lesional tissue: avoid ulcerated areas unless suspicious for malignancy

Table 5.2 Treatment approach based on disease severity

Disease severity	Induction therapy (2–4 weeks)	Maintenance therapy[a]
Severe OVED Pain >8 scale of 10 Signs >80% Involvement	Prednisone (60 mg a.m. QD) until 50–75% remission of signs and symptoms occurs (average time – 3 weeks), together with daily azathioprine 150 mg QD or Cellcept 3 gm QD [14]	Start to phase out prednisone to an intermediate dose (45–50 mg a.m. QD or QOD), with azathioprine 150 mg QD or Cellcept 3 gm QD HPTS BID QD or QOD
Moderate OVED Pain 5 scale of 10 Signs >50%	Prednisone (50 mg a.m. QD.) until 50–75% reduction of signs and symptoms is seen. Consider adjunct therapy if patient shows early side effects. Curcuminoids 6000 mg/d in 3 divided doses [15]	Prednisone 50 or 40 mg a.m. QD or QOD. If patient has a setback, increase dose to 60 mg QD for 2–4 days, and start azathioprine 100 mg or Cellcept 2.5 gm QD. HPTS three times QD
Mild OVED Pain <5 scale 10 Signs <25%	Fluocinonide oint in Orabase 1:1 clobetasol prop. oint. in Orabase 1:1 (0.025%)TID [16] Tacrolimus powder Orabase 1% Prednisone 50 mg am QD for 10 days followed by HPTS [17]	HPTS BID or QD or QOD depending on disease control or Curcuminoids 6000 mg/d in 3 divided doses [15]
Gingival lesions	Use trays if disease is confined to the hard palate and gingival mucosa. Custom-made vinyl trays for HPTC or Tacrolimus powder Orabase 1% to be worn one tray at a time for up to 5 min TID until complete healing is achieved	Custom-made soft or hard trays for HPTS application, to use one tray at a time QOD and QO week

HPTS high-potency topical steroids

Cellcept prescribed to patients unable to tolerate azathioprine

Avoid food known to irritate the mouth

Avoid antimicrobial mouth rinse such as chlorhexidine and Listerine® because of their alcohol content

Monitored for yeast infection while on HPTS

[a]Maintenance therapy should be considered after condition is 80–90% under control

5.6.3 Home Care

- Maintain good oral hygiene.
- Eat a bland-soft diet when mouth flares up, and avoid any food known as irritating the mucosa (spicy, salty, acidic, rough).
- See your dentist once a year and dental hygienist two to three times a year.
- Eat a balanced diet, especially rich in vitamin C.

5.6.4 Pharmacotherapy

- Steroidal anti-inflammatory drugs:
  - Systemic prednisone
    Dose: should be taken as a single dose AM, to minimize side effects. Starts on alternate-date (QOD) therapy as soon as disease is 50% under control.
    Precautions: multiple side effects if taken for prolonged period of time such as headaches, sleep disturbance, increased appetite and weight-gained, depression, bone loss (long-term use), etc. [19–22].
  - High-potency topical steroids:
    Fluocinonide oint 0.05% in Orabase (0.025%) [18].
    Clobetasol oint 0.05% in Orabase (0.025%) [23].
- Azathioprine, a cytotoxic drug:
  - Dose: azathioprine 50 mg tablets QD (up to 150 mg QD).
  - Precautions: several side effects may occur when taken on high doses such as bone marrow suppression and liver toxicity. Always do a base line CBC and liver test, and repeat during the course of therapy. First week after initiating therapy, 2-week later, once a month, every 3 months [14].
- Mycophenolate mofetil is an immunosuppressive drug used for the treatment of severe PV:
  - Dose: Cellcept up to 3 g per day.
  - Precautions: several side effects have been reported such as bone marrow suppression and immunosuppression. Good replacement for azathioprine in patients who show increase of liver enzymes.
- Tacrolimus and pimecrolimus are calcineurin inhibitors, which result in down-regulation of the immune response. Both have been approved by the FDA for use in atopic dermatitis:
  - Dose:
    - Tacrolimus powder in Orabase 0.1% TID [17].
    - Pimecrolimus cream 1%, apply BID on ulcer [24].
  - Precautions: there is a risk of systemic absorption, especially when used on large ulcerated areas. However, it is a relatively safe anti-inflammatory topical medication. Patients may report headaches and local burning sensation.

5.6.5 Treatment Goals and Sequence of Care

- Goals of treatment include:
  1. Reduce or eliminate pain.
  2. Promote healing.
  3. Increase disease-free period.
  4. Restore quality of life.
- Short-term strategy is to restore normal eating habits and quality of life.
- Long-term strategy includes reducing recurrence of signs and symptoms of disease.
- Acute cases of recent onset should be aggressively treated to minimize the need for long treatments and adverse effects.
- Educate patient on home-care strategies such as optimal home care, oral hygiene, healthy eating habits, and bland-soft diet when needed as well as minimize exposure to agents and/or factors that induce flares.

References

1. Chianini Wu N, Silverman S, Lozada-Nur F, Mayer P, Watson J. Oral lichen planus: patient profile, disease progression and treatment responses. J Am Dent Assoc. 2001;132:901–200.
2. Lozada F, Silverman S Jr. Erythema multiforme: clinical characteristics and natural history in 50 patients. Oral Surg Oral Med Oral Pathol. 1978;46:628–36.
3. Lozada-Nur F, Gorsky M, Silverman S Jr. A follow-up study in 96 patients with oral erythema multiforme. Oral Surg Oral Med Oral Pathol. 1989;67:36–41.
4. Ayangco L, Rogers RS 3rd. Oral manifestations of erythema multiforme. Dermatol Clin. 2003;21(1):195–205.
5. Silverman S Jr, Gorsky M, Lozada-Nur F, Liu A. A follow-up study in 65 patients with mucous membrane pemphigoid. Oral Surg Oral Med Oral Pathol. 1986;61:233–7.
6. Chan LS, Ahmed AR, Anhalt GJ, Bernauer W, Cooper KD, Elder MJ, Fine JD, Foster CS, Ghohestani R, Hashimoto T, Hoang-Xuan T, Kirtschig G, Korman NJ, Lightman S, Lozada-Nur F, Marinkovich MP, et al. The first international consensus on mucous membrane pemphigoid: definition, diagnostic criteria, pathogenic factors, medical treatments, and prognostic indicators. Arch Dermatol. 2002;138:370–9.
7. Lozada-Nur F, Miranda C. Oral lichen planus: pathogenesis and epidemiology. Semin Cutan Med Surg. 1997;16:290–5.
8. Chan, L, Olivry, T, Lozada-Nur, F. Oral manifestations of autoimmune blistering diseases from dermatology/diseases of the oral mucosa. e-medicine.com. 2001.
9. Chanaini-Wu N, Lozada-Nur F, Terrault N. Oral lichen planus and hepatitis C. A review. Med Oral Pathol Oral Radiol Endod. 2004;98(2):171–83.
10. Bramanti TE, Dekker NP, Lozada-Nur F, Sauk JJ, Regezi JA. Heat shock (stress) proteins and gdT-lymphocytes in oral lichen planus. Oral Surg Oral Med Oral Path. 1995;80:698–70.
11. Regezi JA, Dekker N, MacPhail L, Lozada-Nur F, et al. Vascular adhesion molecules in oral lichen planus. Oral Surg Oral Med Oral Path. 1996;81:682–90.

12. Ramirez-Amador V, Dekker NP, Lozada-Nur F, Mirowski GW, MacPhail LA, Regezi JA. Altered interface adhesion molecules in oral lichen planus. J Oral Dis. 1996;2:188–92.
13. Mirowski GW, Lozada-Nur F, Dekker NP, MacPhail LA, Regezi JA. Altered expression of epithelial integrins and extracellular matrix receptors in oral erythema multiforme. J Cutan Pathol. 1996;23:473–8.
14. Lozada F. Prednisone and azathioprine in the treatment of oral inflammatory mucocutaneous diseases. Oral Surg Oral Med Oral Pathol. 1981;52:257–60.
15. Chainani-Wu N, Madden E, Lozada-Nur F, Silverman S. High-dose curcuminoids are efficacious in the reduction in symptoms and signs of oral lichen Planus. J Am Acad Dermatol. 2012;66:752–60.
16. Lozada-Nur F, Miranda C. Topical and systemic therapy for oral lichen planus. Semin Cutan Med Surg. 1997;16:295–300.
17. Lozada-Nur F, Stroussi H. Tacrolimus-powder in Orabase 0.1% for the treatment of oral lichen Planus and lichenoid reactions: a open clinical trial. Oral Surg Oral Med Oral Pathol Oral Radiol Endod. 2006;102:744–9.
18. Lozada F, Silverman S Jr. Topically applied fluocinonide in adhesive base in the treatment of oral vesiculoerosive diseases. Arch Dermatol. 1980;116:898–901.
19. Frey FJ, Amend WJC Jr, Lozada F, Frey BM, Benet LZ. Endogenous hydrocortisone, a possible factor contributing to the genesis of Cushingoid habitus in patients on prednisolone. J Clin Endocrinol Metab. 1981;53:1076–80.
20. Benet LZ, Frey FJ, Amend WJC, Lozada F, Frey BM. Endogenous and exogenous glucocorticoids in cushingoid patients. Drug Intell Clin Pharm. 1982;16:863–8.
21. Lozada F, Frey F, Benet L. Prednisone clearance: a possible determinant for gluco-corticoid efficacy in patients with oral vesiculo-erosive diseases. J Dent Res. 1983;62:575–7.
22. Lozada-Nur F, Silverman S Jr, Migliorati C. Adverse side effects associated with prednisone in the treatment of oral inflammatory ulcerative diseases. JADA. 1984;109:269–70.
23. Lozada-Nur F, Miranda C, Maleski R. A double blind clinical trial on the efficacy and toxicity of clobetasol ointment in Orabase and fluocinonide ointment in Orabase for the treatment of chronic oral inflammatory diseases. Oral Surg Oral Med Oral Pathol. 1994;77:598–604.
24. Mc Caughey C, Machen M, Bennet R, et al. Pimecrolimus 1% cream for erosive oral lichen planus: a 6-week randomized, double-blind, vehicle controlled study with a 6-week open-label extension to assess efficacy and safety. J Eur Acad Dermatol. 2011;9:1061–7.

Oral Candidiasis

6

Scott S. De Rossi and Katharine Ciarrocca

Pearls of Wisdom

Important facts about oral candida infections:

- Commonly cause acute or chronic multiple lesions.
- Are caused by an opportunistic unicellular yeastlike fungus, a natural inhabitant of the oral microbial flora in over 50% of healthy individuals.
- Are related to xerostomia, diabetes, immunosuppression, use of broad spectrum antibiotics.
- Clinical diagnosis can be confirmed with gram stain and culture.

6.1 Introduction

Candida infections involving oropharynx and oral mucous membranes are fairly common. The majority of these cases are associated with *Candida albicans*. Frequently, oropharyngeal candida can be asymptomatic or associated with oral soreness, dysgeusia, dysphagia, or odynophagia [1]. Over 50% of individuals carry *Candida albicans* as a normal commensal organism. Oral candida is often considered an opportunistic infection, which grows as either yeasts or hyphae. Candida typically colonizes the mucocutaneous surfaces, but these can be portals of entry

S.S. De Rossi, DMD (✉)
Oral Health and Diagnostic Sciences, UNC School of Dentistry,
Office of the Dean, Koury Health Sciences Building, 385 S. Columbia St, CB 7450,
Chapel Hill, NC 27599, USA
e-mail: scott_derossi@unc.edu

K. Ciarrocca, DMD, MSEd
Oral Health and Diagnostic Sciences, Augusta University Dental College of Georgia,
1120 15th Street GC 2254, Augusta, GA 30912, USA

J.N.A.R. Ferreira et al. (eds.), *Orofacial Disorders*,
DOI 10.1007/978-3-319-51508-3_6

into deeper tissues when host defenses are compromised [2]. Species other than *C. albicans* are seen increasingly in immunocompromised patients. Candida though is more commonly seen in the following groups or associated with:

- Women
- Blood type
- High carbohydrate diets
- Xerostomia
- Broad-spectrum antibiotic use
- Denture wearers
- Smokers
- Immunocompromised patients
- Hospitalized patients [1–3]

6.2 Clinical Presentation

There are six clinical oral presentations of candida (Table 6.1) [1, 3]:

Table 6.1 Summary of common clinical manifestations of candida

Pseudomembranous candidiasis	"Thrush"
	White or yellowish cheese-like plaques, easily removed occasionally leaving a bleeding mucosal base
	Mucobuccal folds most common site
	Usually appears in early stages of immune suppression
	May be accompanied by burning sensation, pain, and difficulty swallowing
Atrophic candidiasis	Generalized erythematous, atrophic areas on any mucosal surface
	"Kissing lesions" affecting the palate and tongue
	May be present the entire course of HIVD but is usually the first to appear during mild immunosuppression
	Usually asymptomatic but can be painful or ulcerative
Hyperplastic candidiasis	A more chronic form of pseudomembranous candida
	White, confluent patches not easily removed
	Associated with severe immunosuppression and xerostomia
	Painful chewing/swallowing and persistent dysgeusia
Angular cheilitis	Inflammation at the commissures of the lip
	Very common; M=F; usually adults
	Predisposing factors: smoking, dry mouth, deficiency states, malabsorption states, immune deficiency
	Candida and staph aureus
	Mechanical factors play a role
Median rhomboid glossitis	Central papillary atrophy at mid-dorsum
	Relatively uncommon
	No age, gender, or geographic predilection
	Rarely sore – usually incidental finding
	Usually incidental finding
Denture-related stomatitis	Mild inflammation of the mucosa beneath a denture
	Papillary erythema on denture-bearing areas
	Usually complete upper denture
	Chronic wear of denture and underlying systemic disease

1. Pseudomembranous candidiasis commonly referred to as "thrush" manifests as white cheese-like plaques, easily removed occasionally leaving a bleeding mucosal base (Fig. 6.1).
2. Atrophic candidiasis manifests as generalized erythematous, atrophic areas commonly resulting in "kissing lesions" affecting both the palate and tongue simultaneously (Fig. 6.2).
3. Hyperplastic candidiasis, which often presents as white, confluent patches, is not easily removed (Fig. 6.3).

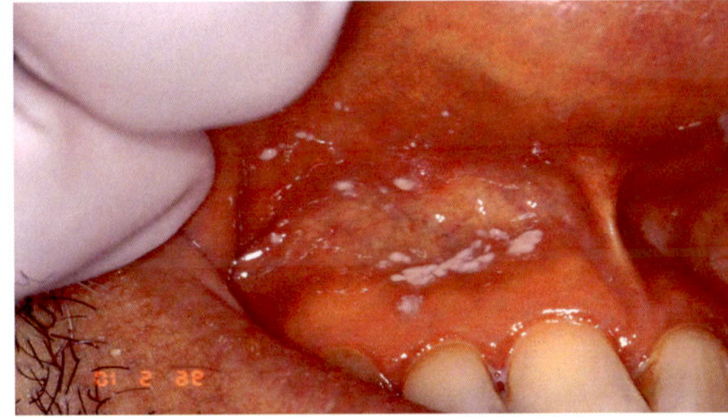

Fig. 6.1 Thrush/pseudomembranous candida

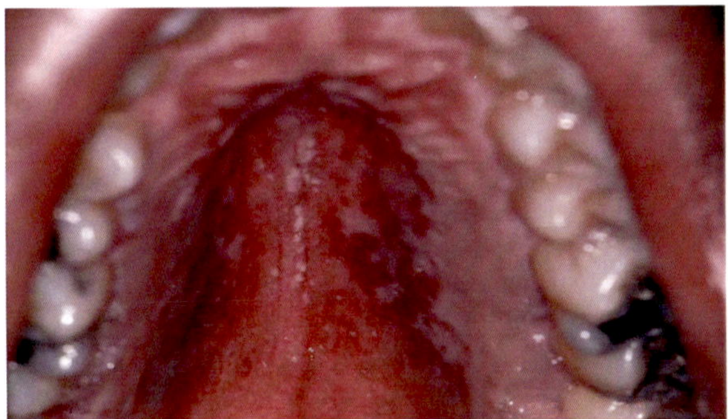

Fig. 6.2 Erythematous candida of the hard palate in HIVD

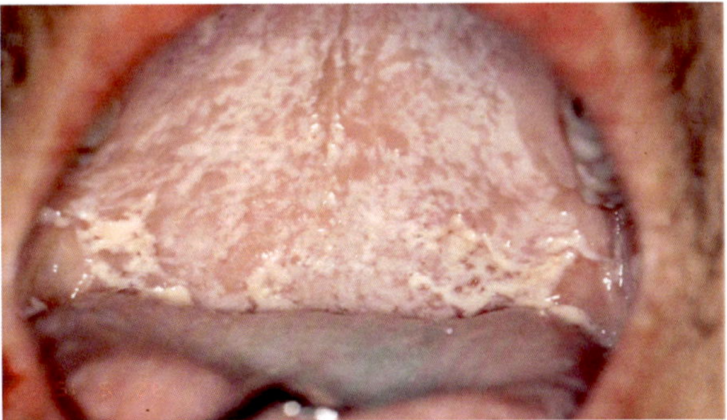

Fig. 6.3 Hyperplastic candida in HIVD

4. Angular cheilitis manifests as erosive, erythematous, painful areas at the lip commissures with bacterial superinfection (e.g., staphylococci and streptococci) (Fig. 6.4).
5. Median rhomboid glossitis presents as a central papillary atrophic area at the middorsal surface of the tongue (Fig. 6.5).
6. Denture-related stomatitis manifests as inflamed red mucosa under denture-bearing areas (Fig. 6.6).

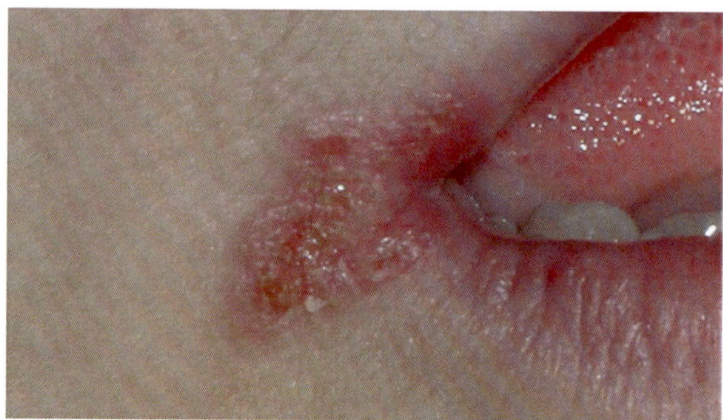

Fig. 6.4 Angular cheilitis

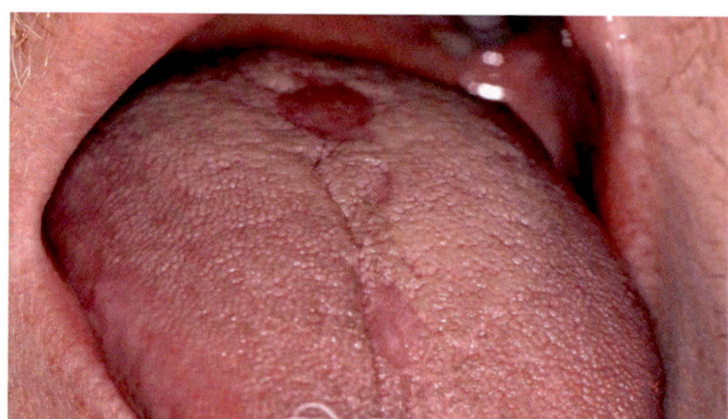

Fig. 6.5 Median rhomboid glossitis

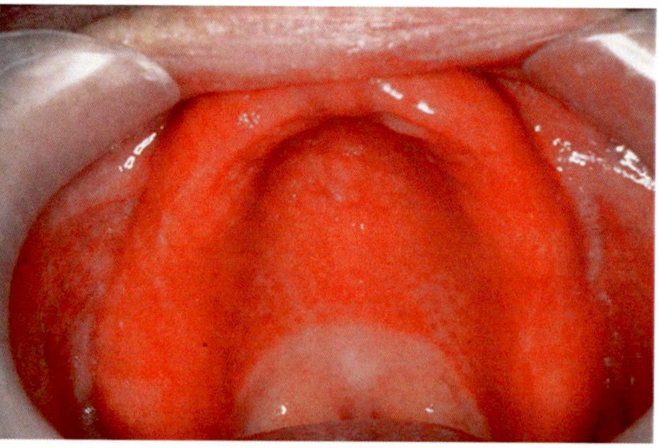

Fig. 6.6 Denture-associated stomatitis

Table 6.2 Prevalence of common candidal species [3–5]

Species	Percent of cases (%)
Candida albicans	50–60
Candida glabrata	15–20
Candida parapsilosis	10–20
Candida tropicalis	6–12
Candida pseudotropicalis	<5
Candida guilliermondii	<5
Candida krusei	<5
Candida lusitaniae	<5
Candida dubliniensis	<5
Candida stellatoidea	<5

6.3 Etiology and Epidemiology

Although candidal carriage in the oral cavity may be a normal occurrence in a majority of individuals, candidiasis infection is a result of candida overgrowth. The most common pathogenic species of candidiasis is *Candida albicans*, occurring in 50–60% of cases. Less commonly identified strains are more frequently found in immunosuppressed populations. Greater than 15% of oral candidiasis is caused by non-albicans species in those with HIV [2]. Similarly, 46% of cases of oral candidiasis in patients with malignancy are caused by non-albicans species [4, 5].

The prevalence of candidal species is listed in Table 6.2.

6.4 Pathophysiology and Mechanisms

Candida albicans can be differentiated serologically into A and B serotypes with equal distribution in healthy individuals with a significant shift to type B in immunocompromised patients. Multiple host defenses, including the oral epithelium barrier, microbial interactions and oral flora competition, salivary nonimmune defenses and salivary components with antimicrobial activity, local and systemic immune defenses, etc., play a role in the development of or resistance to candida infections [1, 3].

Risk factors for active infection can be divided into endogenous and exogenous causes [1–4]:

1. Endogenous causes:
   - Infancy
   - Aging
   - Pregnancy
   - Immunocompromised states
   - Diabetes mellitus
   - Sjögren's syndrome-induced xerostomia
   - Vitamin deficiencies

2. Exogenous causes:
   - Poor nutrition
   - Cigarette smoking
   - Ill-fitting oral prostheses
   - Localized radiotherapy
   - Malignancy with chemotherapy

6.5 Diagnosis and Diagnostic Criteria

Candidiasis of the oral cavity can be broadly categorized as primary or secondary. Primary candida infections involve the oral or perioral tissues, whereas the secondary candida characterizes systemic candidiasis that secondarily involves the oral cavity. Primary oral candidiasis has been traditionally subdivided into acute pseudomembranous candidiasis, acute atrophic candidiasis, chronic hyperplastic candidiasis, chronic atrophic candidiasis, median rhomboid glossitis, angular cheilitis, and linear gingival erythema [2].

Candida infection is usually a clinical diagnosis. However, the diagnosis can be complicated by number of carriers especially when culture is used instead of cytology. Identification of blastospores and pseudo-hyphae in stained smears is effective for a quick diagnosis. Culture, PCR studies, and histology stained with periodic acid-Schiff may occasionally be necessary [2].

Oral manifestations of candidiasis vary greatly. The differential diagnosis for oral candidiasis is broad and includes lichen planus, herpes infection, hairy leukoplakia, erythema multiforme, anemia and other vitamin deficiencies, chemotherapy-related mucositis, and vesiculo-ulcerative diseases [2, 6–7].

6.6 Rationale for Treatment

- Initial management should begin by eliminating predisposing factors identified during the interview and examination. Despite adequate antifungal treatment, recurrences are common in patients in whom the underlying risk factors are not eliminated.
- In cases in which the diagnosis of candidiasis is apparent, empiric treatment can be undertaken.
- In cases resistant to initial therapy, one should consider culture and sensitivity testing.
- If the diagnosis is uncertain, a biopsy for evaluation of the fixed tissue should be obtained.
- Parenteral antifungal agents are generally not used to treat isolated oral candidiasis and should be reserved for more invasive disease.
- Individuals who face an increased risk of invasive fungal infection or suffer from frequent recurrences may be candidates for chemoprophylaxis.

Table 6.3 Common antifungal regimens [3, 6–8]

Topical antifungal therapy	Triamcinolone-nystatin ointment for angular cheilitis
	Nystatin oral suspension 100,000 units/cc
	Clotrimazole troches 10 mg
	Clotrimazole buccal tablet 50 mg
Systemic antifungal therapy	Fluconazole 100 mg qd
	Ketoconazole 200 mg qd
	Itraconazole 100 mg bid

6.7 Treatment Options

Options for treating oral candidiasis are available in several forms (Table 6.3) including rinses, suspensions, powders, creams, ointments, lozenges, capsules, and tablets. The unique environment of salivary dilution and clearance and the action of deglutition result in decreased therapeutic drug concentration, mandating a need for frequent dosing. More frequent dosing schedules along with the unpalatable taste of some formulations may lead to noncompliance and treatment failure.

Treatment choice considerations should include drug effectiveness, infection severity, ease of administration, patient adherence, potential drug interactions, and cost. More detailed treatment options can be reviewed in 3 and 9–12.

6.8 Treatment Goals and Sequencing of Care

1. Address underlying causes or medical conditions
2. Avoid or reduce smoking
3. Treat xerostomia/salivary gland hypofunction
4. Improve oral hygiene (chlorhexidine has some antifungal activity)
5. Use antifungal medications – topical and/or systemic therapies

References

1. Akpan A, Morgan R. Oral candidiasis. Postgrad Med J. 2002;78(922):455–9.
2. Klein RS, et al. Oral candidiasis in high-risk patients as the initial manifestation of the acquired immunodeficiency syndrome. N Engl J Med. 1984;311(6):354–8.
3. Kragelund C, Reibel J, Pedersen AML. Management of patients with oral candidiasis. Oral Infections and General Health. Springer International Publishing; Switzerland. 2016. p. 137–44.
4. Lalla RV, et al. A systematic review of oral fungal infections in patients receiving cancer therapy. Support Care Cancer. 2010;18(8):985–92.
5. Li L, Redding S, Dongari-Bagtzoglou A. Candida glabrata, an emerging oral opportunistic pathogen. J Dent Res. 2007;86(3):204–15.
6. Lyu X, et al. Efficacy of nystatin for the treatment of oral candidiasis: a systematic review and meta-analysis. Drug Des Dev Ther. 2016;10:1161.

7. Marable DR, et al. Oral candidiasis following steroid therapy for oral lichen planus. Oral Dis. 2016;22(2):140–7.
8. Niimi M, Firth NA, Cannon RD. Antifungal drug resistance of oral fungi. Odontology. 2010;98(1):15–25.
9. Patuwo C, et al. The changing role of HIV-associated oral candidiasis in the era of HAART. J Calif Dent Assoc. 2015;43(2):87–92.
10. Salerno C, et al. Candida-associated denture stomatitis. Med Oral Patol Oral Cir Bucal. 2011;16(2):e139–43.
11. Samaranayake LP, Keung Leung W, Jin L. Oral mucosal fungal infections. Periodontol 2000. 2009;49:39–59.
12. Terai H, Shimahara M. Usefulness of culture test and direct examination for the diagnosis of oral atrophic candidiasis. Int J Dermatol. 2009;48(4):371–3.

Part III

Oral Diseases of the Senses

7 Chemosensory Disorders

Joseph A. D'Ambrosio

Pearls of Wisdom

- The majority of flavor perception is derived from odorants. Thus, many patients who present with a complaint of taste loss in actuality have smell loss and require olfactory testing.
- Dysgeusias are typically characterized by qualities identifiable by the taste system and should be described as either salty, sweet, sour, bitter, savory, or possibly metallic. Any other descriptors, such as "foul" or "rancid," are more likely to be associated with the olfactory system and should be classified as parosmias.

7.1 Introduction

There are three chemosensory systems in the nose and mouth. Smell (olfaction) is the ability to detect and identify odors. Taste (gustation) involves the discrimination of five identifiable taste qualities in the mouth: salt, sweet, sour, bitter, and savory (umami). The common chemical sense is the ability to perceive irritating stimuli in the mouth and nose, such as the burn of a chili pepper or the tingle of ammonia. Taste is often confused with flavor, which is the total sensory experience derived from the smell, taste, texture, temperature, and irritating properties of food and beverages.

J.A. D'Ambrosio, DDS, MS
Adjunct Faculty, Pima Community College, Tucson, AZ, USA
e-mail: josephadambrosio@gmail.com

J.N.A.R. Ferreira et al. (eds.), *Orofacial Disorders*,
DOI 10.1007/978-3-319-51508-3_7

7.2 Clinical Presentation

7.2.1 Smell Disorders

- Anosmia – complete loss of smell
- Hyposmia – reduced ability to smell
- Dysosmia – alteration or distortion of smell perception:
  - Parosmia (troposmia) – perception of an odor (usually unpleasant), triggered by a stimulus
  - Phantosmia – perception of an odor, without a stimulus present (olfactory hallucination)

7.2.2 Taste Disorders

- Ageusia – complete loss of taste
- Hypogeusia – reduced ability to taste
- Dysgeusia – alteration or distortion of taste perception. Dysgeusia may occur in conjunction with burning mouth syndrome:
  - Parageusia – altered taste (usually unpleasant), triggered by a stimulus
  - Phantogeusia – perception of a taste, without a stimulus present (gustatory hallucination)

7.3 Etiology and Epidemiology

7.3.1 Prevalence

- The actual prevalence of chemosensory disorders is unknown. It has been estimated that more than two million Americans have some type of smell or taste disorder. Newer estimates of the prevalence of self-reported chemosensory alterations from the 2011–2012 US National Health and Nutrition Examination Survey (NHANES) are 23% for smell and 19% for taste alterations.
- Olfactory disorders occur more frequently than taste losses, due to the anatomical distinctiveness of the olfactory system.
- Dysgeusias are intrusive and more commonly reported than actual taste losses, which are less readily perceived.

7.3.2 Etiologic Factors

- Upper respiratory infection (usually viral)
- Sinonasal conditions:
  - Allergic rhinitis
  - Chronic rhinosinusitis
  - Nasal polyps

- Head and facial trauma
- Neurodegenerative disorders:
  - Alzheimer's disease
  - Parkinson's disease, Parkinsonism
  - Multiple sclerosis
- Aging
- Medications:
  - Chemotherapy
  - Antimicrobials
  - Antihistamines and decongestants
  - Antidepressants
  - Antihypertensives
- Postradiation treatment
- Chronic medical conditions:
  - Cancer
  - Diabetes mellitus
  - Gastroesophageal reflux disease
  - Human immunodeficiency virus
  - Hypothyroidism
  - Renal or hepatic failure
- Psychiatric conditions
- Congenital conditions
  - Kallmann syndrome
  - Congenital anosmia
- Toxic chemical exposures
- Surgical procedures:
  - Middle ear surgery
  - Third molar extractions
- Salivary dysfunction, xerostomia
- Oral infections:
  - Candidiasis
  - Periodontal diseases
- Idiopathic

7.4 Pathophysiology and Mechanisms

- The sense of smell involves the transport of odorant molecules through the nasal cavity to a small patch of receptor cells in the olfactory neuroepithelium. Once the odorants are dissolved in the mucus surface of the epithelium, receptor cells are depolarized, and electrical signals traverse the cribriform plate to the olfactory bulb. From there, neural pathways project to other parts of the brain. The location of olfactory receptors high in the nasal cavity renders them susceptible to changes in nasal patency and airflow patterns that potentially limit the access of stimulus molecules. Also, the vulnerable position of olfactory nerve axons near the cribriform plate makes them subject to tearing or severing from coup-contrecoup forces associated with head injury.

- The neural pathways for taste are more complex. Taste receptor cells are located primarily in taste buds in the circumvallate, foliate, and fungiform papillae of the tongue. Additional taste receptors are found in the soft palate, pharynx, uvula, and epiglottis. Primary sensory neurons enter the base of the taste bud and synapse with taste cells. In contrast to olfaction, which is mediated by a single cranial nerve (I), innervation of the taste buds is supplied by three different cranial nerves: facial (VII), glossopharyngeal (IX), and vagus (X). The lingual branch of the trigeminal nerve (V) also innervates the anterior tongue and provides tactile and temperature sensation which interact with gustation to enhance flavor perception. The superficial placement of taste buds makes them susceptible to direct injury from chemicals, drugs, and viruses. Taste perception is also affected by the quantity and composition of saliva.
- Stimulation of the common chemical sense is through branches of the trigeminal nerve in the nose and oral cavity. The glossopharyngeal nerve provides additional sensory information.
- Most of the etiologic factors associated with chemosensory disorders can thus be divided into two major categories:
  - Transport Dysfunction – the odorant or taste stimulus cannot make contact with functioning olfactory neuroepithelium or taste buds.
  - Sensorineural Dysfunction – the odorant or taste stimulus cannot be processed due to neural injury. Olfactory neurons have a slow turnover rate (30–60 days). In contrast, taste cells have a rapid turnover rate (10–20 days) and have bilateral and multiple innervation. Therefore, complete loss of taste occurs with much less frequency than anosmia.

7.5 Diagnosis and Diagnostic Criteria

- Medical and dental history – documentation and differentiation of the specific chemosensory abnormality (smell, taste, or both) including description of chief complaint, duration, intensity, frequency, past medical history, medications, past treatment, modifying factors, and diagnostic studies.
- Physical examination – including thorough head and neck, neurological, and intraoral exams to rule out etiological factors noted above. A multidisciplinary approach combining internal medicine, neurological, otorhinolaryngological, and dental consultations may be useful.
- Chemosensory tests:
  - Odor discrimination tests determine a patient's ability to identify a series of common odorants such as coffee and chocolate. Commercially available microencapsulated "scratch and sniff" tests such as the University of Pennsylvania Smell Identification Test (UPSIT) can be self-administered by the patient. Although the 40-item UPSIT remains the "gold standard" of olfactory tests, briefer 3-item and 12-item variants have been developed (e.g., Pocket Smell Test, Quick Smell Identification Test, Brief Smell Identification Test).

  - Odor detection threshold tests utilize progressively stronger concentrations of an odorant such as butanol to determine the weakest dilution that a patient can detect. Each nostril must be tested separately to determine if the smell disturbance is unilateral or bilateral.
  - Trigeminal function for the common chemical sense is assessed by a patient's ability to detect a pungent odor such as menthol.
  - Whole mouth and spatial (regional) taste tests are used to assess a patient's ability to identify the quality and intensity of salty, sweet, sour, and bitter stimuli. A magnitude matching method used in specialized chemosensory clinics requires a patient to match the relative intensities of a series of taste solutions with sounds or weights to determine the extent of taste loss.
  - Electrogustometry delivers weak anodal electrical currents to the different areas of gustatory innervation on the tongue in order to assess the integrity of an individual nerve.
- Topical anesthesia or mandibular nerve blocks are useful in determining whether the cause of a taste disorder is due to local or central factors. If the complaint persists after the anesthetic is administered, then the source of the disorder may originate from the central nervous system.
- Somatosensory testing with Semmes-Weinstein monofilaments can be utilized to assess pressure detection thresholds for peripheral nerve fields in the oral cavity.
- Imaging modalities are useful for ruling out intracranial or peripheral nerve abnormalities. The following modalities are suggested:
  - Computed tomography
  - Magnetic resonance imaging
  - Positron emission tomography
  - Single photon emission tomography.
- Laboratory tests may be necessary to diagnose underlying medical or metabolic abnormalities.

7.6 Rationale for Treatment

- Improve the patient's symptoms and quality of life
- Manage identified underlying etiologies
- Reduce the risk of unintentional weight change, malnutrition, and worsening of concomitant medical illnesses (particularly in the elderly)
- Reduce the risk of toxic exposures (e.g., natural gas, smoke, poisons, spoiled food)

7.7 Treatment Options

- Treatment is highly dependent upon the specific etiologic factor.
- Prognosis for olfactory disorders is better when the patient has a reversible cause of intranasal interference, such as nasal polyps, rhinitis, or allergies.

- Medical treatments are not as effective in restoring lost olfactory function that results from an upper respiratory infection or head trauma.
- Factors that make improvement less likely include severity and duration of symptoms, advanced age at onset, and smoking.
- Drug and radiation-induced dysgeusias can be reversed with cessation of the offending agents, and other taste disorders often resolve spontaneously over time in the absence of any treatment.

7.7.1 Pharmacotherapy

- Systemic and topically applied intranasal corticosteroids for reducing mucosal edema and shrinking nasal polyps.
- Antibiotics, decongestants, and antihistamines for chemosensory losses due to bacterial sinus infection and allergic rhinitis.
- Proton pump inhibitors, histamine receptor antagonists, and antacids for management of dysgeusias associated with gastroesophageal reflux disease.
- Antifungal therapy for treatment of dysgeusia associated with oral candidiasis.
- Benzodiazepines, tricyclic antidepressants, and anticonvulsants may also be helpful for patients with dysosmias and dysgeusias. Some examples are:
  - Clonazepam 0.5–2 mg/day
  - Amitriptyline 25–100 mg/day
  - Gabapentin 300–2,000 mg/day
- The efficacy of dietary supplements such as zinc gluconate, alpha-lipoic acid, and vitamin A for chemosensory dysfunction is inconclusive, but may be useful for some patients.

7.7.2 Surgery

- Endoscopic and nasal sinus surgery for obstructive disorders may result in return of normal olfactory function if more conservative approaches are unsuccessful.

7.7.3 Miscellaneous

- Management of underlying disorders such as periodontal disease and xerostomia may improve taste function. Artificial saliva may be helpful for patients with xerostomia.
- Masking techniques such as sugarless chewing gum, lozenges, or topical anesthetics may provide temporary relief for idiopathic dysgeusias.

7.8 Treatment Goals and Sequencing of Care

- Baseline and repeat chemosensory testing are useful in assessing prognosis for recovery of normal function.
- Treatment should include counseling on smoke and natural gas detection, labeling of food to track spoilage, and food preparation to maximize appeal and flavor.
- Nutritional counseling is also essential, as patients may compensate for chemosensory losses by overusing salts and sugars.
- Referral to a multidisciplinary taste and smell center may be necessary when diagnosis of the specific disorder cannot be readily established.
- Patients should be reassured that chemosensory disorders are typically not life-threatening and that recovery of normal function may take several years or may never occur, depending upon the specific etiology.

References

1. Rawal S, Hoffman HJ, Bainbridge KE, Huedo-Medina TB, Duffy VB. Prevalence and risk factors of self-reported smell and taste alterations: results from the 2011–12 US National Health and Nutrition Examination Survey (NHANES). Chem Senses. 2016;41:69–76.
2. Hoffman HJ, Ishii EK, Macturk RH. Age-related changes in the prevalence of smell/taste problems among the United States adult population: results of the 1994 disability supplement to the National Health Interview Survey (NHIS). Ann N Y Acad Sci. 1998;855:716–22.
3. Cowart BJ. Taste dysfunction: a practical guide for oral medicine. Oral Dis. 2011;17:2–6.
4. Bromley SM, Doty RL. Olfaction in dentistry. Oral Dis. 2010;16:221–32.
5. Malaty J, Malaty I. Smell and taste disorders in primary care. Am Fam Physician. 2013;88(12):852–9.
6. Bromley SM. Smell and taste disorders: a primary care approach. Am Fam Physician. 2000;61(2):427–36.
7. Cullen MM, Leopold DA. Disorders of smell and taste. Med Clin N Am. 1999;83(1):57–74.
8. Spielman AI. Chemosensory function and dysfunction. Crit Rev Oral Biol Med. 1998;9(3):267–91.
9. Doty RL. Olfaction. Annu Rev Psychol. 2001;52:423–52.
10. Mann N, Lafreniere D. Anosmia and nasal sinus disease. Otolaryngol Clin N Am. 2004;37(2):289–300.
11. Pribitkin E, Rosenthal MD, Cowart BJ. Prevalence and causes of severe taste loss in a chemosensory clinic population. Ann Otol Rhinol Laryngol. 2003;112(11):971–8.
12. Comeau TB, Epstein JB, Migas C. Taste and smell dysfunction in patients receiving chemotherapy: a review of current knowledge. Support Care Cancer. 2001;9(8):575–80.
13. Mott AE, Grushka M, Sessle BJ. Diagnosis and management of taste disorders and burning mouth syndrome. Dent Clin N Am. 1993;37(1):33–71.
14. Ship JA. Gustatory and olfactory considerations: examination and treatment in general practice. J Am Dent Assoc. 1993;124(6):55–62.
15. Mott AE, Leopold DA. Disorders in taste and smell. Med Clin N Am. 1991;75(6):1321–53.

Oral Malodor

8

Patricia Lenton

Pearls of Wisdom

- Chronic persistent oral malodor is often due to a combination of variables, and a blend of treatment modalities are often required to manage breath odor problems.
- While there are numerous products on the market that claim to effectively treat bad breath, many products either have no published research, or very limited published data to back up those claims. Therefore, it is challenging for dental professionals to make evidence-based treatment recommendations.
- Bad breath treatment recommendations must be individualized for each patient, based on their personal concerns and preferences. It is advisable to begin with tongue and interdental cleaning and then slowly adding in supplemental products based on evidence and patient preferences.
- Product use may require 2–3 weeks of consistent application to determine efficacy.
- Future research of bad breath treatment regimens may provide a better understanding of the factors that contribute to breath odor production and ways in which to interrupt the production of the volatile sulfur compounds known to be the principle components of bad breath.

8.1 Introduction

Oral malodor, also known as bad breath or halitosis, refers to unpleasant odors that come from the mouth. Most bad breath is considered to be transient in nature, for example, morning breath. However, it has been estimated that up to 25% of the population suffer from bad breath on a regular basis in spite of having good physical

P. Lenton, BSDH, MA, CCRP
Oral Health Clinical Research Clinic, School of Dentistry, University of Minnesota, Minneapolis, MN, USA
e-mail: lento001@umn.edu

J.N.A.R. Ferreira et al. (eds.), *Orofacial Disorders*,
DOI 10.1007/978-3-319-51508-3_8

and oral health and after the elimination of offensive foods and beverages. Having chronic offensive breath odor can be detrimental to one's self-image and confidence, causing social, emotional, and psychological anxiety.

Most breath odor experts agree that about 90% of breath odor originates within the mouth. Since the majority of breath odors have an oral origin, the dental office is the most logical place for patients to seek advice and treatment. When patients look to dental professionals for expert advice, it is important that we are prepared to explain the causes of oral malodors, that we are able to assess our patients' breath, and that we can provide recommendations for helping patients manage their breath odor. It is also important for dental professionals to recognize when breath odor might have an extraoral origin because this could signal a potentially serious disease and warrant a referral to a health professional (Tangerman, 2012).

The following information is provided to help dental professionals assess the source of their patients' oral malodors and assist their patients in reducing and managing their breath odor.

8.2 Clinical Presentation

Patients with breath odor and/or breath odor concerns present with varying characteristics. Due to the phenomena of adaptation and habituation, it is difficult for a person to assess their own breath odor or other bodily odors. For this reason, some people have bad breath but are unaware of it. Other patients have bad breath and are aware of it, often because people who are significant in their life have told them so. Still others may complain of bad breath even though others cannot detect it. Many of these aforementioned patients can be reassured and educated in methods to assess and manage their breath odor. However, there is a small segment of the population that can develop a delusional or an exaggerated perception about some aspect of their being, in this case, having bad breath that they believe warrants extreme measures to fix. This is known as a body dysmorphic disorder (BDD) and in the case of breath is characterized by an obsessive preoccupation about having extremely offensive breath odor. The term most often used by dental professionals to describe these persons is halitophobia or olfactory reference syndrome (ORS). Persons with halitophobia are extremely difficult to convince that they don't have bad breath. Treating ORS patients in the dental office is extremely challenging. Fortunately, the overwhelming majority of breath odor concerns can be successfully managed in the general dental practice.

Persons with genuine halitosis need to be evaluated, beginning with a thorough medical history to determine any medications that they are taking and also to find out if they have any medical conditions associated with breath odor.

8.3 Etiology and Epidemiology

Breath odor results from the bacterial breakdown by gram-negative anaerobic bacteria, particularly those residing on the posterior dorsum of the tongue, of sulfur-containing amino acids. The released sulfurs volatize and are expelled from the mouth. The principle volatile sulfur compounds (VSCs) associated with intraoral breath odor are hydrogen sulfide (H_2S), methyl mercaptan (CH_3SH), and to a lesser degree, dimethyl sulfide (CH3)2S.

It is widely accepted that 80 to 90% of all bad breath has an oral origin, and of that, 80 to 90% is produced on the posterior third of the tongue. Other dental problems, such as periodontal disease, over-hanging dental restorations, dry mouth, and tonsilar crypts can also contribute to the generating these offensive gases.

The remaining 10% of breath odor can be attributed to non-oral (extraoral) sources. Extraoral halitosis is classified as being either non-blood borne such as halitosis from the sinuses and/or respiratory tract infection or blood-borne halitosis that can include certain systemic disorders. The majority of extraoral halitosis is from blood-borne causes and is associated with the VSC, dimethyl sulfide [$(CH_3)_2S$]. When assessing breath odor, it is important to distinguish between intra- and extra-oral halitosis because blood-borne halitosis can be indicative of a serious disease.

The easiest way to determine if the odor has an oral origin is to compare the odor coming from the mouth with the odor level that comes from the nostrils. Therefore, once it has been determined that an individual's expelled breath has an odor, you would then assess the odor level when they expel air through their nostrils. If the odor remains, and at the same intensity, as the odor detected from the mouth, then you would refer the affected patient for a medical consultation.

8.4 Pathophysiology and Mechanisms

8.4.1 Oral Pathological Etiology (90% of Chronic Bad Breath)

1. Tongue coating on the dorsum of the tongue (80% of oral malodor):
   - Bacterial-laden tongue coating consisting of anaerobic bacteria.
   - Degradation of sulfur-containing amino acids found in oral fluids, tissue, and food debris produces volatile sulfur compounds (VSCs), primarily hydrogen sulfide and methyl mercaptan resulting in pungent rotten egg smell.
   - Thorough tongue scraping starting in the area of the circumvallate papilla and scraping in a forward motion seven to ten times until tongue coating appears clear and the brushing of all other oral structures and interdental cleaning will reduce VSCs and eliminate most oral malodor for up to 3 h.
   - The use of antibacterial, zinc-containing, and/or oxygenating products, twice daily, have been shown to reduce the production of VSCs and breath odor levels.
   - Regular meal eating and good hydration can reduce VSCs for up to 2 h.
2. Periodontitis:
   - Periodontal pathogens (P. gingivalis, T. denticola, B. forsythus) produce VSCs, primarily methyl mercaptan that has a pungent spoiled cabbage smell.
   - Increased tongue coating is associated with periodontal disease.
   - Generalized periodontitis with moderate to severe bone loss is needed to produce and release adequate concentrations of VSCs from the sulcus to achieve detectable, offensive breath odor.

- Therapeutic periodontal treatments (scaling/root planing, referral for surgical interventions, and thorough daily home care, including thorough tongue scraping) generally reduces/eliminates odor.
- Patients with a breath concern often choose to incorporate mouth rinsing as part of their oral hygiene regimen for reassurance. The use of oral rinses also can assist in reducing the incidence of experiencing the report of having a bad taste that can occur with or without periodontal disease.

3. Unclean dentures and partials:
   - If plaque and calculus are present, clean denture/partials using a brush and water only and place them into a sealed plastic bag for 5–10 min. Smell bag for odor quality and intensity.
   - Compare mouth odor, with dentures removed, to odor of the bagged dentures. Stronger odor in bag is indicative of denture odor origin.
   - If candida is present, oral odor will have a sweetish acid quality, and appropriate antifungal treatment will be required.
   - Daily denture cleaning and soaking with over-the-counter effervescent tablets will generally control most denture/appliance odor.
   - Patient should remove denture(s) out overnight to prevent bacterial accumulation.
   - For persistent odor, appliances can be soaked in Peridex for 10–15 min. Prolonged soaking in Peridex may cause staining. Do not use bleach or peroxide due to bleaching and corrosive nature.
4. Postnasal drip:
   - A significant amount of this mucous does end up in the mouth and provides a substantial amount of cysteine and methionine (amino acid substrate) for bacterial putrefaction.
   - Patient will have the distinctive odor quality of sulfur (rotten eggs).
   - Odor is often intermittent and with varying intensity. Patient may be unaware of the problem since it is difficult to self-assess.
   - Thorough tongue scraping and gargling with a zinc and/or antimicrobial mouth rinse often eliminates most of the offending problem; however, if persistent, the patient can use antimicrobial sprays to reach those areas that cannot be brushed or scraped, such as the throat and tonsils.
   - Patients who regularly use antihistamines, inhalers, or other medications known to result in dry mouth should maintain meticulous home care and drink fluids to improved hydration, and prevent reduced salivary flow, which intensify the level of odiferous compounds into oral cavity.
   - Some patients benefit from use of saline nasal sprays and/or the use of netti pots. Please note, if patients want to use a Netti pot they should be encouraged to use either distilled water, or, water taht has been boiled and allowed to cool.
5. ANUG:
   - Overwhelmingly pungent fetid odor of rotting hay or sulfides associated with necrosis of gingival tissues.
   - Gingival debridement and antibiotic therapy will eliminate odor.
   - Daily and routine professional oral care needed to maintain oral health.
6. Tonsiloliths:
   - Calcified material attached to tonsils with a pungent rotten cabbage smell.

- Patient is often aware of the calcifications and is often very self-conscious of the possibility of offending others.
- Generally odor can only be detected when placed in close proximity of the nose. Others generally cannot smell a person's tonsiloliths when talking at a social-distance apart.

7. Dental abscesses and localized infections:
   - Patients with localized infections will often complain of having a bad taste (sour or bitter) in their mouth. When patients perceive a bad taste in their mouth they often equate this with having a breath odor problem when none exists.
   - Patient would need to have a significant abscess or generalized oral infections before breath odor would be noticeable to others.
   - Off tastes (a.k.a. after or bad tastes) are usually the result of medications, sinus drainage, xerostomia, dental infections, and bacterial putrefaction around defective restorations.
   - If the off taste is due to an infection, treatment of the localized infection together with the use of an antimicrobial mouth rinse will often eliminate off taste sensations and eliminate complaint of bad breath.

8.4.2 Oral Physiological Factors (Not Causal But Contributing Factors to Oral Malodors)

1. Morning breath:
   - Reduced salivary flow during sleep favors bacterial putrefaction and the dryness intensifies odor levels.
   - Unclean mouth gives patient perception of offensive odor.
   - Transient and will disappear after oral stimulation (talking, eating, etc.).
2. Xerostomia caused by medications or salivary dysfunction:
   - Reduction of salivary flow rate and stagnation of saliva contribute to bacterial shift that can increase oral malodor formation (Kleinberg and Westbay).
   - Alkaline environment is also associated in oral malodor production.
   - Lack of wetting of mucosa increases release of offending compounds into the oral air.
   - Patients suffering from reduced salivary flow should frequently drink and rinse oral cavity with water for continued hydration of the oral mucosa.
   - Eating regularly will lower pH, provide some mechanical debridement to help reduce bacterial growth on tongue, and also stimulate salivary flow. Fasting/hunger can has also been associated with oral malodor due to dehydration.
   - Frequent oral stimulation and use of artificial saliva may be helpful.
3. Large carious lesions and or defective restorations:
   - Trapping of food debris by generalized poor or lack of dental care usually does not produce sufficient level of odor to offend others.
   - Patient may experience bad taste and perceives odor exists.
   - Professional dental care and thorough oral home care often eliminates patients concerns.

8.4.3 Non-pathological and Nonphysiological Factors (10%)

Halitosis can be caused by the absorption of malodorous compounds through the digestive system and transferred and released through the respiratory system or can be a symptom of a late stage pathogeneses (e.g., cancer, kidney failure). Professional or home care will not eliminate problem. Patient will need to be referred to physician for diagnosis and treatment.

1. Pulmonary abscesses, pneumonia, and bronchial conditions:
   - Pungent sewer-like odor (diseased tissues) for proliferation of anaerobic bacteria with tissue destruction or decaying blood quality
   - Often associated with other symptoms (cough, difficulty breathing, etc.)
   - Referral for medical treatment of infection or condition
2. Sinusitis and nasopharyngeal infections:
   - Nasal malodor usually has a slightly cheesy odor characteristic.
   - Often it is transient lasting 7–10 days.
   - Chronic persistent problem needs referral to physician.
   - A nasal odor that only occurs during the morning may be indicative of a concentrated nasal mucous accumulation during sleep. Odor may last for 1–2 h until mucous has been discharged. The use of nasal sprays or drinking hot liquids can be helpful in eliminating the mucus buildup.
3. Diet: strong spicy foods (garlic, curry, onions, etc.) and alcohol consumption:
   - Odorant will have a specific quality similar to offending food/beverage.
   - High protein low carbohydrate can induce ketosis with a characteristic acetone smell.
   - Large quantities of protein supplements above recommendation can produce distinctive musty and stale-like odor and bad taste.
   - Can last for up to 36 h; however, odor will typically disappear after abstinence, and the compounds are metabolized and released into the lungs.
   - Frequent use of flavored rinses, gums, mints, and sprays will mask odor.
4. Medications:
   - Disulfiram (alcoholism) metabolized to carbon disulfide (slight fecal odor).
   - Dimethyl sulfoxide (muscle pain) and cysteamine (nephropathic cystinosis) metabolized to dimethyl sulfide (garlic odor).
   - Frequent use of flavored rinses, gums, mints, and sprays reduces odor intensity by masking odorant.
   - Medications can alter taste sensations and is not associated with malodor.
   - Referral to physician for evaluation of prescription change or if odor perception has psychological concerns.
5. Tobacco use – distinctive nicotine odorant quality from lungs:
   - Occasional smoker – Frequent use of flavored rinses, gums, mints, and sprays will mask odor until gone (5–8 h).
   - Heavy smoker – Frequent use of flavored rinses, gums, mints, and sprays will not completely mask odor. Complete abstinence is required for several weeks to remove offending nicotine tars in lungs.

6. Metabolic disorders will have distinctive odor quality:
    - Trimethylaminuria (TMA) enzyme insufficiency to metabolize trimethylamine. Distinctive fishy amine odor in urine, sweat, and breath with a constant presence of odor 24/7. Referral to primary physician for evaluation is recommended.
    - Hypermethioninemia involves high levels of methionine with an overwhelmingly sweet odor in urine and breath. Referral to primary physician for evaluation is recommended.
7. Systemic conditions/diseases will have characteristic odor quality:
    - Diabetes, incomplete carbohydrate metabolism (ketoacidosis):
        - Distinctive acetone scent in breath (rotting apples)
        - Usually intermittent unless uncontrolled
        - Referral to primary physician for evaluation
    - Liver failure/cirrhosis, shunting of portal blood around the liver:
        - Distinctive musty garlic-like odor in breath and blood
        - Referral to primary physician for evaluation
    - Kidney disease/failure:
        - Accumulation of dimethylamine and trimethylamine
        - Distinctive stale urine/fishlike odor in breath, blood, and urine
        - Referral to primary physician for evaluation
    - Gastric reflux, H. pylori, or stomach conditions:
        - Odor expelled during intermittent belching or vomiting.
        - Patient may complain of heartburn.
        - Heavy acidic sour odor.
        - Rinsing with water or product use for foul taste.
        - Referral to primary physician for evaluation.

8.4.4 Undetectable Malodor (Oral and Non-oral)

1. Halitophobia or olfactory reference syndrome – Clinician should suspect the patient has an exaggerated fear they suffer from bad breath if:
    - Clinician cannot smell any odor at three to four separate odor evaluation appointments.
    - Patient cannot provide a confirmation from a confidant stating they have personally noticed mouth odor from the patient.
    - Objective instruments do not record detectable levels VSCs or microbes.
    - Patient believes they can smell the odor and indicates it lasts all day.
    - Patient indicates that it interferes with social life and ability to work, and they avoid interacting with others.
    - Patient practices concealment by frequent use of gum chewing, eating mints, toothbrushing, keeps at safe distance, and/or covers mouth when talking to others.
    - Patient has sought treatment and evaluation from several other health professionals (ENT, gastroenterologist, etc.).

    - Patient shows signs of anxiety and depression and/or express unhappiness with life overall.
2. Provide patient with reassurance that their perceived odor is not offensive:
    - Give patient permission to talk to you freely about this embarrassing topic and their concerns.
    - Encourage discussion and give information about the causes of malodor formation and perceptions others may have about bad breath.
3. Provide strategies for self-assessment:
    - Self-assessment techniques (wrist lick, spoon, syringe collection test).
    - Encourage identification of a confidant to help patient monitor changes in odor over time (trusted friend, family member, co-worker).
4. Consider referral for psychological assessment and counseling if suspicious of body dysmorphic dysfunction (BDD), which is a subclass of obsessive-compulsive disorders. Antipsychotic chlorpromazine and tricyclic antidepressants have had some success in treating BDD in malodor patients.

8.5 Diagnosis and Diagnostic Criteria

8.5.1 Clinical Examination

Patient needs to present having prepared for odor evaluation by refraining from:

- Taking antibiotics at least for 1 month prior to examination.
- Eating strong spicy foods for 48 h before examination.
- Eating or drinking flavored beverages for 6–8 h before examination. Water is permitted up to 2 h before examination.
- Wearing scented personal care products (colognes, hair spray, aftershave, etc.) on examination day.
- Using oral care products for 10–12 h before evaluation.

8.5.2 Subjective Sensory Evaluation Methods

The human nose provides the best test to determine if a patient has a bad breath problem; therefore, it is important to simply smell and assess their breath. It is important that the person who is conducting the evaluation has a good sense of smell and that they are not overly sensitive to malodors so that they are able to accurately evaluate the breath odor quality and intensity. This is a good protocol for assessing a person's breath:

1. Patient keeps mouth closed for 2 min and then repeats "Pat's Puppy" several times while the practitioner uses an index card to waft the breath toward their own nose and directly sniffs the breath for odor intensity and quality. (Pronouncing words that begin with the letter "P" helps to project the breath.)

2. Patient closes their mouth and exhales through their nasal passages while the practitioner evaluates nostril breath for intensity and quality and compares to the odor intensity of the patient's oral breath.
3. Oral origin – If odor is stronger from mouth than nasal passages then:
   - Comprehensive dental examination for oral pathology is performed (e.g., periodontal disease, plaque retentive restorations and large carious lesions, ulcerations and acute oral infections).
   - Assess cleanliness of dentures and partials. Place in plastic bag for 10 min then smell bag odor. Clean appliances with brush and tap water and place in plastic bag for another 10 min. Open bag and smell for odor. Compare odor form oral cavity to odor in bag.
   - Evaluate levels of gingival plaque and bacterial tongue coating. Scrape posterior dorsum with plastic spoon and smell plaque accumulation for odor for similarity to mouth odor.
   - Assess salivary flow. Saliva and soft tissues may have the capability to store large quantities of VSCs.
   - Characteristic oral odor will be rotten egg (sulfur) or sweet fecal (mercaptans).
4. Non-oral origin – If odor emitted from the nasal passages is equal to or stronger than the odor from the oral cavity, then a systemic condition should be considered:
   - Obtain a thorough medical history and review for possible metabolic disturbances or diseases.
   - Frequency and types of prescription and OTC medications used.
   - Frequency of acute respiratory infections or conditions.
   - Dietary evaluation for characteristic food odors and dramatic dietary changes for metabolic processes (Atkins, vegetarian high in sulfur, hunger/starvation, dehydration).
   - Medications and systemic conditions will have a characteristic odor quality (fishy, acetone, ammonia, etc.) and is generally different from typical bacterial plaque odor.
5. History of odor onset and intensity:
   - Equal intensity from the nose and mouth – systemic origin and will usually have a distinctive quality.
   - Quick onset and strong intensity – acute infection in respiratory system.
   - Intermittent odor – gastrointestinal, habits, and will have characteristic quality (garlic, onions, alcohol).
   - Rapid onset and progressively intensifying breath malodor is suggestive of an infective process, possibly secondary to carcinomas or other localized pathologies in the airway.
   - Slow gradual onset with varying intensity with periodic absence – chronic condition and/or disease progression.
   - Quick onset or periodic and regular occurrence – gastric conditions, hormonal (puberty, menses), and/or routine medication use.
   - Regular daily occurrence associated with medication, poor eating habits, and lack of fluid intake.
   - Time of onset and relationship to major changes in life – stress, social, and psychological events.

- Duration of problem – Patient states that the odor is every day, 24 h day, and extremely offensive patient is probably halitophobic.

6. Personal practice questionnaire:
   - Patient's perception of problem – intensity, duration, starting date, taste.
   - Dietary practices – type and amount of fluids and foods, special diets.
   - Habits – smoking, alcohol.
   - Frequency of use of oral care products.
   - Illness and attitude questions to identify anxiety, phobias, and compulsive activities.
   - How did patient determine they have a malodor problem? Third-party verification.
   - What is the patient's belief as of the cause of their malodor?
   - Previous examinations by health professionals and their findings and recommendations. What is the patient's perception of these findings?

8.5.3 Objective Evaluation Instruments

In addition to subjective assessment of breath odor levels, it is ideal if you also have an "objective" method for assessing breath odor. This is especially true if you plan to offer ongoing breath odor assessment and treatment in your practice.

1. Halimeter® is used for evaluating nasal and oral breath:
   - Only measures total sulfur level; typically, over 100 parts per billion (ppb) indicates offensive odor level.
   - Correlated to sensory odor judges.
   - Requires large sample volume.
   - Sensor measures total VSCs and is more sensitive to hydrogen sulfide than methyl mercaptan. Sensor easily contaminates with alcohol- and/or essential oil-containing products. Need to follow the manufacturer's instruction to wait for a defined period of time following usage of such rinses to avoid contaminating the sensor.
   - Fast, portable, easy to use, and good for measuring improvement over time.
2. OralChroma™ is used for evaluating nasal and oral breath:
   - Measures hydrogen sulfide, methyl mercaptan, and dimethyl sulfide individually. (If over 80 ppb, it indicates offensive odor.)
   - Requires less than 5 ml of sample and 8 min per analysis time.
   - Correlated to sensory odor judges.
   - Portable, easy to use, and works well to measure improvement over time.
   - Expensive and requires some training for use.
3. Gas chromatography used for evaluating nasal and oral breath (gold standard). This analytical method is usually reserved for large institutions due to the cost and specialized technical skills involved in using the equipment:
   - Can identify specific compounds in addition to VSCs.
   - Requires little time and small sample volumes.
   - Excellent sensitivity, specificity, and reliability.

- Expensive and needs trained personnel.

4. BANA test (benzoyl-DL-arginine-2-napthylamide synthetic peptide):
    - Analysis for microbes producing trypsin-like enzyme T. denticola, P. gingivalis, and B. forsythus associated with periodontal disease and oral malodor
    - Small chair side incubator with 5 min analysis time
    - Correlates well sensory odor judges
    - Can be used before and after treatment to visually show the patient the differences following treatment

8.6 Rationale for Treatment

Given that the majority of bad breath has an oral origin and that the majority of breath odor emitted from the mouth results from the bacterial coating on the posterior dorsum surface of the tongue, the most important treatment recommendation is for patients to mechanically clean their tongue. Some oral malodor researchers have raised concerns about patients becoming overzealous about cleaning their tongue and scraping too hard so that they actually traumatize the tongue's surface. For this reason, it is important to give detailed oral hygiene instructions to patients for whom tongue cleaning is recommended.

8.7 Treatment Options

As mentioned previously, fully comprehensive oral hygiene instructions are key to patients for whom tongue cleaning is recommended.

In addition to mechanical debridement, chemotherapeutic methods are often employed. The following methods outline several options:

8.7.1 Mechanical Debridement

1. Tongue cleaning with scrapers:
    - Tongue scrapers come in a variety of shapes and sizes.
    - Smaller working ends allow for better access to the most posterior regions of the tongue.
    - If gagging is a problem, have patient rinse with very cold water before scraping or pant while scraping the tongue.
    - To prevent curling of tongue, patient can hold end with clean cloth to flatten tongue during cleaning.
    - Starting at the most posterior region of the tongue dorsum, the scraper is drawn to the anterior while maintaining a gentle pressure. Pressing hard may damage tongue surface.
    - Tongue should be scraped seven to ten times cleaning the entire dorsal surface.
2. Tongue cleaning with brushes
    - Tongue brushes come in a variety of shapes and sizes.

- Brushes are generally used after scraping to apply antimicrobial agents to the tongue surface.
- Use short circular motions with light pressure to work chemical agent into the fissures and between the tongue papillae.
- Scraping of residual agent is required after application, and refraining from rinsing after scraping will allow the chemical agent prolonged access to offending compounds and bacteria.

8.7.2 Localized Chemical/Antibacterial Methods

Mouth rinsing is often used as a chemical approach to treat chronic and persistent oral malodor cases. Mouth rinse efficacy must balance the elimination/reduction of the pathogenic bacteria while maintaining the balance of the normal oral flora and preventing an overgrowth of opportunistic pathogens. If rinses are not used in conjunction with oral debridement, their effect will only be temporary since they are unable to penetrate thick layers of bacterial plaque and mucus.

1. Antimicrobial agents
   (a) Chlorhexidine – can be used for a defined period of time:
      - Very effective broad-spectrum bactericidal agent.
      - Does reduce anaerobic bacteria on the tongue dorsum.
      - Substantivity increases efficacy.
      - Long-term use is not recommended due to adverse effects of staining and altered taste.

   (b) Peroxides:
      - Oxygenating mechanisms are effective against anaerobic microbes.
      - Able to oxidize and reduce sulfur compounds.
      - Use of full-strength hydrogen peroxide is not recommended due to possible soft tissue effects. There are peroxide products on the market that use an attenuated level of hydrogen peroxide.

   (c) Zinc-containing products:
      - Zinc ions bind to protein receptors on the surface of the bacteria prohibiting proteins from binding and preventing protein metabolism, therefore preventing production of new VSCs.
      - Zinc ion also binds to sulfur radicals inhibiting the expression of the VSCs.
      - Zinc rinses (in chloride, citrate, or acetate form) used twice daily have been found to reduce oral VSC concentrations for greater than 3 h.
      - Zinc-based products usually have strong flavoring agents to mask the zinc taste.
      - Mainly used in rinses but also found in tongue-cleaning gels, chewing gums, and lozenges.

   (d) Chlorine dioxide – most widely promoted rinse for the control of oral malodor:

- Chlorine dioxide (ClO_2) is a strong oxidizing agent that has a high affinity for sulfur-containing compounds and can oxidize some amines and phenols.
- Has affinity for cell surfaces and concentrates in plaque and soft tissues.
- Bacterial effect may be interference with protein synthesis and alterations in cell wall permeability.
- ClO_2 has a short shelf life therefore needs to be mixed just before using. Sodium chlorite is stabilized chlorine dioxide and has a longer shelf life but less ClO_2 availability in the solution.

(e) Cetylpyridinium chloride (CPC) in many OTC rinses:
- Cationic quaternary ammonium compound with antiseptic
- In vitro as effective as CHX however not as effective in vivo which is due to low substantivity

(f) Triclosan (2,4,4′-trichloro-2′-hydroxydiphenyl ether):
- Broad-spectrum nonionic lipid soluble antimicrobial agent.
- Effective against most types of oral cavity bacteria.
- A mouth rinse system combining zinc and triclosan has been shown to have a cumulative effect, with the reduction of malodor increasing with the duration of the product use.
- Formulation mainly in toothpastes but also found in some rinses. (Note: effective September, 2017, the United States Food & Drug Administration (FDA) has banned the use of Triclosan in rinses and other products due to a lack of evidence of efficacy).

8.8 Treatment Goals and Sequencing of Care

A flowchart is displayed in Fig. 8.1, which will help guide clinicians to manage halitosis.

- The primary goal is to assist the patient in managing their breath odor level so that is below the level of detection by the human nose.
- Improving patients' quality of life, especially the psychosocial aspects, is of utmost importance.
- Reassurance that everyone suffers from bad breath and it is often not as intense as one imagines is an important concept to explain.
- Provide patient with strategies for determination of oral malodor presence and self-assessment of odor intensity are important.
- Treatment sequence:
  - Dietary counseling is an important consideration, especially if the patient eats abundant sulfur-producing foods (e.g., onions, garlic, horseradish, etc.).
  - Must include daily debridement of the tongue. If tongue cleaning reduces odor but there is some detectable offensiveness, then chemotherapeutic agents should be added to the treatment regimen.

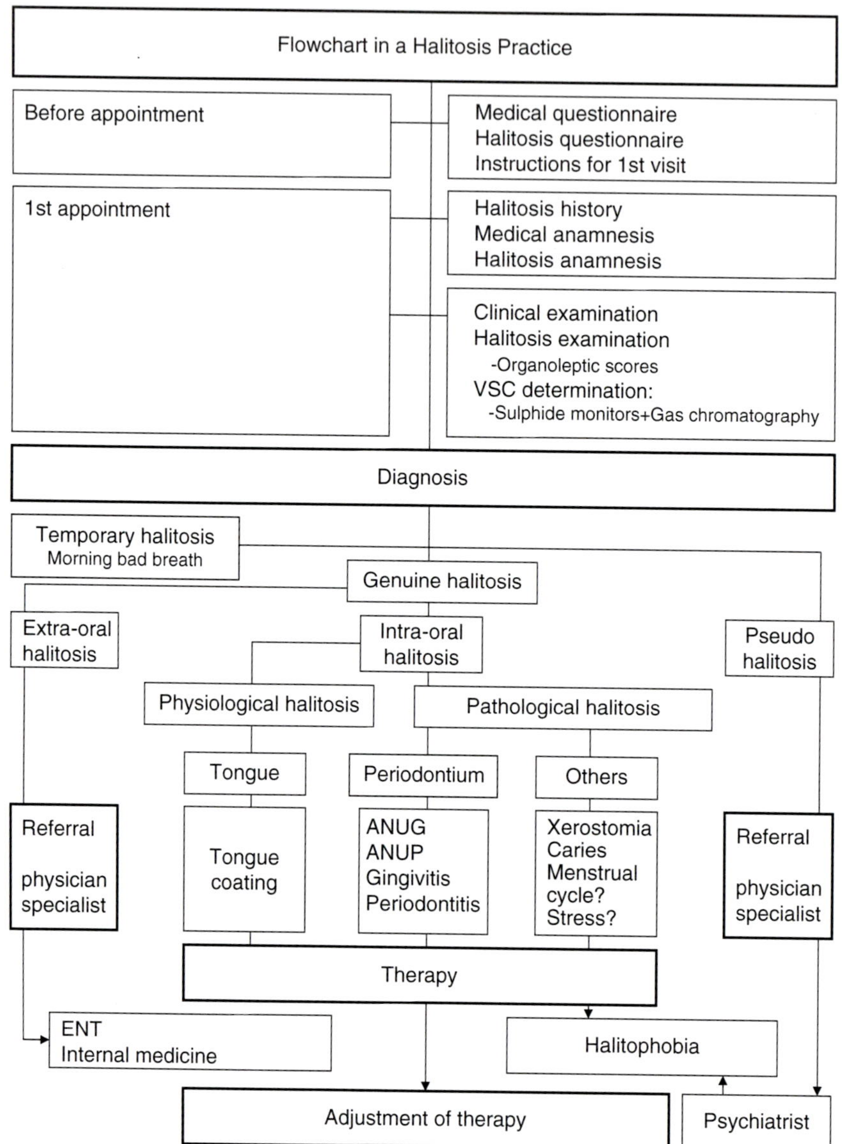

Fig. 8.1 Flowchart for halitosis management (Permission to reproduce needs to be requested to Winkel et al. [16].)

- Products containing zinc, chlorine dioxide, or cetylpyridinium chloride have been shown to be helpful.
- Product must reach source of odor and remain long enough to have an effect. Therefore, sprays may be indicated for the throat and far posterior regions of the tongue, tongue-cleaning gels for thick tongue coatings and rinses, and lozenges and gums for reduced salivary flow which may be beneficial for odor control.

References

1. Furne J, Majerus G, Lenton P, Springfield J, Levitt D, Levitt M. Comparison of volatile sulfur compounds measured with a sulfide detector vs gas chromatography. J Dent Res. 2002;81(2):140–3.
2. Kawaguchi Y. Psychological management of halitosis. In: Yaegaki K, editor. Clinical guidelines for halitosis. Tokyo: Quintessence Publishing; 2000. p. 87–96.
3. Kleinberg I, Westbay G. Salivary and metabolic factors involved in oral malodor formation. J Perinatol. 1992;63:768–75.
4. Lenton P, Majerus G, Bakdash B. Counseling and treating bad breath patients: a step-by-step approach. J Contemp Dent Pract. 2001;2(2):1–13.
5. Morita M, Wang HL. Association between oral malodor and adult periodontitis: a review. J Clin Periodontol. 2001;28:813–9.
6. Nakano Y, Yoshimura M, Koga T. Correlation between oral malodor and periodontal bacteria. Microbes Infect. 2002;4:679–83.
7. Quirynan M, Mongardini C, van Steenberghe D. The effect of a 1-stage full-mouth disinfection on oral malodor and microbial colonization of the tongue in periodontitis patients. A pilot study. J Periodontol. 1998;69:374–82.
8. Seemann, Rainer, et al. "Effectiveness of mechanical tongue cleaning on oral levels of volatile sulfur compounds." The Journal of the American Dental Association 132.9 (2001): 1263–1267.
9. Suarez F, Jurne J, Springfield J, Levitt M. Morning breath odor: influence of treatments on sulfur gases. J Dent Res. 2000;79(10):1773–7.
10. Tangerman A. Halitosis in medicine: a review. Int Dent J. 2002;52(3):201–6.
11. Van Steenberghe D. Breath malodor. Curr Opin Periodontol. 1997;4:137–43.
12. Winkel E, Roldan S, Winkelhoff A, Herrera D, Sanz M. Clinical effects of a new mouthrinse containing chlorhexidine, cetylpyridinium chloride and zinc-lactate on oral halitosis. J Clin Periodontol. 2003;30:300–6.
13. Yaegaki K, Coil JM. Tongue brushing and mouth rinsing as basic treatment measures for halitosis. Int Dent J. 2002;52(3):192–6.
14. Tangerman A, et al. Halitosis and Helicobacter pylori infection. J Breath Res. 2012;6(1):017102.
15. Tangerman A, Winkel EG. Volatile sulfur compounds as the cause of bad breath: a review. Phosphorus Sulfur Silicon Relat Elem. 2013;188(4):396–402.
16. Seemann R, Conceicao MD, Filippi A, Greenman J, Lenton P, Nachnani S, Quirynen M, Roldan S, Schulze H, Sterer N, Tangerman A, Winkel EG, Yaegaki K, Rosenberg M. Halitosis management by the general dental practitioner—results of an international consensus workshop at BREATH ANALYSIS Summit 2013—International Conference of Breath Research, 9th of June 2013—Saarbrücken/Wallerfangen, Germany. J Breath Res. 2014;8(1):017101.

Part IV

Salivary Gland Dysfunctions

Salivary Gland Dysfunction and Xerostomia

9

Mahvash Navazesh

Pearls of Wisdom

- Saliva plays an important role in oral and systemic health.
- Dry mouth or xerostomia is a common complaint among patients of different ages in general and among geriatric and medically complex patients in particular.
- Salivary gland disorders are caused by a variety of etiologic factors.
- Salivary gland dysfunction may lead to irreversible intraoral hard and soft tissue changes and ultimately may reduce the quality of life.
- Oral healthcare providers play a significant role in risk assessment, early detection, management, and prevention of salivary gland disorders. These are essential for maintaining a proper oral and systemic health in this patient population.

9.1 Introduction

Saliva plays a significant role in oral and systemic health. The major functions of saliva include, but are not limited to, lubrication, intraoral hard and soft tissue protection, remineralization of teeth, and digestion.

Qualitative and quantitative changes associated with salivary gland disorders could affect the quality of life of an individual. Recurrent dental caries and oral fungal infection are the most common complications associated with chronic salivary gland dysfunction.

M. Navazesh, DMD
Division of Diagnostic Sciences, Herman Ostrow School of Dentistry, University of Southern California, Los Angeles, CA, USA
e-mail: navazesh@usc.edu

J.N.A.R. Ferreira et al. (eds.), *Orofacial Disorders*,
DOI 10.1007/978-3-319-51508-3_9

Saliva contains more than 2,000 proteins that are involved in different biologic functions to maintain oral homeostasis. Salivary biomarkers have received significant recognition by different scholars in recent years for their potentials in the detection of early stages of oral and systemic diseases.

Firstly, it is important to define these two key concepts:

- Xerostomia: the subjective complaint of dry mouth.
- Salivary gland dysfunction: objective evidence of alterations (qualitative and/or quantitative) in saliva output. Dysfunction may include a decrease (hypofunction) or an increase (hyperfunction) of the saliva output.

9.2 Clinical Presentation

9.2.1 Symptoms

- Asymptomatic (no dry mouth complaint)
- Difficulty chewing, speaking, swallowing, wearing removable intraoral prostheses
- Dry, sore, or burning symptoms in the eyes, mouth, tongue, lips, throat, nose
- Bad breath
- Taste abnormalities including salty, metallic, bitter sensations (dysgeusia)
- Facial swelling or pain, ear pain
- Frequent need to sip water with food or awakening at nighttime with dry mouth
- Drooling due to excessive salivation (sialorrhoea)

9.2.2 Signs

- Salivary gland enlargement
- Lack of saliva upon palpation of salivary glands
- Atrophic mucosal changes involving orifices of major salivary glands
- Blood or pus contaminated saliva upon palpation of major glands
- Dry, inflamed intraoral mucosa
- Inflamed, lobulated tongue mucosa
- Rampant dental caries
- Recurrent dental caries
- Extensive restorative experience
- Recurrent oral fungal infection

9.3 Etiology and Epidemiology

9.3.1 Etiological Factors

- Genetic disorder (salivary gland aplasia).
- Inflammation (sialadenitis) is the most common cause of salivary gland dysfunction. Most common causes of sialadenitis:

  - Sialoliths
  - Bacterial and viral infections
  - Polypharmacy
- Neoplasm (adenoma, carcinoma type).
- Noninflammatory, nonneoplastic enlargement (sialadenosis).

9.3.2 Prevalence

The prevalence of salivary gland dysfunction and xerostomia varies in different population and age groups based on ethnicity, gender, medical conditions, medications, severity of the medical conditions, and type, dosage, and frequency of medication usage.

9.4 Pathophysiology and Mechanisms

Salivary gland dysfunction and xerostomia may be transient or permanent, acute or chronic in nature based on the etiologic factor(s). Common systemic conditions associated with salivary gland dysfunction are:

- Autoimmune (Sjogren's syndrome, scleroderma, lupus erythematous)
- Cardiovascular (hypertension)
- Endocrine (hypothyroidism, unstable diabetes)
- Neurologic (Alzheimer's disease)
- Psychiatric (depression, anxiety disorders)
- Infectious (HIV, HCV, paramyxovirus)

Salivary gland function altered by autoimmune diseases is often irreversible in nature. Sjogren's syndrome affects mostly women and involves the exocrine glands' function leading to dry mouth and dry eyes. The lymphocytic infiltration of normal tissue by the disease process is permanent in nature and leads to major clinical complications if not addressed in a timely manner.

Common pharmacotherapeutic approaches associated with complications of salivary gland dysfunction:

- Irradiation to the head and neck regions
- Chemotherapy
- Anticholinergic medications
- Selected antiretroviral medications, sedatives, analgesics, antihypertensives, anticonvulsives, cytotoxics, and antidepressants

Radiation-induced salivary gland damage is often permanent in nature in about 40% of patients. New treatment modalities such as intensity-modulated radiation therapy (IMRT) and gland-sparing techniques may help present such irreversible damage.

The severity and reversibility of the salivary gland changes caused by pharmacotherapeutic agents vary significantly. However, inflammatory changes caused by most other categories of drugs are transient and could be reversible if the medications are discontinued or salivary changes are compensated for in a timely manner.

9.5 Diagnosis and Diagnostic Criteria

The risk assessment and diagnostic workup is key when a patient complains of dry mouth and/or positively answers the dry mouth questionnaire. In Fig. 9.1, a flowchart is displayed to better understand how to evaluate and manage xerostomia.

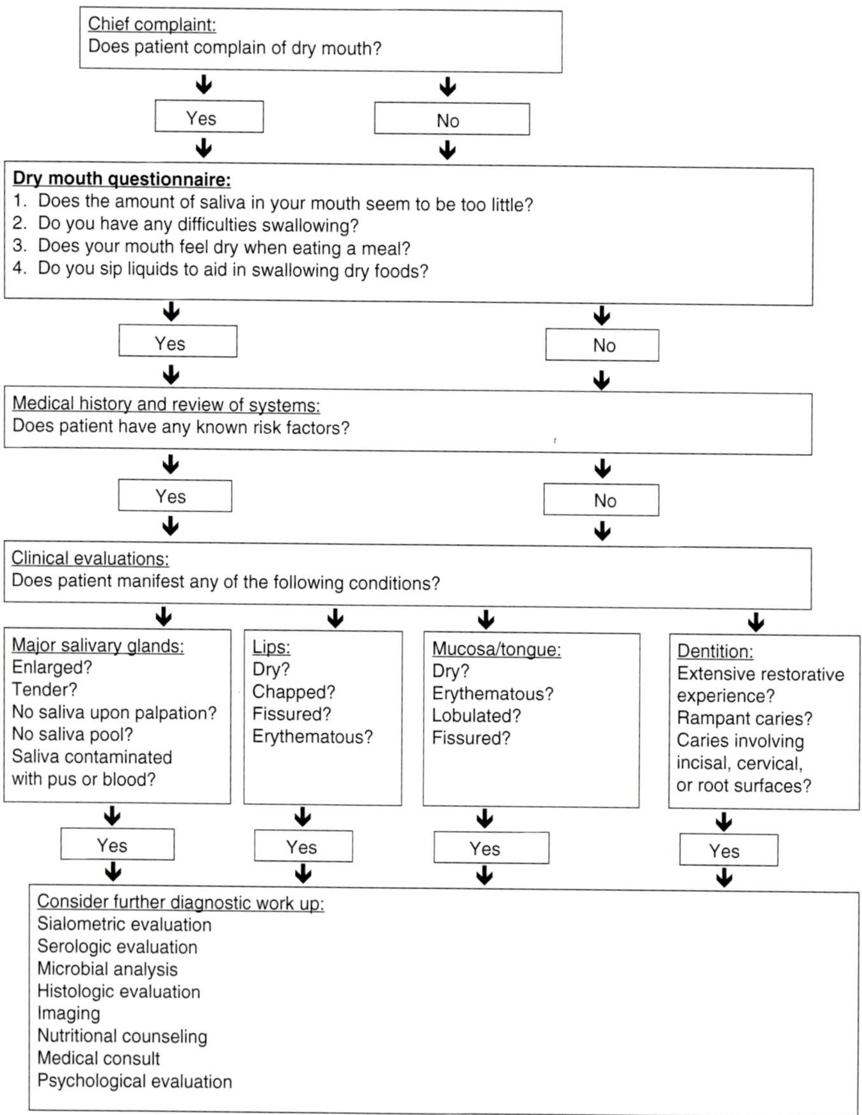

Fig. 9.1 Identifying patients with or at risk for chronic salivary gland hypofunction

9.6 Rationale for Treatment

- Identify patients at risk of development of xerostomia and/or salivary gland dysfunction.
- Identify patients with existing xerostomia and/or salivary gland dysfunction.
- Assess the severity of existing or evolving complications associated with salivary gland dysfunction.
- Identify and, if possible, eliminate the risk and/or etiologic factors.
- Make referrals to other healthcare providers if needed for the management of systemic conditions.
- Utilize evidence-based decision making and evolving scientific information.
- Implement patient-centered individualized strategies to prevent onset or progression of complications associated with salivary gland dysfunction.
- Restore form and function of affected structures and manage other existing complications caused by salivary gland dysfunction.
- Monitor management outcomes and reassess efficacy of implemented plan and treatment. Revise plan accordingly if needed.

9.7 Treatment Options

Treatment modalities vary based on the etiology and severity of existing conditions and may include:

- Stimulation of saliva secretion: non-cariogenic sialagogues
- Hydration
- Lubrication
- Saliva replacement (saliva substitute)
- Dietary modifications
- Psychiatric and behavioral counseling for coping strategies and to reduce behavioral and lifestyle factors associated with the condition
- Pharmacotherapeutic interventions
- Surgical approaches

Several potential treatment approaches have been explored and studied recently (e.g., gene therapy, cell therapy), and these will be discussed in detail in the following two chapters.

9.8 Treatment Goals and Sequence of Care

The above treatment options are aimed for increasing the oral cavity moisture by lubricating the intraoral soft and hard tissues with stimulated saliva or by taking saliva substitutes.

The first line of treatment should focus on improving oral hygiene consistently with non-cariogenic sialagogues in the form of topical, gel, spray, or mouthrinses.

The use of cholinergic medications should be carefully evaluated if patient has a complex medical history or is under a polypharmacy treatment regimen.

Suggested Readings

1. Jensen SB, Pedersen AML, Vissink A, et al. A systematic review of salivary gland hypofunction and xerostomia induced by cancer therapies: prevalence, severity and impact on quality of life. Support Care Cancer. 2010;18(8):1039–60. doi:10.1007/s00520-010-0827-8.
2. Villa A, Wolff A, Aframian D, et al. World workshop on oral medicine VI: a systematic review of medication-induced salivary gland dysfunction: prevalence, diagnosis, and treatment. Clin Oral Invest. 2015;19:1563–80. doi:10.1007/s00784-015-1488-2.
3. Löfgren CD, Wickström C, Sonesson M, et al. A systematic review of methods to diagnose oral dryness and salivary gland function. BMC Oral Health. 2012;12:29. doi:10.1186/1472-6831-12-29.
4. Luciano N, Valentini V, Calabrò A, et al. One year in review 2015: Sjögren's syndrome. Clin Exp Rheumatol. 2015;33(2):259–71.
5. O'Connor R, David MA, Peter BA. Focused review of investigation, management and outcomes of salivary gland disease in specialty-specific journals. Br J Oral Maxillofac Surg. 2014;52(6):483–90. doi:10.1016/j.bjoms.2014.03.016.
6. Turner L, Mupparapu M, Akintoye SO. Review of the complications associated with treatment of oropharyngeal cancer: a guide to the dental practitioner. Quintessence Int. 1985;44(3):267–79. doi:10.3290/j.qi.a29050.
7. Spolarich AE. Risk management strategies for reducing oral adverse drug events. J Evid Base Dent Pract. 2014;14:87–94. doi:10.1016/j.jebdp.2014.04.009.
8. Davies A, Bagg J, Laverty D, et al. Salivary gland dysfunction ('dry mouth') in patients with cancer: a consensus statement. Eur J Cancer Care. 2010;19(2):172–7. doi:10.1111/j.1365-2354.2009.01081.x.
9. Jensen SB, Pedersen AML, Vissink A, et al. A systematic review of salivary gland hypofunction and xerostomia induced by cancer therapies: management strategies and economic impact. Support Care Cancer. 2010;18(8):1061–79. doi:10.1007/s00520-010-0837-6.
10. Kałużny J, Wierzbicka M, Nogala H, et al. Radiotherapy induced xerostomia: mechanisms, diagnostics, prevention and treatment–evidence based up to 2013. Otolaryngol Pol. 2014;68(1):1–14. doi:10.1016/j.otpol.2013.09.002.
11. Hanchanale S, Adkinson L, Daniel S, et al. Systematic literature review: xerostomia in advanced cancer patients. Support Care Cancer. 2015;23(3):881–8. doi:10.1007/s00520-014-2477-8.

For Further Information Visit the Following Websites

12. http://www.nidcr.nih.gov
13. http://www.sjogrens.org
14. http://www.nci.org

Gene Therapy for Radiation-Induced Salivary Hypofunction

10

Bruce J. Baum

Pearls of Wisdom

- Often patients who have radiation-induced salivary hypofunction are told by their surgeons or oncologists that they should be happy "they are cured" and not complain about a "minor side effect," i.e., a small problem such as having too little saliva due to their cancer treatment. Even patients for whom gene or pharmacological therapy are not options benefit greatly from a clinician's attention and careful instructions on how to care for their oral health and how to chew and swallow deliberately.
- It must be recognized that gene therapy is still in its developmental stages. The vectors used now to transfer genes into salivary glands and other tissues doubtless will be viewed as primitive in one to two decades.
- Indeed, it may be feasible within a decade or so to prevent radiation damage to healthy salivary glands using gene transfer technology alone or in conjunction with improved advanced radiotherapy techniques and/or pharmacological agents.

10.1 Introduction and Diagnostic Subtypes

This chapter primarily will focus on the use of gene therapy to correct radiation-induced salivary hypofunction but of necessity addresses how a clinician would determine that a patient with this condition is a candidate for gene therapy.

B.J. Baum, DMD, PhD
National Institutes of Health Scientist Emeritus, Molecular Physiology and Therapeutics Branch, National Institute of Dental and Craniofacial Research, National Institutes of Health, Department of Health and Human Services, Bethesda, MD, USA
e-mail: bbaum@dir.nidcr.nih.gov

J.N.A.R. Ferreira et al. (eds.), *Gene Therapy for Radiation-Induced Salivary Hypofunction*, DOI 10.1007/978-3-319-51508-3_10

Salivary hypofunction refers to a reduction in salivary flow [1, 2]. It is an objective term, i.e., determined by measuring salivary fluid output from individual glands (gland saliva) or from the entire mouth (whole saliva, i.e., expectoration). Salivary flow can be measured in the absence or presence of stimulation. Typical stimuli used include swabbing the tongue with 2% citric acid, sucking a sugarless lemon drop, or chewing dental wax. *Xerostomia* refers to a subjective complaint, a symptom, reported by a patient that indicates the individual is having the sensation of a dry mouth [1, 2]. It most frequently, but not always, is associated with salivary hypofunction. Both salivary hypofunction and xerostomia are commonly seen in patients following radiation therapy for head and neck cancers, but also frequently observed in patients with the autoimmune disorder Sjögren's syndrome, and in patients using certain commonly prescribed medications, e.g., opiates, anticholinergics, antidepressants, or common over-the-counter drugs, e.g., antihistamines.

10.2 Clinical Presentation

Whatever the etiology of the salivary hypofunction, patients typically present with one or more of the following symptoms or signs:

- Dry mouth
- Difficulty swallowing (inability to form and translocate a food bolus in the mouth)
- Oral mucosal sores (due to the absence of growth factors and antimicrobial proteins from saliva that help heal oral sores)
- Burning tongue (often associated with Candida infections because of the absence of saliva's antifungal proteins)
- Bad breath (inability to clear food and microbial debris due to too little salivary fluid)
- Pain (often related to increased caries activity due to the loss of salivary antimicrobial proteins and remineralizing proteins)

True salivary hypofunction is accompanied by a reduction in saliva flow [1, 2]. If a clinician does not already have salivary flow information for their patient prior to any complaints, then the saliva output determined following a patient's complaint must be compared with population values. However, for an individual patient, the use of population standards may not be helpful. For example, normal values for both unstimulated and stimulated saliva output from glands can easily vary by an order of magnitude [3]. Similarly, for whole saliva, there is wide variance. Thus, the normal output for some people may be 1.25 mL/15 min, while for others it may be 3 mL/15 min (or much more). If the latter individuals experience a reduction in whole saliva output from 3.0 to 1.5 mL/15 min, for whatever cause, they will likely experience a dry mouth, even though their saliva output is greater than the former individuals, who are comfortable and accommodated to producing lower levels of saliva in their mouth.

10.3 Etiology and Epidemiology

As noted earlier, this chapter is focused on the use of gene therapy to treat radiation-induced salivary hypofunction, i.e., the etiology is clear. Each year in the United States, there are 40,000–50,000 individuals diagnosed with head and neck cancers [4], while worldwide there are ~500,000 persons affected by this condition. For almost all of these patients, treatment typically includes radiotherapy, and salivary glands in the field of radiation are significantly damaged. Most of these patients will experience salivary hypofunction, and for a great many of them, the damage will be permanent [5].

10.4 Pathophysiology and Mechanisms

Salivary glands are like a bunch of grapes. The latter have fruit (berries) and stems, while the former have, analogously, the acinar cells and the duct cells. Acinar cells are like the berries and are the sole site of exocrine fluid movement in these glands [6], secreting a so-called primary fluid that is then modified by the ducts. When acinar cells are damaged or lost, for whatever reason, it is impossible for salivary glands to secrete fluid. Duct cells are like the stems. In addition to functioning to modify the primary fluid (reabsorb or secrete ions, secrete some proteins), the ducts convey the saliva to the mouth. The exact mechanism of acinar cell damage following radiation is not entirely clear, but it apparently involves multiple sites of injury [7]. Whatever the mechanism (s), the absence of saliva leads to all the negative signs and symptoms mentioned above under clinical presentation.

10.5 Diagnosis and Diagnostic Criteria

- Positive history of radiation therapy to the head and neck region, most likely for the treatment of a malignancy.
- Visually low levels of whole saliva, which has a sticky or viscous consistency.
- A test of salivary stimulation, e.g., with 2% citric acid, which fails to elicit a significant visual increase in salivary flow or sublingual pooling (this suggests it is likely that all or most acinar cells have been lost or damaged).
- Oral signs such as increased dental caries, *candidal* infections, and/or frequent oral sores.
- No noticeable improvement in the sensation of oral moisture following the above salivary stimulation.
- Complaints of a having dry mouth and/or a reported difficulty in swallowing.
- Additional testing, such as various types of diagnostic imaging and clinical laboratory analyses, is typically not necessary.

10.6 Rationale for Treatment

The key factor in managing a patient with radiation-induced salivary hypofunction is appreciating the relative amount of surviving acinar cells present [6, 8]. The abovementioned test of stimulation is a simple yet helpful tool for this determination. If there is good stimulation, and the patient notices an improvement in oral moisture, then in all likelihood there are a significant number of acinar cells that have survived the radiotherapy. Conversely, if there is no increase in saliva output following stimulation, it is reasonable to assume that most or all acinar cells have been lost or damaged. In between these two extremes lies a range of possibilities that can be evaluated empirically when treatment options are considered (below).

10.7 Treatment Options

There are three general treatment options based on the above-described test of salivary stimulation:

1. When there is good stimulation, the patient is not a candidate for gene therapy, even if they complain of a dry mouth and have signs of salivary hypofunction. It is clearly preferable to treat such a patient pharmacologically using either of two well-established secretagogues, pilocarpine (Salagen) or cevimeline (Evoxac), assuming there are no medical contraindications to their use. If there are such contraindications, or if preferable to the patient, the clinician can consider using an intraoral electrostimulation device [9].
2. When there is absolutely no stimulation detected and no improvement in oral moisture noted, the patient likely has had almost all of their acinar cells lost and a gland substantially replaced with fibrotic tissue. Currently, little can be done for such a patient, other than palliative care, e.g., use of an artificial saliva, and counseling related to careful oral hygiene and attentive chewing and swallowing, to prevent choking and aspirations.
3. Between these extremes lie patients with some modest response to stimulation, but one that is insufficient to provide much symptomatic or practical relief. These patients likely have some acinar, and many ductal cells present, i.e., a reasonable amount of epithelial tissue able to be "reengineered" to secrete fluid via a gene therapy approach [6, 10].

10.7.1 Gene Transfer Strategies

There are two general ways to transfer genes into cells or intact animals, including humans, using (i) viral vectors or (ii) nonviral methods (Table 10.1).

All of the above-indicated examples have been utilized in the salivary glands of preclinical animal models, while at the time of this writing (March 2016) only an

Table 10.1 Methods used to transfer genes

Method of gene transfer	Examples	Advantage	Disadvantage
Viral vector	Adenoviral, adeno-associated viral	Relatively high level of gene transfer	Safety concern due to immune reactivity
Nonviral	Plasmids ± liposomes ± polyethylenimine ± nanoparticles ± microbubbles and ultrasound	Generally considered to be quite safe	Generally lower level of gene transfer

adenoviral vector has been used in human salivary glands (see below). For the clinical trial that my colleagues and I conducted using gene therapy to "repair" radiation-damaged parotid glands, we previously described in great detail the reasons for choosing the viral vector strategy employed, including gene selection and delivery method (see [6, 8]). Thus, only the key points are listed below:

- Gene (cDNA) used encodes human aquaporin-1 (hAQP1), a water channel.
- Method to transfer the hAQP1 cDNA into the surviving salivary epithelial cells used an adenoviral vector (AdhAQP1) via intraductal cannulation.
- The approach was beneficial in preclinical studies in rats and miniature pigs.
- Importantly, it was beneficial in a first-in-human clinical trial when administered to a single parotid gland through Stensen's duct [10].
- In the trial, 11 subjects were treated with AdhAQP1 at four escalating doses (4.8×10^7, 2.9×10^8, 1.3×10^9, 5.8×10^9 vector particles).
- Efficacy was dose dependent, and, at the first three doses, five of the nine subjects treated showed positive objective responses, i.e., increased parotid saliva secretion, and improved subjective responses, e.g., reduced mouth dryness (1, 2, and 2 at each respective dose; see Fig. 10.1).

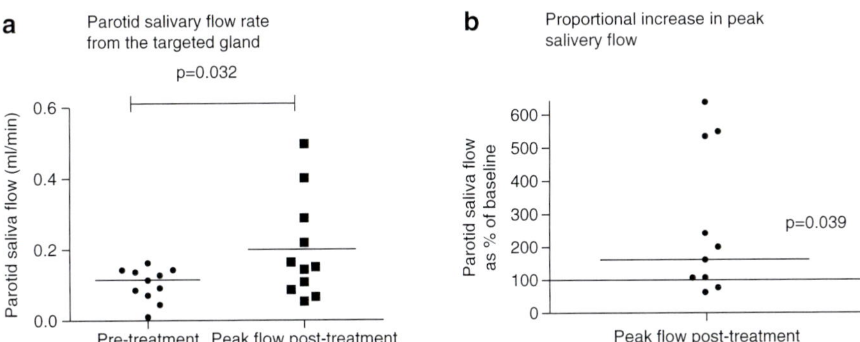

Fig. 10.1 AdhAQP1 trial clinical response data. Clinical responses following AdhAQP1 vector delivery as measured by (**a**) absolute parotid salivary flow rate from the targeted gland and (**b**) the proportional increase in peak parotid salivary flow are shown as the percent of baseline. Significance was determined using the Wilcoxon matched pair rank test for the change in absolute values. The Wilcoxon signed rank test was used to test if the peak proportional increase in parotid salivary flow was significantly different from the baseline (100%). Individual changes in parotid salivary flow are shown in (**c**) for absolute salivary flow rates and in (**d**) for proportional changes compared to baseline. Coding for individual subjects is shown as indicated in the panel (**c**) insert. All subjects shown in *black* were considered nonresponders (<50% increase in salivary flow rate). All subjects shown in colors were considered responders (six; at least a 50% increase in parotid salivary flow following AdhAQP1). The days indicated to the right of each peak data point in panel (**c**) correspond to the days on which that peak parotid flow rate was observed. Visual analogue scale (VAS) results from all subjects, at baseline and peak time of parotid salivary flow, are shown for both the amount of saliva perceived ((**e**); rate how much saliva is in your mouth) and dryness of their mouth ((**f**); rate the dryness in your mouth). Note that lower VAS results indicate an improvement in symptoms. The colors and symbols used to identify individual subjects are identical to those shown in panel (**c**). Five of the six subjects considered responders by flow rate increases (mentioned above) showed improvement in their symptoms (This figure is reprinted from, and the legend slightly modified from, Fig. 2, originally published in Baum et al. [10])

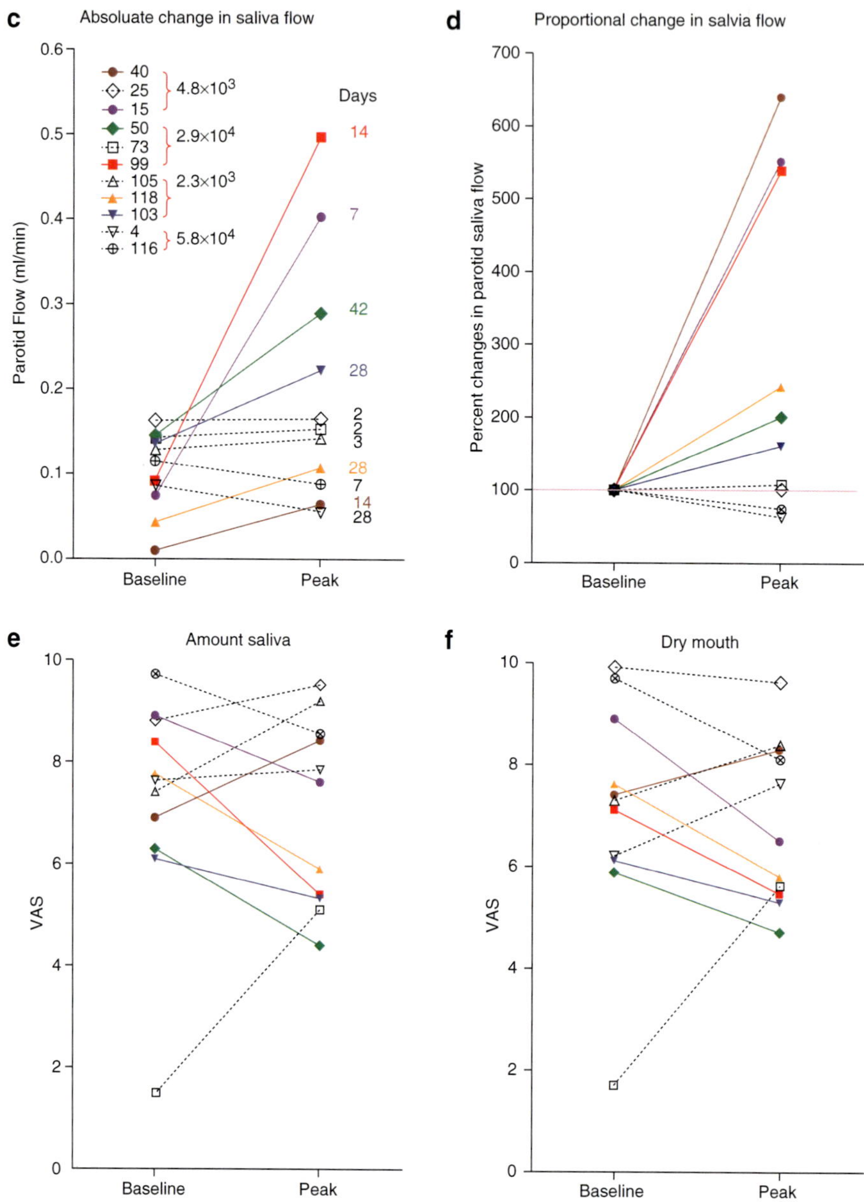

Fig. 10.1 (continued)

- At the highest dose, both treated subjects exhibited significant immune reactivity to the adenoviral vector and no positive objective or subjective response to gene delivery.
- Of particular import, there were no significant side effects to adenoviral vector delivery in all 11 trial subjects (see Table 10.2).

At present, there are no other genes being tested to correct existing radiation damage in salivary glands. However, the hAQP1 gene also can be successfully transferred via an adeno-associated viral vector [11] and a nonviral vector (ultrasound-assisted gene transfer; UAGT [12]) to parotid glands of miniature pigs. Of note, UAGT employs suspending the hAQP1 cDNA in microbubbles and delivery in a similar retroductal infusion manner as used in the AdhAQP1 study. After gene administration, an ultrasound pulse leads to disruption of the microbubbles and facilitates entry of the gene to all cells with which it has contact.

There are two distinct approaches that have been reported in preclinical animal models using gene transfer to *prevent* radiation damage to salivary glands, both shown to work in rodents after retroductal delivery to submandibular glands. As yet, these have not been tested in humans. In the first strategy (viral-based) [13], they used rats as a model and transferred the tousled kinase 1B (TK1B is involved in chromatin rearrangement) gene with an adeno-associated viral vector. In the second approach (nonviral-based) [14], researchers used mice as a model and transferred a short interfering RNA (siRNA) that blocks radiation-induced apoptosis; they have used nanoparticles for siRNA transfer.

Table 10.2 Summary of adverse events

Dose tier (n)	Grade 1 (mild)	Grade 2 (moderate)	Grade 3 (severe)
1 (3)	18[a]	2	0
2 (3)	19[b]	3	0
3 (3)	19[c]	1	0
4 (2)	3	0	0
Total (%)	59 (90.8%)	6 (9.2%)	0 (0%)

Data shown are the number of adverse events (grades 1, 2 or 3) recorded in each dosing tier. Dosing tiers are numbered 1–4 for convenience and correspond, respectively, to 4.8×10^7, 2.9×10^8, 1.3×10^9, and 5.8×10^9 vector particles. The percentages shown are of the total number of adverse events seen, i.e., 65

[a]Five were judged possibly related to treatment

[b]Three were judged possibly related to treatment

[c]Two were judged possibly, four probably, and one definitely related to treatment (all with a single subject)

All other adverse events (50/65; 76.9%) were judged as unlikely related or unrelated to treatment. This table is slightly modified from one originally published in Baum et al. [10]

10.8 Treatment Goals and Sequencing of Care

The primary objective of treating any patient with radiation-induced salivary hypofunction, regardless of the treatment approach, is to increase their salivary output and decrease the typical symptoms and signs associated with this disorder. The first of these can be assessed objectively by measuring saliva flow before and after treatment [1, 2]. Symptoms related to oral dryness can be quantified using a validated visual analogue scale [15]. Another important patient complaint, difficulty swallowing, can be readily assessed by examining the oropharyngeal phase of swallowing with dynamic ultrasound imaging [16].

Acknowledgment I am extremely grateful to the Intramural Research Program of the National Institute of Dental and Craniofacial Research for supporting my research and enabling everything that is mentioned in this chapter. I am also extremely grateful to my many wonderful colleagues at NIH and elsewhere who worked so hard to make a 1991 vision into a clinical reality.

References

1. Fox PC, van der Ven PF, Sonies BC, et al. Xerostomia: evaluation of a symptom with increasing significance. J Am Dent Assoc. 1985;110:519–25.
2. Ship JA, Fox PC, Baum BJ. How much saliva is enough? Normal function defined. J Am Dent Assoc. 1991;122:63–9.
3. Heft MW, Bruce BJ. Unstimulated and stimulated parotid salivary flow rate in individuals of different ages. J Dent Res. 63:1182–5.
4. Siegel R, Ma J, Zou Z, Jemal A. Cancer statistics, 2014. CA Cancer J Clin. 2014;64:9–29.
5. Cox JD, Stetz J, Pajak TF. Toxicity criteria of the Radiation Therapy Oncology Group (RTOG) and the European Organization for Research and Treatment of Cancer (EORTC). Int J Radiat Oncol Biol Phys. 1995;31(5):1341–6.
6. Baum BJ, Zheng C, Alevizos I, et al. Development of a gene transfer-based treatment for radiation-induced salivary hypofunction. Oral Oncol. 2010;46:4–8.
7. Vissink A, Mitchell JB, Baum BJ, et al. Clinical management of salivary gland hypofunction and xerostomia in head-and-neck cancer patients: successes and barriers. Int J Radiat Oncol Biol Phys. 2010;78:983–91.
8. Samuni Y, Baum BJ. Gene delivery in salivary glands: from the bench to the clinic. Biochim Biophys Acta. 1812;2011:1515–21.
9. Strietzel FP, Lafaurie GI, Mendoza GR, et al. Efficacy and safety of an intraoral electrostimulation device for xerostomia relief: a multicenter randomized trial. Arthritis Rheum. 2011;63:180–90.
10. Baum BJ, Alevizos A, Zheng C, et al. Early responses to adenoviral-mediated transfer of the aquaporin-1 cDNA for radiation-induced salivary hypofunction. Proc Natl Acad Sci U S A. 2012;109:19403–7.
11. Gao R, Yan X, Zheng C, et al. AAV2-mediated transfer of the human aquaporin-1 cDNA restores fluid secretion from irradiated miniature pig parotid glands. Gene Ther. 2011;18:38–42.
12. Wang Z, Zourelias L, Wu C, et al. Ultrasound-assisted nonviral gene transfer of AQP1 to the irradiated minipig parotid gland restores fluid secretion. Gene Ther. 2015;22:739–49.
13. Timiri Shanmugam PS, Dayton RD, Palaniyandi S, et al. Recombinant AAV9-TLK1B administration ameliorates fractionated radiation-induced xerostomia. Hum Gene Ther. 2013;24:604–12.

14. Arany S, Benoit DS, Dewhurst S, Ovitt CE. Nanoparticle-mediated gene silencing confers radioprotection to salivary glands in vivo. Mol Ther. 2013;21:1182–94.
15. Pai S, Ghezzi ES, Ship JA. Development of a visual analogue scale questionnaire for subjective assessment of salivary dysfunction. Oral Surg Oral Med Oral Pathol Oral Radiol Endod. 2001;91:311–6.
16. Chi-Fishman G, Sonies BC. Effects of systematic bolus viscosity and volume changes on hyoid movement kinematics. Dysphagia. 2001;17:278–87.

Salivary Hypofunction in Aging Adults

11

Catherine Hong and João N.A.R. Ferreira

Pearls of Wisdom

- Rapid progression to an edentulous status due to rampant tooth decay, opportunistic infections, inability to retain removable prostheses, discomfort during eating and speaking, burning sensation of the mouth, and diminished taste acuity are some of the reported signs and symptoms of dry mouth in aging adults.
- A variety of symptomatic measures are available to alleviate dry mouth symptoms in the elderly, but these largely fall under two categories: (1) saliva substitutes and lubricants and (2) saliva stimulants for local or systemic application.

11.1 Introduction

Saliva is essential for the function and preservation of oropharyngeal health. Xerostomia and salivary gland hyposalivation are used interchangeably to describe dry mouth; however, it is important to distinguish between terms as persons suffering from xerostomia may not necessarily have hyposalivation. Salivary gland dysfunction is a condition in which either the chemical properties of saliva is altered or when the unstimulated or stimulated salivary flow is significantly reduced. Salivary hypofunction is generally defined as an unstimulated flow rate of less than 0.1–0.2 ml/min and a stimulated saliva flow rate of less than 0.7 ml/min. Xerostomia refers to the subjective perception of dry mouth and is sometimes but not always accompanied by salivary gland dysfunction [1–3].

C. Hong, DDS, MS, Dip. AAOM
Orthodontics and Paediatric Dentistry, Faculty of Dentistry, National University of Singapore, Singapore, Singapore

J.N.A.R. Ferreira, DDS, MS, PhD, Dip. ABOP (✉)
Oral and Maxillofacial Surgery, Faculty of Dentistry, National University of Singapore, Singapore, Singapore
e-mail: denjnarf@nus.edu.sg

J.N.A.R. Ferreira et al. (eds.), *Orofacial Disorders*,
DOI 10.1007/978-3-319-51508-3_11

11.2 Epidemiology

Clinical experts and researchers have proposed that salivary gland dysfunction and xerostomia be considered as separate entities as studies conducted on prevalence of xerostomia and salivary gland dysfunction have demonstrated that both conditions existed together only about 2–5% of the time [3, 4]. In this chapter, for the purpose of ease, the term dry mouth will be used when referring to both salivary gland dysfunction and xerostomia.

In patients with Sjögren's syndrome and those who are undergoing head and neck radiotherapy, the prevalence of dry mouth is almost 100%. However, the prevalence data of xerostomia and salivary gland hypofunction in the general population is more difficult to ascertain and ranges widely due to both the heterogeneity of sampled populations and varying definitions of dry mouth in the literature [5–7].

In a systematic review by Orellana et al. [8], it was reported that the prevalence of xerostomia is approximately 20% in the community, but appears to be higher in the elderly and institutionalized individuals. Ship et al. [3] estimate the prevalence of xerostomia in adults aged 65 years and over to be 30% and up to 50% in institutional elders. Presently, there is no convincing evidence that age is a significant cause of dry mouth, and polypharmacy is still believed to be the leading cause of dry mouth in this population. There are over 400 medications that cause dry mouth as a side effect and with the increase of prescription medications with age; the prevalence of medication-induced dry mouth is expectedly higher in older individuals. There are many other causes of dry mouth (e.g., Sjögren's syndrome, head and neck radiation, dehydration), which will not be discussed in this chapter as these have been reviewed in Chaps. 9 and 10.

Although non-life-threatening, dry mouth can adversely affect oral health status and has been associated with a myriad of subjective and clinical problems. Rampant dental decay, opportunistic infections, inability to retain removable prostheses, discomfort during eating and speaking, burning sensation of the mouth, and diminished taste acuity are some of the reported signs and symptoms of dry mouth in aging adults [9, 10]. These can consequently impact the quality of general and oral health and well-being particularly in the elderly.

11.3 Diagnosis and Diagnostic Criteria

A systematic approach should be used to distinguish and diagnose patients with xerostomia and those with salivary gland hypofunction [11]. To begin, in-depth exploration of the *chief complaint* with questions pertaining to oral dryness during eating (e.g., need to sip liquids to swallow dry foods, difficulty swallowing) and self-perception of amount of saliva must be elicited. Other questions pertaining to feeling of dryness on awakening and during the night, speech difficulties, taste disturbances, burning sensation, and intolerance to acidic and spicy foods may also be elicited. For a comprehensive assessment, the Xerostomia Inventory (XI) is a useful 11-item validated instrument for assessing changes in symptoms over time [12].

Next, a thorough medical history to identify and rule out conditions (e.g., Sjögren's syndrome), medical drug therapies (e.g., polypharmacy), and treatment (e.g., head and neck radiation therapy) should be obtained. This should be followed by a physical examination of the extra- and intraoral structures to identify signs of hyposalivation. Extraoral findings include dry and cracked lips and enlarged unilateral or bilateral salivary glands due to salivary obstructions or infections. Glossy and sticky oral mucosa, depapillated, fissured, and erythematous tongue and lack of salivary pooling in the floor of the mouth are some of the common findings intraorally. Saliva expression from the parotid ducts in the buccal mucosa and the submandibular ducts situated in the floor of the mouth should be performed routinely. Cloudy or purulent discharge from the ducts may indicate an infection in the salivary glands.

Due to the loss of the various protective functions of saliva (e.g., lubrication, immunologic, buffering capacity, oral clearance), individuals with salivary gland hypofunction are at high risk for trauma, all forms of oral candidiasis (pseudomembranous, erythematous, median rhomboid glossitis, and angular cheilitis), and dental caries.

The objective measure of salivary production is essential to differentiate between xerostomia and salivary gland hyposalivation. There are several methods of measuring unstimulated (UWS) and stimulated whole saliva (SWS); the most common collection method for unstimulated salivary flow rate in clinical practice is the spitting or drooling method [11]. This method is favored as it does not require special equipment, is easily administered, and is reproducible [13]. The UWS rate is measured by the patient allowing saliva to accumulate in the mouth for 5 min and spitting into a collection tube and then repeating this for a 15 min period. Alternatively, the patient may incline his or her head forward and drool into a receptacle for the same amount of time. For SWS rate, this can be measured by having the patient chew on a piece of paraffin wax or using a sialagogue such as 4–10% citric acid. There are other methods for measuring salivary flow such as the use of suction cups over the parotid gland; however, these tend to be used for experimental studies to obtain measurements of flow from selected major salivary gland. A UWS of less than 0.1–0.2 ml/min and a SWS flow rate of less than 0.5–0.7 ml/min are considered indicative of hyposalivation [11, 14].

Salivary gland abnormalities can also be identified by a variety of imaging techniques. Plain radiography is an inexpensive and simple investigative tool to evaluate the salivary gland; however, its use is limited due to its ability to only provide a two-dimensional view of a three-dimensional structure. Scintigraphy involves the injection of a radiopaque compound (^{99m}technetium pertechnetate) into the blood. Tc is then selectively taken up into the salivary glands which can then be visualized and graded for disease process. Another technique that has been traditionally used is sialography which involves a radiopaque compound medium being directly introduced in the duct of the major salivary gland and the resulting image (sialogram) used to visualize anatomy and integrity of ducts and acinar as well as obstructions from calcifications and tumors. However, conventional sialography has fallen out of use due to the improved ability of modern imaging procedures such as ultrasonography and MRI (magnetic resonance imaging) to assess salivary gland abnormalities. These methods are noninvasive as they do not possess the risks associated with conventional sialography (e.g., rupture of ductal system, allergy to contrast agent, radiation exposure). MRI sialography can define the ductal system of a salivary gland without injection of a contrast agent and is able to demonstrate characteristic changes in parotid glands (typically a nodular pattern, characterized by multiple hypo- and hyperintense areas of varying size) associated with Sjögren's syndrome (SS). However, the imaging modality uses patient's own saliva as a contrast agent as such resulting image resolution may be poor in patients with no or minimal saliva production. Ultrasonography has been shown to demonstrate characteristic salivary gland changes (e.g., multiple hypoechoic areas with convex borders, hyperechoic linear bands, cysts and calcifications in advanced disease) in SS with diagnostic value comparable to traditional methods such as scintigraphy and salivary gland biopsy. Computed tomography can also be used to evaluate structural abnormalities of salivary gland; however, its use is limited compared to ultrasonography and MRI due to the involvement of ionizing radiation [15].

Salivary gland biopsy provides a definitive diagnosis of gland pathology. Biopsy of labial minor salivary glands is commonly preferred over biopsy of a major gland for the diagnosis of Sjögren's syndrome as it is more accessible with fewer complications [16]. The presence of at least one focus area of periductal lymphocytic infiltration is consistent with the diagnosis of Sjögren's syndrome. A focus is defined as an agglomerate of at least 50 mononuclear cells in 4 mm^2 of tissue.

Other investigations include blood tests to assess for hematinic deficiencies and serological tests to identify antibodies to diagnose diseases with salivary gland pathology.

11.4 Treatment Rationale and Goals

After the diagnosis of dry mouth has been made, a stepwise management approach is often taken. The primary goals are alleviation of symptoms, avoidance strategies, and prevention of complications (e.g., dental caries, oral candidiasis) arising from dry mouth.

11.5 Sequencing of Care

11.5.1 Alleviation of Symptoms

There are a variety of symptomatic measures available to alleviate symptoms in aging adults, and these largely fall under two categories: (1) saliva substitutes and lubricants and (2) saliva stimulants for local or systemic application.

Salivary substitutes and lubricants (e.g., Biotene Oral Balance Moisturizing Gel®, Caphosol®, GC Dry Mouth Gel®, Oramoist®, Oasis®) frequently contain a mix of carboxymethylcellulose, mucopolysaccharides, polythene gycol, natural mucins, sorbitol, and electrolytes to provide more viscosity and lubrication than water. In general, these products have been shown to improve the subjective complaint of xerostomia but not salivary flow. Additionally, saliva substitutes and lubricants are rarely effective beyond a few hours, and patients need to use them repeatedly over the course of the day for continued comfort. Frequent sips of water can relieve symptoms, but water does not provide lubricating properties, and excessive sipping of water may strip the mucosa of the mucus film and increase symptoms.

Local stimulation of saliva through sugar-free gums and mints has also been demonstrated to increase saliva production in individuals with residual secretory function [17]. However, there is no strong evidence to support a specific type of salivary substitute or stimulant, as such patients should try several agents and use agent/s (singly or in combination) that provide them the greatest relief [17].

In patients who do not achieve sufficient symptomatic relief with saliva substitutes/lubricants and topical stimulants, systemic saliva stimulants can be prescribed. Muscarinic agonists such as pilocarpine nonspecific muscarinic agonist) and cevimeline (specific muscarinic agonist with higher affinity for receptors on the lacrimal and salivary epithelium) have been demonstrated in several clinical trials to improve salivary flow and complaints of xerostomia compared to placebo [18–20]. Both medications have not been compared directly to each other but appear equally efficacious. Adverse effects are frequent in both medications, though cevimeline being a selective muscarinic agonist may have a more favorable adverse effects profile than that of pilocarpine, which is desirable in elderly patients. The typical dose for pilocarpine is 5–7.5 mg orally four times daily; for cevimeline, the usual dose is 30 mg orally, three times a day. It is recommended that the medications be taken about a half-hour before meals. When initiating therapy, it is advisable to slowly titrate the dose of pilocarpine or cevimeline upward (e.g., one dose daily for the first week) to minimize side effects such as sudden onset of sweating and nausea. In patients who are prone to dyspepsia and gastric bloating, taking the medication with food or using a proton pump inhibitor may minimize symptoms. In patients who are unable to tolerate the side effects of the full dose, a reduced pilocarpine dose of 2.5 mg three times a day or 5 mg once a day may still provide some benefit. Alternatively, the capsule or tablet can be dissolved in water and be used as a rinse and spit regimen to minimize systemic absorption. As the response is frequently delayed, patients should be placed on the drug for at least 3 months' duration to assess for therapeutic benefit and side effects. Due to the cholinergic side effects, pilocarpine and cevimeline may be contraindicated in patients with pulmonary and cardiovascular conditions, gastric ulcers, glaucoma, and urethral reflex and in patients on ß-blockers [18–20].

11.5.2 Avoidance Strategies

Elderly patients should be advised to avoid caffeine-containing, acidic, and alcoholic beverages as these may be dehydrating locally or systematically and could worsen oral dryness symptoms. Other measures that can alleviate symptoms of xerostomia, dry eyes, and dry nasal mucosa include avoidance of medications that may worsen oral dryness and use of humidifiers by the bedside during the night.

In oncological treatment for head and neck cancer, modern advances in radiotherapy (e.g., intensity-modulated radiotherapy and image-guided radiotherapy) have allowed for restriction of high-dose radiation region to the target volume thus minimizing radiation dose to neighboring tissues. In the PARSPORT trial, whereby 94 patients with head and neck cancer were randomly assigned to intensity-modulated radiation therapy or conventional radiotherapy, with a dose of 60–65 Gy, severe xerostomia was significantly less common with those patients in the IMRT at both 12 and 24 months [21].

11.5.3 Prevention of Complications

Dry mouth predisposes patients to dental caries and opportunistic infections (e.g., candidiasis) due to the loss of the protective functions of saliva. Thus, it is imperative that patients maintain meticulous home care (tooth brushing, flossing) and a non-cariogenic diet (e.g., avoid cariogenic sweet and sticky foods and frequent snacking). Patients should visit their dentist every 3–6 months for oral cleanings and hygiene; the frequency is dependent on the extent of dryness. Dentists should consider frequent professional fluoride applications and formulate a customized preventive plan for their patients which may include the following:

(i) Fluoride supplementation with prescription strength (0.5% fluoride or 1.1% sodium fluoride) fluoride toothpaste (Prevident®) or fluoride gels in custom fitted trays daily
(ii) Topical antimicrobial agents such as chlorhexidine [22]
(iii) Adjunct agents such as supersaturated calcium phosphate rinses or bland mouth rinses containing baking soda, bicarbonate, or xylitol [23]

11.5.4 Submandibular Gland Transfer

A small multicenter trial found that surgical transfer of the submandibular gland from an uninvolved side of the neck to the submental space in head and neck cancer patients prior to radiation is superior to the use of pilocarpine. However, this technique has not gained popularity due to the need for an elective invasive procedure and has not been evaluated against newer radiation techniques (e.g., IMRT—intensity-modulated radiation therapy) [24].

11.5.5 Investigational and Other Agents

Amifostine has been shown to reduce dry mouth in patients undergoing head and neck radiation by acting as a scavenger of free radicals generated in tissues exposed to radiation [25]. However, the value of amifostine is still unclear due to the paucity of studies, mixed results, high cost, and side effects (potential increase in tumor survival).

In summary, the management of salivary hypofunction and xerostomia in the elderly is currently based on pharmacological approaches to alleviate the oral dryness symptoms. These approaches largely fall under two main categories: (1) saliva substitutes and lubricants and (2) saliva stimulants for local or systemic application.

Intraoral electrical stimulation in the mouth (e.g., tongue and palate, oral mucosa), acupuncture, use of hydroxychloroquine (antimalarial drug), nizatidine (histamine receptor antagonist) in Sjögren's syndrome patients, and hyperbaric oxygen therapy have shown some benefit on dry mouth, but there are very few studies with mixed results and a high risk of bias when these approaches are used [26–28]. As such, results need to be confirmed in larger-scale randomized clinical trials. The following novel strategies are also being studied in animal models and in preclinical trials:

- Gene therapy to increase endogenous levels of water channels via ductal cannulation of viral and nonviral vectors (siRNA). These have been discussed in detail in Chap. 10.
- Use of other cytoprotective agents (e.g., tempol) [29].
- Autologous stem/progenitor cell transplantation and other stem cell therapies [30, 31].

References

1. Ship J, et al. How much saliva is enough? "Normal" function defined. J Am Dent Assoc. 1991;122:63–9.
2. Thomson WM, et al. The xerostomia inventory: a multi-item approach to measuring dry mouth. Community Dent Health. 1999;16:12–7.
3. Ship JA. Xerostomia and the geriatric patient. Prog Geriatr. 2002;50:535–43.
4. Dawes C. Physiological factors affecting salivary flow rate, oral sugar clearance and the sensation of dry mouth in man. J Dent Res. 1987;66:648–53.
5. Liu B, et al. Xerostomia and salivary hypofunction in vulnerable elders: prevalence and etiology. Oral Surg Oral Med Oral Pathol Oral Radiol. 2012;114:52–60.
6. Schein OD, et al. Dry eye and dry mouth in the elderly: a population-based assessment. Arch Intern Med. 1999;159:1359–63.
7. Sreebny LM, et al. A reference guide to drugs and dry mouth – 2nd edition. Gerodontology. 1997;14:33–47.
8. Orellana MF, et al. Prevalence of xerostomia in population based samples: a systematic review. J Public Health Dent. 2006;66:152–8.
9. Matear DW, et al. Associations between xerostomia and health status indicators in the elderly. J R Soc Health. 2006;126:79–85.
10. Navazesh M, et al. Relationship between salivary flow rates and *Candida albicans* counts. Oral Surg Oral Med Oral Pathol Oral Radiol Endod. 1995;80:284–8.
11. Navazesh M, et al. Clinical criteria for the diagnosis of salivary gland hypofunction. J Dent Res. 1992;71:1363–9.
12. Thomson WM. Measuring change in dry-mouth symptoms over time using the xerostomia inventory. Gerodontology. 2007;24(1):30–5.

13. Jones JM, et al. Comparison of three salivary flow rate assessment methods in an elderly population. Community Dent Oral Epidemiol. 2000;28:177–84.
14. Heintze U, et al. Secretion rate and buffer effect of resting and stimulated whole saliva as a function of age and sex. Swed Dent J. 1983;7:227–38.
15. Pia A, et al. Imaging of the major salivary glands. Clin Physiol Funct Imaging. 2016;36:1–10.
16. Teppo H, et al. A follow-up study of minimally invasive lip biopsy in the diagnosis of Sjögren's syndrome. Clin Rheumatol. 2007;26:1099–103.
17. Furness S et al. Interventions for management of dry mouth: topical therapies. Cochrane Database Syst Rev. 2011;(12):CD008934.
18. Ramos-Casals M, et al. Treatment of primary Sjögren's syndrome: a systematic review. JAMA. 2000;304(4):452.
19. Fife RS, Chase WF, Dore RK, Wiesenhutter CW, Lockhart PB, Tindall E, Suen JY. Cevimeline for the treatment of xerostomia in patients with Sjögren syndrome: a randomized trial. Arch Intern Med. 2002;162(11):1293.
20. Papas AS, Sherrer YS, Charney M, Golden HE, Medsger Jr TA, Walsh BT, Trivedi M, Goldlust B, Gallagher SC. Successful treatment of dry mouth and dry eye symptoms in Sjögren's syndrome patients with oral pilocarpine: a randomized, placebo-controlled. Dose-Adjust Study J Clin Rheumatol. 2004;10(4):169.
21. Nutting CM, et al. Parotid-sparing intensity modulated versus conventional radiotherapy in head and neck cancer (PARSPORT): a phase 3 multicentre randomised controlled trial. Lancet Oncol. 12(2):127.
22. Banting DW, Papas A, Clark DC, Proskin HM, Schultz M, Perry R. The effectiveness of 10% chlorhexidine varnish treatment on dental caries incidence in adults with dry mouth. Gerodontology. 2000;17(2):67.
23. Hay KD, Thomson WM. A clinical trial of the anti-caries efficacy of casein derivatives complexed with calcium phosphate in patients with salivary gland dysfunction. Oral Surg Oral Med Oral Pathol Oral Radiol Endod. 2002;93(3):271.
24. Jha N, et al. Phase III randomized study: oral pilocarpine versus submandibular salivary gland transfer protocol for the management of radiation induced xerostomia. Head Neck. 2009;31(2):234.
25. Wasserman TH, Brizel DM, Henke M, Monnier A, Eschwege F, Sauer R, Strand V. Influence of intravenous amifostine on xerostomia, tumor control, and survival after radiotherapy for head-and- neck cancer: 2-year follow-up of a prospective, randomized, phase III trial. Int J Radiat Oncol Biol Phys. 2005;63(4):985.
26. Strietzel FP, et al. Electrostimulating device in the management of xerostomia. Oral Dis. 2007;13(2):206–13.
27. Fomer L, et al. Does hyperbaric oxygen treatment have potential to increase salivary flow rate and reduce xerostomia in previously irradiated head and neck cancer patients? A pilot study. Oral Oncol. 2011;47(6):546.
28. Kruize AA, et al. Hydrochloroquine treatment of primary Sjögren's syndrome: a two year double blind crossover trial. Ann Rheum Dis. 1993;52(5):360.
29. Mizrachi A, Cotrim AP, Katabi N, Mitchell JB, Verheij M, Haimovitz-Friedman A. Radiation-induced microvascular injury as a mechanism of salivary gland hypofunction and potential target for radioprotectors. Radiat Res. 2016;186(2):189–95.
30. Lombaert I, Movahednia MM, Adine C, Ferreira JN. Salivary gland regeneration: therapeutic approaches from stem cells to tissue organoids. Stem Cells. 2017;35(1):97–105.
31. Ferreira JN, Rungarunlert S, Urkasemsin G, Adine C, Souza GR. Three-dimensional bioprinting nanotechnologies towards clinical application of stem cells and their secretome in salivary gland regeneration. Stem Cells Int. 2016;2016:7564689. doi: 10.1155/2016/7564689. Epub 2016 Dec 20.

Part V

Oral Parafunctions and Sleep Disorders

Oral Parafunctional Behaviors

12

Alan G. Glaros and James Fricton

Pearls of Wisdom

- Many oral parafunctional habits and their consequences will improve or get worse with the passage of time as life circumstances change.
- To address patient requests for relief from suffering, the conservative, reversible approaches recommended by the National Institute of Dental and Craniofacial Research will speed relief without subjecting patients to complex or irreversible dental treatments that have little evidence of efficacy.
- Splints are "cueing" devices that improve patients' awareness of parafunctions and help decrease their occurrence.
- Simple self-care strategies are easy to describe to patients but may be difficult for them to understand and implement. Providers will have greater success recommending these techniques when their approach uses a committed, personalized approach to their patients and a willingness to engage patients in finding workable strategies for implementing change.
- Online patient cognitive-behavioral training programs are available to support clinicians in finding the time and skills to teach patients to reduce these risk factors and encourage normal healing and function.

12.1 Introduction

Oral parafunctional behaviors are a broad class of behaviors that can occur during the day and at night. They are characterized by activation of the masticatory muscles for purposes other than chewing, swallowing, and speaking. They can be distinguished from the functional behaviors of the masticatory muscles by their often

A.G. Glaros, PhD (✉)
University of Missouri-Kansas City, Kansas City, MO, USA
e-mail: GlarosA@umkc.edu

J. Fricton, DDS, MS, Dip. ABOP
University of Minnesota, Minneapolis, MN, USA

J.N.A.R. Ferreira et al. (eds.), *Orofacial Disorders*,
DOI 10.1007/978-3-319-51508-3_12

repetitive, non-goal-oriented actions. Behaviors such as clenching, grinding, and tapping of teeth are clearly oral parafunctional behaviors.

Other common behaviors involving the masticatory muscles may also qualify as oral parafunctional behaviors. These could include:

- Chewing gum
- Biting/chewing oral tissues (e.g., buccal mucosa, lips)
- Biting/chewing on nonfood objects (e.g., pens, pencils, erasers, fingernails)

Dr. Richard Ohrbach's Oral Behavior Checklist can be used to assess a broad range of oral parafunctional behaviors: http://www.rdc-tmdinternational.org/Portals/18/Translations_other/Oral%20Behaviors%20Checklist%20v1-1%20-%20English.pdf.

In addition, repetitive behaviors that are goal oriented but continuous can also strain the teeth, jaw, and neck musculature. These behaviors may include playing musical instruments with the mouth, scuba diving, and cradling a phone between the head and the shoulders.

There is no formal nosology for diagnosing oral parafunctional behaviors that accounts for the broad spectrum of behaviors involved. Some authors distinguish between oral parafunctional behaviors that occur at night ("sleep bruxism") and those that occur during the day ("awake bruxism") [1]. This distinction ignores some commonalities in behavior between the two times. Grinding, extended tooth contact ("clenching"), and tapping of the teeth can occur during sleep, whereas awake bruxism is most likely to consist of extended tooth contact and other behaviors noted above.

12.2 Clinical Presentation

Self-report and clinical signs are the two main methods by which patients present with oral parafunctional behaviors. Both can provide useful information, but both must be approached cautiously in a clinical setting.

A patient self-report of oral parafunctional behaviors may be limited to a small number of such behaviors. To get a more complete sense of the breadth of these behaviors, clinicians should ask patients about each type of oral habit and the frequency of oral habits (Table 12.1).

Most patients can readily detect whether or not their teeth are touching at any given time [2]. However, self-report of "clenching" or "bruxism" can produce unreliable results, as the terms have different meanings for different individuals. For this reason, clinicians should use terms that have clear behavioral referents such as "holding your teeth together," not summary terms such as "clenching."

Family members, friends, and colleagues may be reliable sources of information about some oral parafunctional behaviors. For example, individuals who engage in sleep-related grinding also create noise when they sleep. Bed partners or others who

Table 12.1 Screening questionnaire for self-report of oral habits

Have you or others noticed yourself doing any oral habits regularly (more than once a week)?	Yes	No
Chewing on one side	☐	☐
Leaning on the jaw	☐	☐
Grinding the teeth at night	☐	☐
Grinding your teeth when awake	☐	☐
Waking up with sore jaws	☐	☐
Clenching your teeth when awake	☐	☐
Clenching your teeth at night	☐	☐
Holding your jaw forward	☐	☐
Chewing gum	☐	☐
Playing a musical instrument with the mouth	☐	☐
Sleeping on stomach	☐	☐
Touching or holding your teeth together	☐	☐
Holding or pressing the tongue against your teeth	☐	☐
Holding your jaw in a rigid or tense position	☐	☐
Biting objects (pens, toothpicks, etc.)	☐	☐
Biting your cheeks	☐	☐
Biting your nails or cuticles	☐	☐
Biting your lips	☐	☐
Biting tongue	☐	☐
Bracing the phone with the shoulder or jaw	☐	☐

Table 12.2 Objective indicators of oral habits

	Yes	No
Tooth wear on front teeth	☐	☐
Tooth wear on posterior teeth	☐	☐
Mucosal ridging	☐	☐
Tongue ridging	☐	☐
Masseter hypertrophy	☐	☐
Cheek biting	☐	☐
Lip biting	☐	☐

sleep nearby may provide useful information on sleep-related grinding, but patients themselves are highly unreliable sources of information about their own sleep-related grinding [3].

The signs of oral habits include tooth wear and fracture, masticatory muscle and TMJ tenderness, tongue or cheek ridging, and other extra- and intraoral changes (Table 12.2). When sleep-related oral parafunctions involve grinding, the teeth will show atypical wear facets, fracture, or crazing of the enamel (Fig. 12.1). However, because the presence of abnormal wear patterns is a historical record, the presence of such patterns cannot be used as a reliable indicator of current, ongoing clenching and grinding.

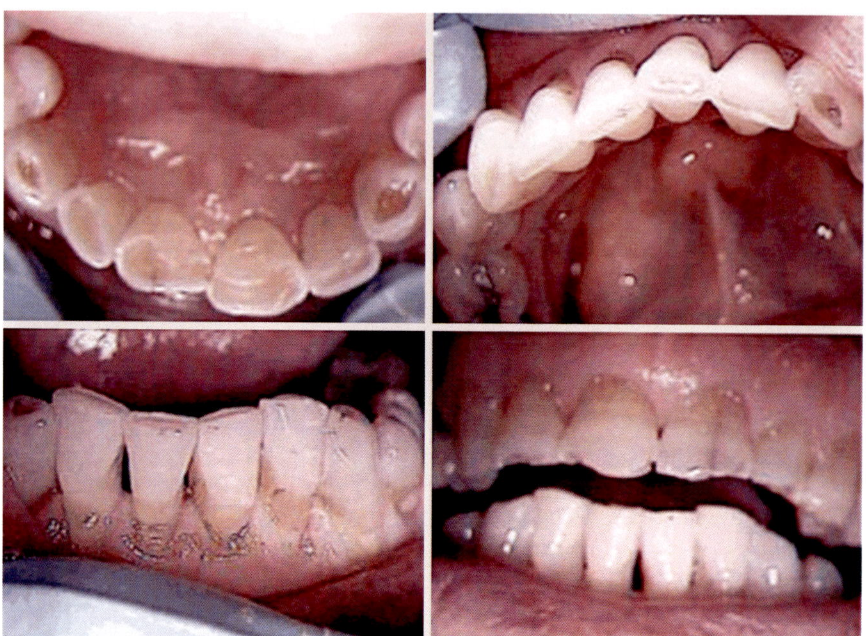

Fig. 12.1 Abnormal tooth wear caused by tooth grinding

Masticatory muscle and TMJ tenderness are more strongly related to extended tooth contact, gum chewing, fingernail biting, and other day activities [4] than nocturnal habits. Morning muscle soreness is not a reliable sign of sleep-related grinding.

In some individuals, oral parafunctional habits manifest themselves extraorally as hypertrophy of the masticatory muscles, especially the masseters or temporalis. In some individuals, direct visualization of the buccal mucosa or inner lips will indicate whether patients chew on their tissues. Evidence of such parafunctions will often present as a thin line of lacerated tissue or a patch of shredded tissue about where the teeth meet. Bracing of the tongue against the teeth will contribute to a scalloping ridge on the lateral border of the tongue. Likewise, oral suction will compress the buccal mucosa against the teeth and contribute to scalloping ridge at the teeth line on the buccal mucosa.

12.3 Epidemiology

Worldwide studies show that about 8% of the adult population engage in sleep-related tooth grinding. Nocturnal grinding can occur as teeth erupt in children and is often, though intermittently, reported in children. The proportion of children who continue teeth grinding into adulthood is small.

Tooth contact is orders of magnitude more frequent than the 17.5 min commonly reported in some dental textbooks [5]. Studies suggest that tooth contact occurs in normal control subjects between 25% and 45% of the day (i.e., 4 h to more than 7 h while awake), while those reporting temporomandibular disorder pain report tooth contact nearly 75% of the day (i.e., as much as 12 h while awake). Other forms of oral parafunctional behaviors appear to be relatively frequent, although most of the studies use retrospective questionnaire data to estimate frequencies of these behaviors. Little is known about prevalence rates of these behaviors across the life-span.

12.4 Pathophysiology and Mechanisms

Nocturnal tooth grinding is a sleep-related disorder [6]. Patients who grind differ from those who do not on a variety of sleep variables, particularly those involving microarousals. Some medications, including stimulants used for ADHD or selective serotonin re-uptake inhibitors (SSRIs) for depression, may produce sleep-related grinding. In some individuals, tooth grinding may protect against acid reflux during sleep.

The etiology of other diurnal oral parafunctional behaviors is less clear. Some findings have associated daytime oral parafunctional behaviors with stress and anxiety, the development of adjunctive behaviors, and deficits in proprioceptive awareness. Some parafunctions may simply represent behaviors that that were learned in childhood and have persisted into adulthood. Some individuals with variations in gene coding for COMT are at higher risk for facial pain.

Older theories focusing on abnormal occlusion have not been substantiated as valid causal factors in most oral parafunctional behaviors. Most individuals who engage in oral parafunctional behaviors are no different occlusally than those who do not engage in parafunctions. Studies reporting occlusal differences between individuals who engage in oral parafunctional behaviors and those who do not typically fail to replicate.

12.5 Diagnosis and Diagnostic Criteria

There are no criteria for establishing a diagnosis of oral parafunctional behaviors. Indeed, some authors argue that even sleep bruxism, the most well-studied of the oral parafunctions, does not meet recognized criteria for being a diagnosable condition. If oral parafunctions are viewed as behaviors that can be measured, both clinicians and researchers can access questionnaires and devices that can provide useful information about the parafunctions:

1. A simple questionnaire can act as screening tool for identifying different types of behavioral patterns (Table 12.1).
2. Sleep polysomnography is the "gold standard" for identifying sleep-related oral parafunctional activity. During sleep polysomnography, electroencephalographic activity, electromyographic activity, electrooculographic activity (to record eye movement), respiration, pulse oximetry, electrocardiogram, blood pressure, and body temperature are typically collected, along with video or audio recordings. Polysomnographic criteria for sleep-related grinding have good sensitivity and specificity for identifying sleep-related grinding when examining those with a

very clear, current history of the behavior vs. those without any evidence of grinding. Sleep polysomnography is expensive and time-consuming.

3. The "Bruxcore" monitoring plate is an alternative to the cost and intrusive characteristics of sleep polysomnography. The Bruxcore monitoring plate is an intraoral appliance fabricated from four layers of plastic laminated to a total thickness of 0.02 in., with microdots printed on the top surface. Grinding on the Bruxcore plate wears away the microdots and exposes the colored layers (Fig. 12.2). A quantitative score can be developed to express the degree of grinding [7].
4. Portable EMG devices specifically designed to capture tooth grinding show some promise, although the quality of information from these devices is not equivalent to information obtained from sleep polysomnography. For example, these devices can presently detect intensive tooth contact but may not be able to distinguish between oral parafunctional behaviors and sleep-related artifacts such as turning in bed [8]. Advances in miniaturization make it increasingly likely that devices will be manufactured that reliably accomplish all these tasks.
5. Experience sampling methods (ESM), also known as ecological momentary assessment, can be used to diagnose the frequency and intensity of oral parafunctional behaviors (Fig. 12.3). ESM is characterized by repeated measurement of a behavior in a person's natural environment. Data collection occurs several times per day, preferably on a random schedule to avoid behavior changes due to the anticipation of a

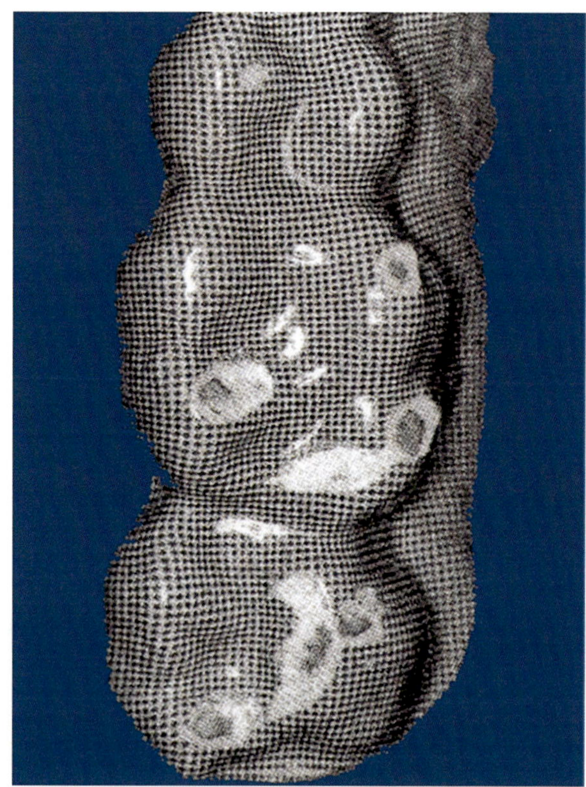

Fig. 12.2 Evidence of grinding as measured by the Bruxcore device (Reprinted from Isacsson et al. [3])

data collection. ESM can assess the frequency and intensity of tooth contact, gum chewing, cheek biting, and other activities that occur during the day.

The mechanism used to trigger recording can vary from the very low-tech (e.g., brightly colored stickers) to sophisticated electronic strategies. An example of the latter is the Participation in Everyday Life (PIEL) Survey tool (https://pielsurvey.org). This free application, available only for Apple products at the present time, takes advantage of smartphone/tablet interfaces and can be readily programmed to

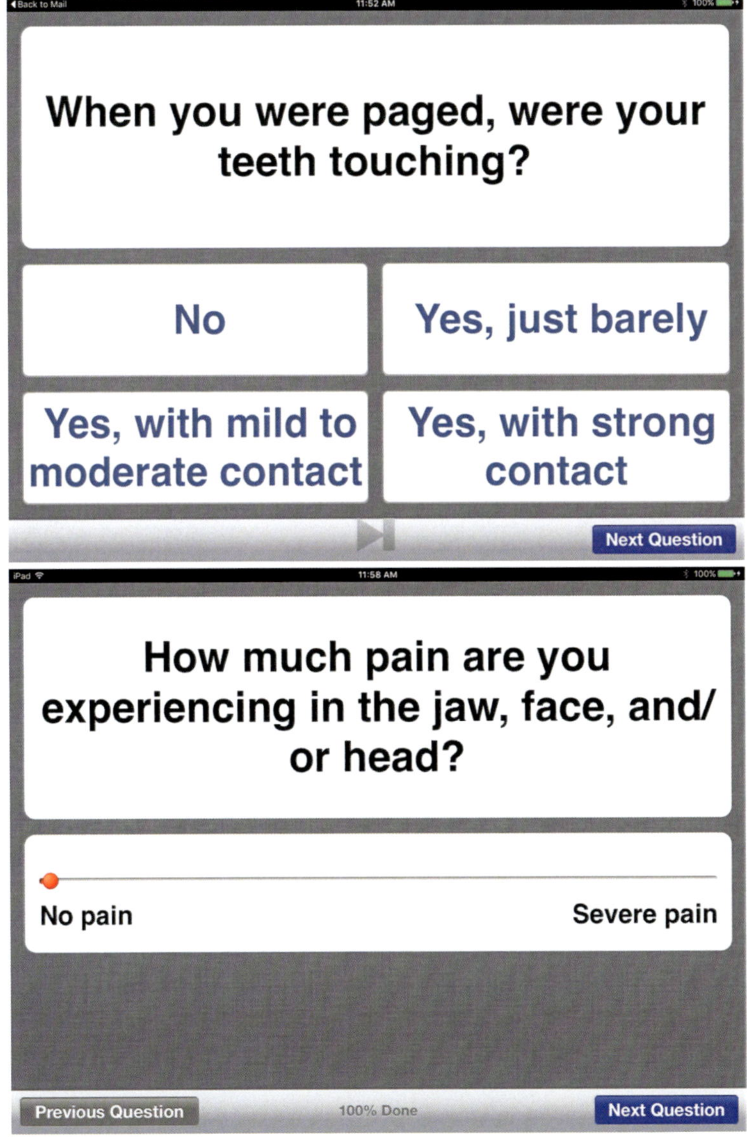

Fig. 12.3 Screenshots of sample ESM questionnaire items using PIEL survey tool

present push buttons, check boxes, sliders, etc. for assessment purposes. The amount of time needed to train patients to use a smartphone-based ESM assessment strategy is typically quite short, as patients are already used to interacting with their devices.

12.6 Rationale for Treatment

Treatment for teeth grinding is designed primarily to prevent further damage to the teeth. There is no evidence that teeth grinding behaviors can be permanently altered by dental, behavioral, or pharmacological interventions.

Treatment for other oral parafunctional behaviors such as extended tooth contact ("clenching") and cheek biting has reduction of injury to the masticatory system and other oral tissues and their subsequent signs and symptoms as the primary goals. This may include reducing pain, jaw dysfunction, soft tissue lesions, tooth fractures, and other consequences.

12.7 Treatment Options

Splints For sleep-related grinding, the use of an intraoral stabilization-type ("flat plane") appliance is suggested. These devices cover all the occlusal surfaces of a dental arch and are typically fabricated from acrylic. This design allows grinding motions to occur and does not "lock" the jaw into a fixed position. Grinding patients only need to wear the device during when the likelihood of grinding is high (i.e., typically during sleep, but not during awake times). The appliance does not permanently reduce grinding, and patients may need to use the device for many years.

For oral parafunction-related pain, a wide range of intraoral appliances have been devised, including anterior/canine guidance, flat plane, anterior repositioning, posterior group function, pivot, neuromuscular, and soft splints have been used. There is no consensus on the amount of time that patients should wear these devices or what the mechanism of action that accounts for their apparent utility in treating pain. Depending on the behaviors involved, splints may be used during the day and/or at night. As pain diminishes, patients can gradually reduce the amount of time that they wear the devices.

Partial coverage splints such as those covering only the anterior or posterior teeth or are worn full time must be carefully monitored to avoid super-eruption in the non-covered teeth and resultant malocclusion. Appliances that are too thick may cause remodeling of the TMJ and should therefore be used with caution.

Self-Care In all cases, splint use for oral parafunction-related pain should be accompanied by provider counseling in self-care. Self-care methods can be quite helpful to reduce habits. These include asking the patient to follow one or more of these self-care strategies:

- Keep the tongue up, teeth apart, and jaw relaxed. Ask patients to closely monitor the jaw position during their waking hours to maintain a relaxed comfortable jaw position. This involves placing the tongue lightly on the palate (roof of the mouth) where it is most comfortable and relaxing the jaw muscles. This tongue position can be achieved by softly saying "n" with the tongue on the roof of the mouth. The upper and lower teeth should never be touching/resting together except occasionally when they touch lightly with swallowing. Similarly, patients should not be encouraged to clench against splints but to use the splint as a reminder to initiate self-care strategies.

- Avoid oral habits and oral parafunctional behaviors. Reducing or avoiding habits such as gum chewing and biting on pencils or pens can help reduce the consequences of these behaviors. The responses patients provide to the oral habits checklist (Table 12.1) will offer multiple possibilities for intervention on oral habits.
- Practice relaxation with diaphragmatic (abdominal) breathing. One simple way to teach this skill is to ask patients to recline and place one hand on the chest and one on the stomach. Instruct patients to breathe so that the stomach hand moves up and down with each inspiration and exhalation, respectively, while chest hand does not move. Daily practice of this relaxation technique will reduce patients' reactions to stressful (and not so stressful) life events and help patients reduce muscle tension, including tension in the masticatory muscles.
- Avoid caffeine. Caffeine is a "muscle-tensing" drug and can make muscles tighter and contribute to rebound headaches. Caffeine and caffeine-like drugs can be found in in coffee, tea, soda, chocolate, and some aspirin compounds.

Nocturnal alarms have been used to treat sleep-related masticatory muscle activity (Fig. 12.4). Typically, these devices monitor masticatory EMG activity or sounds. When the activity exceeds a threshold for a given period of time, an alarm sounds and wakes the patient to terminate the grinding/clenching behaviors. Some devices use a mild electrical stimulus in place of an alarm. Other strategies, including release of a liquid with an aversive taste, have also been used.

Nocturnal alarms can temporarily reduce bruxing behaviors. However, the alarms disrupt sleep. Patients who use nocturnal alarms may report sleepiness and difficulty concentrating while the alarm is being used. Discontinuation of the alarm may lead to "rebound" in the level of grinding.

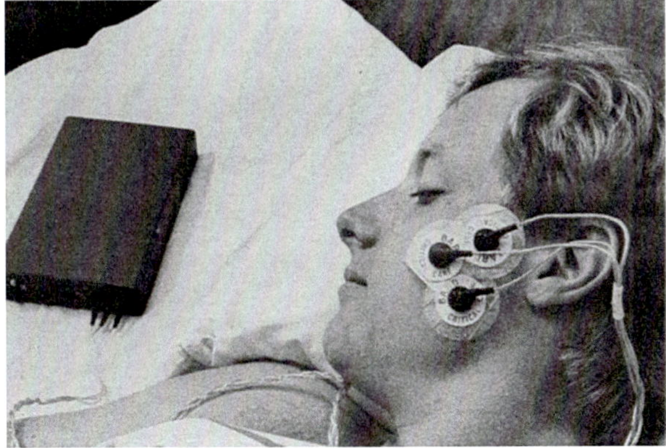

Fig. 12.4 Nocturnal alarm

Medication Pharmacologic approaches are used to manage both oral parafunctions and parafunctional-related pain [9]. These include muscle relaxants for muscle-tensing habits, Botox injections, and nonsteroidal anti-inflammatories (NSAIDs), over-the-counter analgesics, and low doses of tricyclic antidepressants for pain.

Muscle relaxants and anxiolytics are used to manage anxiety, muscle tension, and to improve sleep. Common side effects of sedation are rash and dependency on benzodiazepines. Examples include:

- Cyclobenzaprine 10 mg HS
- Clonazepam 0.5 mg HS

Botulinum toxin ("Botox") injections have been successfully used to treat patients presenting with "bruxism" and orofacial pain. However, the long-term efficacy, side effects, and impact on the functioning of the masticatory system of this treatment are unknown.

NSAIDs often begin with high doses of the drug (400–800 mg dose QID, or two to four times the maximum amount recommended for their over-the-counter equivalents), with monitoring for gastrointestinal side effects such as pain or bleeding. Providers must pay careful attention to other medications that patients are taking and make sure that drug combinations do not inadvertently result in untoward side effects. COX-2 inhibitors are often better tolerated by patients and have fewer gastrointestinal effects. The relationship of COX-2 use with cardiovascular events is an area of concern.

Examples of NSAIDs that can help with jaw pain include:

- Naproxen 250 mg TID with meals
- Ibuprofen 400 mg TID with meals
- Celecoxib (Celebrex) 25 mg BID

Low doses of tricyclic antidepressants (TCAs) can successfully be used for oral parafunction-related pain. Extrapyramidal effects, especially sleepiness and dry mouth, can be mitigated by taking the medications before sleep or through the use of TCAs with a lower incidence of extrapyramidal effects (e.g., nortriptyline). Extrapyramidal effects often diminish with longer-term use. Among the conditions that providers should attend to when using TCAs are cardiovascular diseases. Examples include:

- Amitriptyline 25–50 mg HS
- Nortriptyline 25–50 mg HS

Cognitive-Behavioral Therapy Behavioral interventions can successfully treat oral parafunction-related pain (Table 12.3). The goals of these interventions are to reduce parafunctional activity directly, reduce activity of the masticatory muscles, identify and manage triggers for increased habits and pain, and develop alternative methods for managing the experience of pain. These interventions include relaxation training, biofeedback, cognitive-behavioral pain management, and habit reversal. Online cognitive-behavioral training programs can be found at www.preventingchronicpain.org and other sites.

Table 12.3 Three steps involved in cognitive-behavioral treatment of oral habits [10]

1. *Understanding why to change the old habit.* Oral parafunctional habits place repetitive strain on the muscles and joints that over time that can lead to tension, tenderness, and pain
2. *Knowledge of new habit.* The new habit to learn involves relaxing the jaw muscles, joints, and tongue by keeping the tongue up, teeth apart, and jaw dropped and relaxed. Correct the head and neck posture as well and take a deep breath or two to help with general relaxation
3. *Practice.* Take pauses throughout the day to check if the upper and lower teeth are together. If they are, correct it with the new habit of tong ue up and teeth apart. Practice the new habit two to three times per hour for 2 weeks. Routine awareness of incorrect oral habits will increase the automatic replacement with the new habits. Permanent correction with new habit will generally occur within 2 to 4 weeks

12.8 Treatment Goals and Sequencing of Care

Following the recommendations of the National Institute of Dental and Craniofacial Research (NIDCR), conservative treatments are recommended first. These include self-care strategies, intraoral appliances, medications, and behavioral interventions. Direct demonstration of the impact of tooth contact on the activity of the masticatory muscles helps patients understand the need to minimize parafunctional activity.

If first stage approaches are not adequate, cognitive therapies focusing on pain management and more intensive behavioral and psychophysiological interventions may be needed. If these are not successful, more extensive cognitive therapy, the use of alarm systems, and a reevaluation of the presenting complaint may be needed.

References

1. Lobbezoo F, Naeije M. Bruxism is mainly regulated centrally, not peripherally. J Oral Rehabil. 2001;28:1085–91.
2. Glaros AG. Temporomandibular disorders and facial pain: a psychophysiological perspective. Appl Psychophysiol Biofeedback. 2008;33:161–71.
3. Isacsson G, Bodin L, Seldén A, Barregård L. Variability in the quantification of abrasion on the Bruxcore device. J Orofac Pain. 1996;10:362–8.
4. Glaros AG, Marszalek JM, Williams KB. Longitudinal multilevel modeling of facial pain, muscle tension, and stress. J Dent Res. 2016;95:416–422.
5. Glaros AG, Williams K, Lausten L. The role of parafunctions, emotions and stress in predicting facial pain. J Am Dent Assoc. 2005;136:451–8.
6. Manfredini D, Ahlberg J, Castroflorio T, Poggio CE, Guarda-Nardini L, Lobbezoo F. Diagnostic accuracy of portable instrumental devices to measure sleep bruxism: a systematic literature review of polysomnographic studies. J Oral Rehabil. 2014;41:836–42.
7. Lobbezoo F, Ahlberg J, Glaros AG, Kato T, Koyano K, Lavigne GJ, de Leeuw R, Manfredini D, Svensson P, Winocur E. Bruxism defined and graded: an international consensus. J Oral Rehabil. 2013;40:2–4.
8. Raphael KG, Janal MN, Sirois DA, Dubrovsky B, Klausner JJ, Krieger AC, Lavigne GJ. Validity of self-reported sleep bruxism among myofascial temporomandibular disorder patients and controls. J Oral Rehabil. 2015;42:751–8.
9. Hersh EV, Balasubramaniam R, Pinto A. Pharmacologic management of temporomandibular disorders. Oral Maxillofac Surg Clin North Am. 2008;20(2):197–210.
10. Litt MD, Shafer DM, Kreutzer DL. Brief cognitive-behavioral treatment for TMD pain: long-term outcomes and moderators of treatment. Pain. 2010;151(1):110–6.

Obstructive Sleep Apnea and Snoring

13

Antonio G. Romero and João N.A.R. Ferreira

Pearls of Wisdom

- Moderate-to-severe sleep-disordered breathing (SDB) is common in the general population, particularly between ages 50 and 70.
- Obstructive sleep apnea (OSA) is a major public health concern presenting a high associated risk for hypertension, cardiovascular disease, type II diabetes, and motor vehicle accidents. The dentist should always evaluate for the presence of risk factors in patients with any signs of SDB.
- PSG is the gold standard for the diagnosis of OSA and sleep disorders.
- The CPAP device is still considered the most effective therapeutic approach for the management of SDB in both adults and children; however, their side effects and low adherence make clinicians look for alternative treatment options.
- Oral appliances (OA), especially mandibular advancement devices (MAD), have become viable option for patients with mild-to-moderate OSA or with primary snoring.
- The sleep physician should be the one providing an accurate diagnosis and prescribe OA when indicated. The dentist is considered a key part of the multidisciplinary management team for OSA.
- When using OA, then dentist should use custom-made ones allowing for the titration of the device and should monitor closely the resolution of OSA symptoms and possible side effects.

A.G. Romero, DDS, PhD, Dipl. ABOP (✉)
Member American Academy of Dental Sleep Medicine and Fellow American Academy of Orofacial Pain, Valencia, Spain

Invited professor University of Valencia, Valencia, Spain

Invited Professor Mini-residency of Dental Sleep Medicine, Tufts University, Boston, USA
e-mail: Antonio.Romero@uv.es

J.N.A.R. Ferreira, DDS, MS, PhD, Dipl. ABOP
Faculty of Dentistry, National University of Singapore, National University Hospital, University Dental Cluster, Singapore, Singapore

J.N.A.R. Ferreira et al. (eds.), *Orofacial Disorders*,
DOI 10.1007/978-3-319-51508-3_13

13.1 Introduction and Diagnostic Subtypes

Sleep-related breathing disorders in adults are a heterogeneous group of disorders characterized by different abnormalities of respiration during sleep. The term *sleep-disordered breathing* (SDB) has been used interchangeably with the term *obstructive sleep apnea* (OSA), which has been now supplanted by the term *obstructive sleep apnea–hypopnea* (OSAH) syndrome. However, in strict terms, we should use the term SDB to encompass the entire group of respiratory abnormalities occurring during sleep, not only just the obstructive sleep events. Taking these terms in consideration, the ICSD-3 classifies the sleep-relating breathing disorders as in Table 13.1 below.

Although classically the spectrum of sleep-disordered breathing ranged from primary snoring to severe sleep apnea (Fig. 13.1) and that can be even considered the better approach for the dentist to understand these types of disorders, it is important to point out this aspect in order to keep a balance between the clinical presentation and the rigor of the nomenclature in the sleep medicine field. The term obstructive sleep apnea–hypopnea (OSAH) syndrome should only be applied when making reference to the spectrum of disorders in the family of obstructive respiratory events, including OSA among others.

Firstly, it is important to differentiate the terms OSA and central sleep apnea (CSA) since it will have a definite impact in the treatment that we can provide to our patients. Further, it will also define the role of the dentist or the orofacial pain/oral medicine practitioner on the management of these conditions. Nevertheless, OSA is the most common and serious medical condition and is characterized by recurrent cessation or substantial reduction in breathing during sleep. OSA is

Table 13.1 Sleep-disordered breathing disorders' classification

1. Obstructive sleep apnea disorders (OSA)
2. Central sleep apnea disorders
3. Sleep-related hypoventilation disorders
4. Sleep-related hypoxemia disorders
5. Isolated symptoms and normal variants

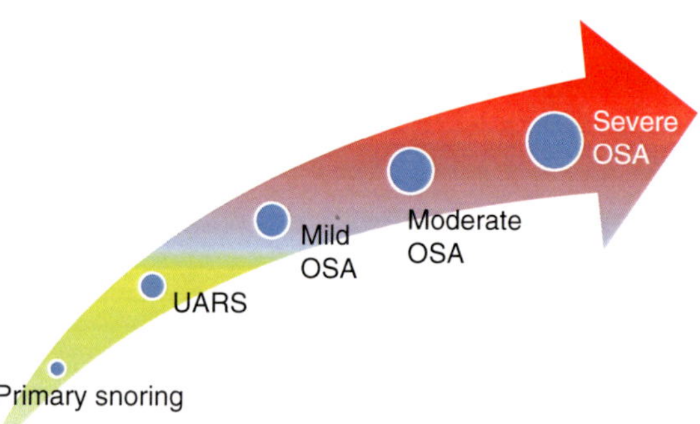

Fig. 13.1 Disease severity spectrum of sleep-disordered breathing

Table 13.2 Types of sleep apnea conditions

Type of sleep apnea	Definition	Comment
Obstructive sleep apnea	Normal ventilation is reduced or obstructed due to a partial or total occlusion of the upper airway Respiratory effort is maintained	It requires to measure the presence of respiratory effort (esophageal manometry or induction plethysmography required) Thoracic and abdominal belt sensors required in home sleep testing devices
Central sleep apnea	Normal ventilation is reduced, but because the brain temporarily stops to send signals to muscles controlling breathing activity, the effort to breathe is reduced or completely abolished during the whole event	It is a central nervous system phenomenon. Thus it is not related to the presence of the same predisposing factors (leading to anatomic obstruction of the upper airway) than the obstructive type
Mixed apnea	When in the same patient we have a combination of central and obstructive sleep apnea episodes	Usually, the central apnea event is followed by the obstructive one

characterized by repeated cessation of breathing during sleeping, due mostly to complete or partial oropharyngeal obstruction; therefore, it is a serious, potentially life-threatening condition. OSA is usually found in severe snorers, in which there are periods of decreased breathing or a complete cessation of breathing during sleep due to an obstruction of airflow. The differences in the definition of OSA, CSA, and a combination of these two (referred as "mixed apnea") are displayed in Table 13.2.

The term "upper airway resistance syndrome" (UARS) was coined by Guilleminault et al. In 1993 UARS is usually defined as the presence of daytime sleepiness associated to a sleep-disordered breathing and microarousals related to respiratory effort (RERA) but without sufficient apneas/hypopneas episodes for meeting the criteria for OSA. The diagnosis is based on both the association of clinical symptoms and polysomnographic findings. UARS patients usually complain of snoring associated with daytime sleepiness.

13.2 Clinical Presentation

Several types of events can occur during sleep-disordered breathing (SDB) and a detailed description of them can be found in Table 13.3.

The clinical spectrum of SDB conditions tends to progress with aging as seen on Fig. 13.1.

Firstly, the *primary snoring* condition is primarily a "social" problem where no excessive daytime sleepiness is present, and the sleep study is within normal observations. Primary snoring can be further categorized as intermittent, mild chronic, and heavy chronic as it increases in severity.

Secondly, as for *UARS*, snoring and excessive daytime sleepiness are present though sleep study is found normal.

Table 13.3 Definition of events during SDB

Type of event	Definition	Comment
Snoring	Loud sound during sleep generated at the level of the upper airway and associated with the vibration of the soft palate and the restriction of the air passage with noisy air turbulences	The hallmark presenting symptom of OSA in up to 95% of patients Snoring alone is a poor predictor of OSA The absence of it makes OSA unlikely but doesn't exclude it
Apnea	Complete cessation or decrease in nasal airflow by ≥90% of baseline for at least 10 s	At least 90% of the event's duration must meet the amplitude reduction criteria for apnea
Hypopnea	Decrease in nasal airflow by ≥90% of baseline for at least 10 s plus ≥4% oxygen desaturation from pre-event baseline	At least 90% of the event's duration must meet the amplitude reduction criteria for hypopnea
Hypopnea (alternative)	Decrease in nasal airflow ≥50% of baseline for at least 10 s plus ≥3% oxygen desaturation from pre-event baseline or the event is associated with an arousal	At least 90% of the event's duration must meet the amplitude reduction criteria for hypopnea
RERA (respiratory effort-related arousal)	Increased respiratory effort for at least 10 s, on esophageal pressure recording to maintain a normal airflow leading to an arousal from sleep shown in the EEG recording	REPA events are not usually associated with oxygen desaturation An event meeting the criteria of apnea/hypopnea cannot be a REPA. REPA events are better detected by esophageal manometry, but nasal pressure and respiratory-induced plethysmography belts can also be used

Table 13.4 Definition of OSA severity stages

Type of OSA	Definition	Alternative
Mild OSA	AHI ≥5 and <15 in an overnight PSG study	Not usually related to high oxygen desaturation degrees
Moderate OSA	AHI ≥15 and <30 in an overnight PSG study	Or when the lowest oxygen saturation is ≥50%
Severe OSA	AHI ≥30 in an overnight PSG study	Or when the lowest oxygen saturation levels are <50%

Lastly, *obstructive sleep apnea* (OSA) is the most common condition with three severity stages (Table 13.4) according to the apnea–hypopnea index (AHI), which is the number of apnea and hypopnea events per hour of sleep. This condition is usually associated with:

- Profound snoring, gasping, snoring, and cessation of breathing during sleep
- Excessive daytime sleepiness

Table 13.5 Clinical differences between OSA and UARS

Clinical/PSG characteristics	OSAHS	UARS
Presence of daytime sleepiness	Common	Common
Arterial hypertension	Common	Uncommon
Orthostatic hypotension	Uncommon	Common
Allergic rhinitis	Uncommon	Common
Headache	Uncommon	Common
Irritable bowel and functional somatic syndromes	Uncommon	Common
Sleep onset insomnia	Uncommon	Common
Mid-sleep insomnia	Common	Common
AHI	≥5 by definition	<5 by definition
RERA events/hour of sleep	<10 per hour/sleep	≥10 per hour of sleep
Lowest oxygen saturation	<92% average	Usually 92%
a-Delta sleep	Uncommon	Common

- An abnormal sleep study
- Multiple systemic effects (life-threatening potential)

More clinical differences between OSA and UARS can be found in Table 13.5, according to polysomnography (PSG) and presence of other signs, symptoms, and medical conditions.

13.3 Epidemiology and Etiology (Risk Factors)

Primary Snoring:

- Occurs in all age groups, but increases with age (40–60% of adults over 40 report snoring).
- In children, it is usually related to the presence of enlarged tonsils or adenoids.
- More prevalent in males, particularly in Hispanic, Asian, and African American.
- Three times more common in obese people.

Obstructive Sleep Apnea (OSA): Overall prevalence is 9% in females and 24% in males

- Symptomatic OSA in 2% of females and 4% of males.
- Have signs of potential sleep-disordered breathing (SDB) since RDI >5.
- Moderate-to-severe SDB is frequent in the general population, affecting 17% of males and 9% of females between ages 50 and 70.

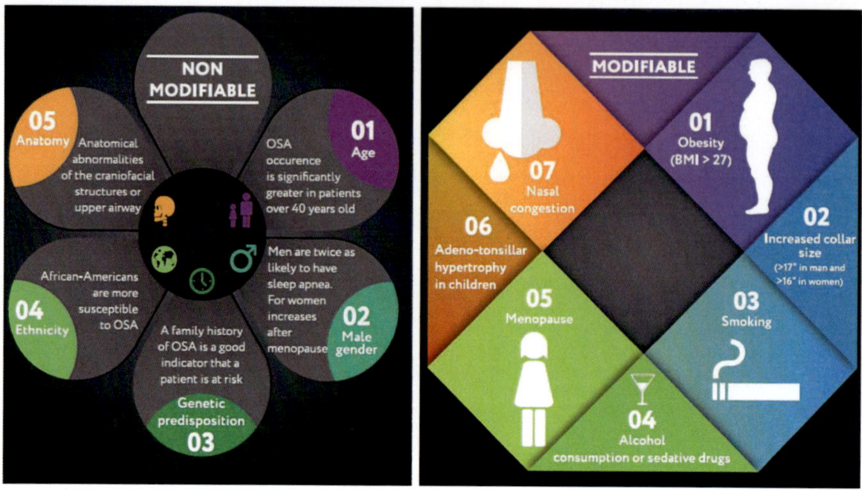

Fig. 13.2 Non-modifiable and modifiable risk factors in OSA

OSA Risk Factors

Several risk factors have been described of being responsible for the development and progression of OSA. These can be categorized as modifiable and non-modifiable OSA risk factors and are presented in Fig. 13.2.

13.4 Pathophysiology and Mechanisms

The critical abnormality in OSA is the repetitive complete or partial collapse of the upper airway during sleep. Because of the relationship between form and function, upper airway anatomy must be taken into consideration in OSA pathophysiology. The upper airway has a collapsible segment that extends from the hard palate to the vocal cords. Thus, the size and the shape of the upper airway will determine the probability of suffering OSA. When there is a restriction in the size of the bony compartment, and excess of soft tissue around the airway or a combination of the two, there will be an excess of extraluminal tissue pressure, producing subsequently a reduction in the caliber and thus affecting negatively the degree of patency (Fig. 13.3).

Certain skeletal conditions as retrognathia; retro-positioning of the maxilla, mandibular, and hypoplasia; or an inferiorly positioned hyoid bone reduce the volume of the bony compartment. In addition, deposition of fat tissue around the upper airway as seen in obesity, macroglossia, adenotonsillar enlargement, thickening of the lateral pharyngeal walls, enlargement of the soft palate, and edema/inflammation are among the soft tissue factors that can favor the airway collapse.

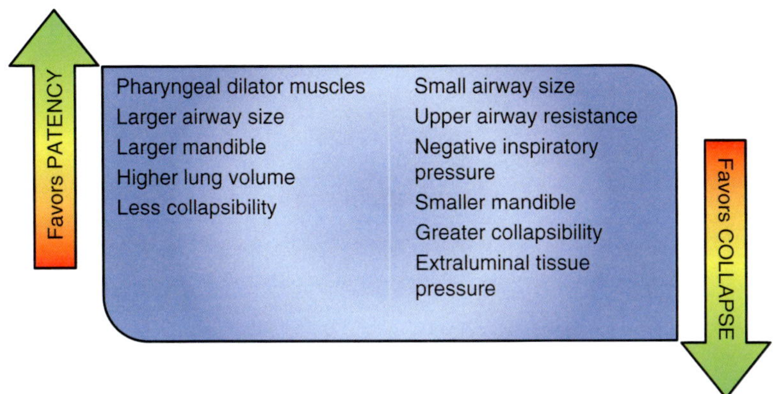

Fig. 13.3 The unbalance between upper airway collapse and patency in OSA pathophysiology

However, the activity of the pharyngeal dilatator muscles and the central control of the ventilation are also key factors in the pathophysiology of OSA. The impairment of mechanoreceptor sensitivity, of the upper airway neuromuscular reflexes, and of the strength and endurance of pharyngeal dilatator muscles can produce a decrease in the pharyngeal dilator muscle activity. The dysregulation of the upper airway neuromuscular reflexes can be a consequence from a neuro-sensorial injury due to inflammation and trauma on the upper airway caused by snoring.

13.4.1 Systemic Effects of OSA

Obstructive sleep apnea (OSA) is a potential life-threatening condition since apnea may trigger a cascade of primary events and physiological consequences involving dysfunctions in respiratory, cardiovascular, and central nervous systems (Figs. 13.4 and 13.5). Hence, these OSA events may lead to increased heart rate and blood pressure (hypertension), cardiovascular disease, type 2 diabetes, neurocognitive impairment, and increased risk to suffer motor vehicle accidents. The risk of heart failure is increased by 140%, the risk of stroke by 60%, and the risk of coronary heart disease by 30% in OSA patients.

Some community studies showed evidence that OSA is a predisposing factor for cardiovascular mortality, independently of traditional cardiovascular risk factors. The increase in morbidity and mortality is likely to involve intermediate pathways that include dyslipidemia, glucose intolerance, and hypertension along with central obesity which defines the so-called metabolic syndrome. This is the reason why OSA is thought to contribute to the development of type 2 diabetes. Out of the two phenotypic components of OSA, hypoxemia is the one more closely associated with glucose intolerance and cardiovascular disease, whereas sleep microarousals are more closely associated with incident hypertension.

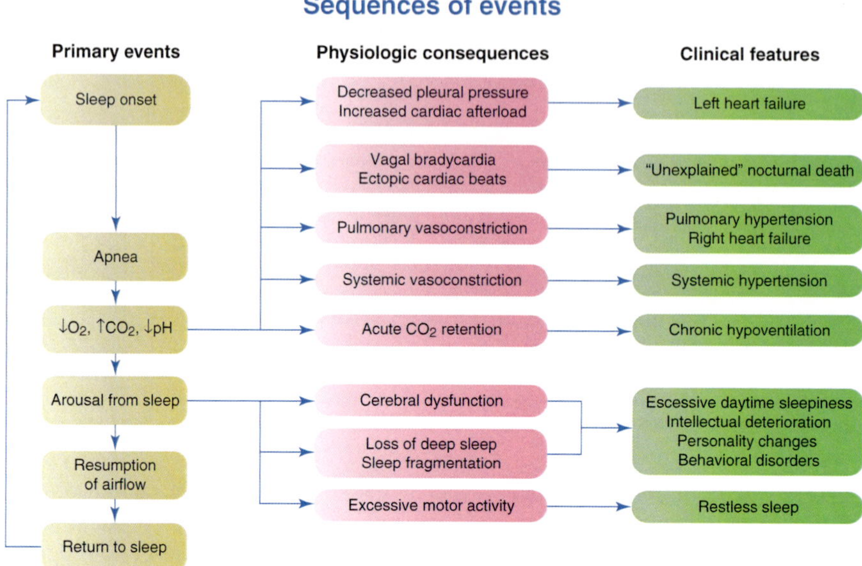

Fig. 13.4 Sequence of events in OSA together with their physiological consequences and associated clinical features

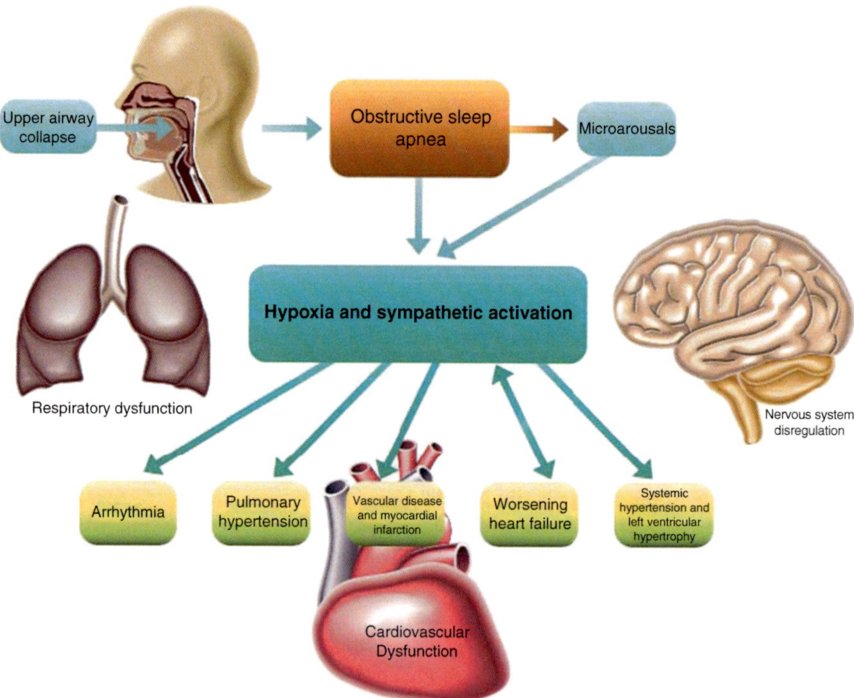

Fig. 13.5 Dysfunctional consequences of OSA in respiratory, cardiovascular, and central nervous systems

The neurocognitive deficits associated with OSA include a decrease in vigilance, memory, and executive function and can be a result of the effects of sleep loss in the prefrontal cortex. Although daytime sleepiness is easily recovered after OSA treatment, it seems that permanent injury to the brain's cognitive centers is secondary to the chronic intermittent hypoxia. Hence, incomplete recovery of those initial neurocognitive deficits does occur even after an appropriate OSA treatment. It is also important to note that in children, OSA-driven neurocognitive effects can be related to cognitive–behavioral problems, attention-deficit/hyperactivity disorder (ADHD) and subsequently impaired academic performance.

13.5 Diagnosis and Diagnostic Criteria

The diagnosis of OSA and SDB is made based on the recognition of typical clinical signs and symptoms, the clinical examination, and the evaluation of sleep studies. Although overnight full PSG is the gold standard for the diagnosis of OSA and sleep disorders according to the American Academy of sleep medicine, the use of home sleep monitors along with a comprehensive clinical evaluation may be used as an alternative to PSG for patients who have a high pretest probability for OSA.

The suspicion of having OSA is based on the presence of clinical signs and symptoms. Those can be divided in daytime (e.g., excessive daytime sleepiness, restless sleep, morning headaches, neurocognitive impairment, depression) and nighttime symptoms (e.g., snoring, choking or gasping, GERD).

The use of different questionnaires can be of help, and they are used mainly as a screening tool to detect the presence of excessive daytime sleepiness, which is a main finding in patients with OSA. The Epworth Sleepiness Scale (ESS) is one example of a quantifiable subjective measure of sleepiness. In this scale, the individual is asked to rate on a scale of 0–3 (0, no chance; 3, high likelihood) the chance of dozing in a series of eight situations. This score has a modest correlation with physiological measures of sleep but has a better correlation with the respiratory disturbance index in patients with obstructive sleep apnea.

In addition, a set of four basic questions represented by the acronym STOP can also be used. A positive response to two or more questions represents an increased risk for sleep apnea. The expanded version, the STOP–BANG questionnaire, has been demonstrated to highly predict sleep apnea's presence (Table 13.6). This questionnaire can have four more questions represented by the acronym BANG. If the score is eight, the probability for severe sleep apnea is nearly 82%.

A comprehensive clinical examination also provides the clinician with the anatomical risk factors that may lead to the diagnosis of OSA. The Table 13.7 below displays a summary of the most common physical findings and signs and symptoms in OSA patients.

Imaging plays a role in the anatomic assessment of the airway and adjacent structures. Although imaging techniques for the head and neck are not regularly used to diagnose OSA, the use of certain techniques can help to (1) visualize the airway, (2) detect anatomic abnormalities, and (3) ultimately predict the risk for upper airway obstruction that may contribute to the presence of a SBD. Thus, cephalometric analysis,

Table 13.6 STOP and BANG questionnaires

STOP questionnaires	Questions	Comments
S for snoring	Does the patient snore loudly?	Snoring is one of the highest OSA indicators
T for tiredness	Does the patient often feel tired?	Indicator of non resting sleep
O for observed	Has someone observed that the patient´s breathing stop durin sleep	Witnessed apneas are always a clue for suffering OSA
P for pressure	Does the patient have high blood pressure?	Hypertension frequently associated to OSA
Bang questionnaire		Comments
B for Body Mass Index	BMI > 28	
A for age	Age > 50 years	OSA increases with age
N for neck size	Male ≥ 17 in; Female ≥ 16″	Neck size is a strong predictor of airway collapsability
G for gender	Are you a male?	OSA more frequent in males

Table 13.7 Common physical findings and signs and symptoms in OSA

Obstructive sleep apnea	
Common physical findings	*Common signs and symptoms*
1. Enlarged uvula	1. Snoring
2. Soft palate hyperplasia	2. Stop breathing at night
3. Nasal congestion	3. Excessive daytime sleepiness
4. Nasal polyps	4. Morning headaches
5. Enlarged tonsils	5. Nightime gasping
6. Enlarged tongue	6. Restless sleep
7. Retruded mandible	7. Poor sleep quality
8. Receded chin	8. Irritability
9. Neck size >17"	9. Short-term memory loss
10. Overweight and obese	10. Decreased attention and concentration
	11. Performance deficiencies
	12. Depression
	13. GERD
	14. Nocturnal enuresis
	15. Impotence
	16. Weight gain

MRI, acoustic reflections, and computed tomography scans are used as part of the patient comprehensive exam. Cone beam computed tomography (CBCT) scans are becoming more and more popular in the dental field, and since these techniques include the teeth, jaws, spine, cranial base, and facial soft tissues, they provide an excellent opportunity to evaluate the functional and developmental relationships between these structures. Furthermore they allow us to visualize and calculate the airway dimension.

Sleep studies are the basic diagnostic tools to provide the definite diagnosis of SDB and OSA, where a complete collection of physiological data from the wake/sleep stages is required for interpretation by a trained sleep medicine specialist.

The American Academy of Sleep Medicine (AASM) defined four levels of sleep studies from which an objective-based assessment is made. These four levels are differentiated per the number of physiological signals recorded as well as if the sleep study is attended or not by a sleep technologist.

Type I sleep study or polysomnography (PSG) is an overnight sleep study performed in a sleep center and monitored by a sleep technologist in a nearby control room with the record and registration of at least seven physiological measures. The PSG is considered to be the "gold standard" in sleep medicine relative to objective-based sleep studies. In Table 13.8 a description of the different types of sleep studies and monitors, with comments about the clinical application of each one, is showed.

Table 13.8 Types of sleep studies and monitors

	Type I	Type II	Type III	Type IV
Definition	Attended PSG	Unattended PSG	Modified portable sleep apnea testing	Continuous single or dual bioparameter recorder
Signals	Minimum of 7 including EEG, EOG, chin EMG, ECG, airflow, respiratory effort, and oxygen saturation	Minimum of 7 including EEG, EOG, chin EMG, ECG, airflow, respiratory effort, and oxygen saturation	Minimum of 4 including chest movement, air flow, heart rate or ECG, and oxygen saturation	Minimum of 1 channel including oxygen saturation, airflow, or chest movement
Attended	Yes	No	No	No
Body position	Objectively documented	Possible	Possible	No
Leg movements	EMG or motion sensor desirable but optional	Optional	Optional	Optional
Interventions	Possible	No	No	No
Clinical application	Diagnosis of OSA and other sleep-related disorders Efficacy of OSA treatments (CPAP or appliance titrations) Research studies	Primarily used for research studies	OSA diagnosis in patients with moderate-to-high pretest probability Test efficacy of oral appliances (controversial) Research studies	OSA diagnosis in patients with moderate-to-high pretest probability if monitor has ≥3 channels Test efficacy of oral appliances Research studies

13.6 Rationale for Treatment

The treatment of snoring and OSA will depend on the severity of the disease (particularly in OSA), and this will determine the treatment options and sequence of care.

13.7 Treatment Options, Goals, and Sequencing of Care

This section will focus on OSA and primary snoring conditions. These are the only conditions that can be managed by an experienced dentist in collaboration with a sleep medicine specialist. Ideally, an effective treatment approach for OSA is to reverse excessive daytime somnolence and fatigue, reduce the risks associated with this condition, minimize the impact of cardiovascular effects, and improve quality of life. In many cases the participation of other healthcare professionals such as the ENT, pneumologists, cardiologists, and maxillofacial surgeons, among others, is mandatory. In fact, the ideal treatment plan is to always establish different patient's needs depending on the severity of the apnea and other health issues related to the patient's condition. Below is a description of cognitive–behavioral, medical devices, pharmacological, and surgical options for OSA management:

1. *Cognitive–behavioral:* We should never underestimate the importance of patient education, especially those items addressed to have an impact on risk factors' modification. Weight loss, changes on sleep position, smoking cessation, alcohol and sedative drug intake avoidance, and sleep hygiene measures are included among the most common approaches.
2. *Medical devices:* The most successful medical modalities for the management of OSA are the use of *positive airway pressure (PAP) devices* and *oral appliances*:
   2.1. *PAP devices:* The most successful medical treatment for OSA is the use of positive airway pressure devices, which maintain upper airway patency during sleep simply by providing a pneumatic splint. PAP devices can be delivered by continuous (CPAP), bi-level (BPAP), or auto-titrating (APAP) modalities. CPAP supplies a flow of positive air pressure adjusted to the level needed to keep the airway open, delivered through a facial device. It reduces AHI, blood pressure, and cardiac arrhythmias and improves oxygen saturation levels, sleep efficiency, self-reported sleep, and well-being. The main disadvantage is that CPAP devices are sometimes difficult to use, thus affecting compliance. Despite CPAP being highly efficacious in preventing upper airway collapse, patients' acceptance, tolerance, and adherence are often low, thereby reducing effectiveness. Several risk factors and comorbid conditions seem to be associated with decreased compliance, especially depression. PAP therapy is considered the first line of treatment for those patients suffering from moderate-to-severe OSA. The success rate with CPAP therapy is considered around 95% of cases.

2.2. *Oral appliances:* In those cases where patient is intolerant to CPAP, when the level of compliance to CPAP therapy is low, and in those cases with primary snoring or mild-to-moderate OSA, the use of oral appliances (OAs) should be considered. There are two main types of oral appliances: tongue retaining devices and mandibular repositioning devices (a.k.a. mandibular advancement devices). It is important to clarify that their level of efficacy is always lower than the CPAP therapy.

While mandibular advancement devices (MADs) increase the anteroposterior dimensions of the oropharynx and velopharynx by repositioning and maintaining the lower jaw in a forward position during sleep, tongue retaining devices (TRDs) provide a forward movement of the tongue producing more favorable changes in the retroglossal region. Anyway the positive effect is attributed to changes in airway configuration. Due to comfort and compliance issues, MADs are usually the first choice unless the patient is edentulous where tongue retaining devices seem to be the first option. There are numerous types of MAD available whose differences rely on material of fabrication, design, advancement mechanisms, size, and thickness.

The level of efficacy of OA for the management of OSA is estimated in 76% in cases of mild OSA (5–15 events/hour sleep), 61%i in moderate cases (15–30 events/hour), and 40% in severe cases (more than 30 events/hour). Different studies have shown that therapy with OA is usually more successful in younger patients and female gender and patients with small neck, lower body mass index (BMI), and retrognathic mandible and positional OSA cases.

The complications and side effects with the use of OA are frequent but usually minor and temporary and include increase or decrease in salivation, tooth movement, tooth soreness, masticatory muscles or TMJ pain, worsening in OSA (around 13% of patients), bite discomfort, and occlusal changes (posterior open bite). There are relative contraindications for the use of OA. These are usually severe or active periodontal disease, active TMD pathology, inadequate dentition (less than six teeth remaining), central sleep apnea, growing children, morbid obesity, unmotivated patients, severe hypoxemia, severe OSA, and concomitant severe cardiovascular pathology.

The use of OA in the treatment of OSA in mild-to moderate cases as well as severe cases intolerant to CPAP therapy is recommended as the current practice parameter. OA also can be used as a part of combination therapy with CPAP and/or upper airway surgery. The flowchart and decision tree for the management of snoring or OSA with a CPAP or MAS are shown in Fig. 13.6 for a better understanding.

3. *Pharmacological:* A large range of pharmacological approaches have been explored over the years, but their effectiveness to treat OSA has been proved minimal, and research is undergoing to find better options. Nasal corticosteroids can reduce AHI index and can help with allergic nasal congestion and vasomotor rhinitis associated with CPAP. Only modafinil (200–400 mg/day) or armodafinil (150–250 mg/day) has shown mild-to-moderate positive effects in specific OSA cases.

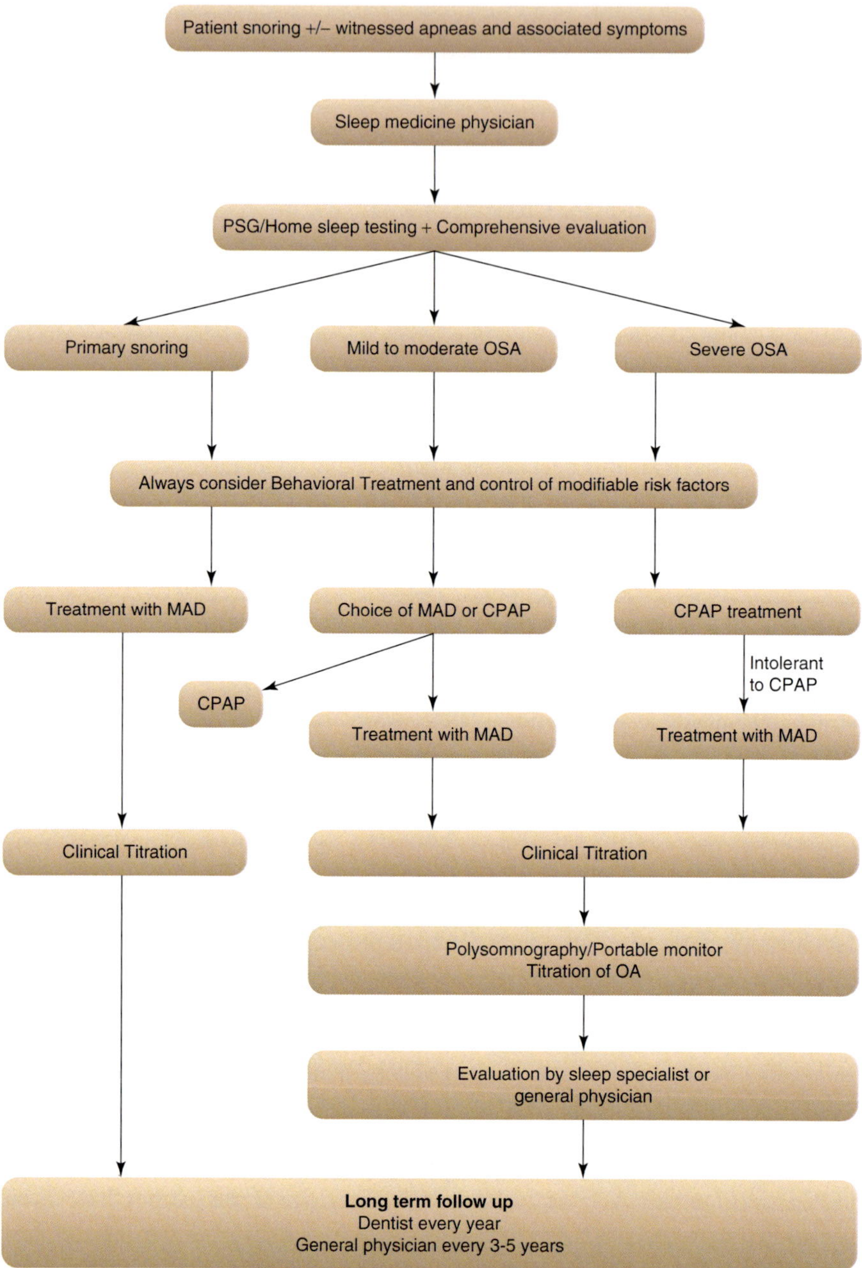

Fig. 13.6 Treatment algorithm for the management of primary snoring and OSA with OA (Modified from Pliska and Almeida [34]. Permission to modify and reproduce was granted)

4. *Surgical:* This is only indicated in severe OSA clinical scenarios when patients have an anatomic obstruction. There are different surgical techniques for treating OSA, whose aim is to relieve the obstruction by removing or bypassing it or increasing airway size. The selection of what modality to use depends on patient's anatomy and physiology. The selection process only comes after a full evaluation by an ENT or a maxillofacial surgeon specialized in OSA management. The most common surgical procedures for OSA treatment are tracheostomy, tonsillectomy/adenoidectomy (for children mainly), septoplasty/turbinate reduction, uvulopalatopharyngoplasty (UPPP), tongue base reduction, hyoid suspension, genioglossus advancement, maxillomandibular advancement, or a combination of these techniques.

Suggested Reading

1. Kryger M, Roth T, Dement W. Principles and practice of sleep medicine. 3rd ed. Philadelphia: W B Saunders Co; 2000.
2. Ramar K, Dort LC, Katz SG, Lettieri CL, Harrod CG, Thomas SM, Chervn RD. Clinical practice guideline for the treatment of obstructive sleep apnea and snoring with oral appliance therapy: an update for 2015: an American Academy of Sleep Medicine and American Academy of Dental Sleep Medicine Clinical Practice Guideline. J Clin Sleep Med. 2015;11(7):773–827.
3. Jordan AS, McSharry DG, Malhotra A. Adult obstructive sleep apnea. Lancet. 2014;383(9918):736–47.
4. Epstein LJ, Kristo D, Strollo PJ, et al. Clinical guideline for the evaluation, management and long term care of obstructive sleep apnea in adults. J Clin Sleep Med. 2009;5(3):263–76.
5. Satela MJ. International classification of sleep disorders-third edition highlights and modifications. Chest. 2014;146(5):1387–94.
6. Rules for scoring respiratory events in sleep: update of the 2007. AASM Manual for the Scoring of Sleep and Associated Events. J Clin Sleep Med. 2012;8(5):597–619.
7. Thomas RJ. Multimodality therapy for sleep apnea syndromes. J Clin Sleep Med. 2012;8(5):565–7.
8. Gharibeh T, Mehra R. Obstructive sleep apnea syndrome: natural history, diagnosis, and emerging treatment options. Nat Sci Sleep. 2010;2:233–55.
9. Punjabi NM. The epidemiology of adult obstructive sleep apnea. Proc Am Thorac Soc. 2008;5:136–43.
10. Gold AR, Dipalo F, Gold MS, O'Hearn D. The symptoms and signs of upper airway resistance syndrome. A link to the functional somatic syndromes. Chest. 2003;123:87–95.
11. Bao G, Guilleminalult C. Upper airway resistance syndrome-one decade later. Curr Opin Pulm Med. 2004;10:461–7.
12. Palombini L, Lopes M, Tufik S, Guilleminault C, Bittencourt LR. Upper airway resistance syndrome: still not recognized and not treated. Sleep Sci. 2011;4(2):72–8.
13. Scherr SC, Dort LC, Almeida F, et al. Definition of an effective oral appliance for the treatment of obstructive sleep apnea and snoring. A report of the American Academy of Dental Sleep Medicine. J Dent Sleep Med. 2014;1(1):39–50.
14. del Campo MF, Ruiz Albi T, Zamarrón SC. Upper airway resistance syndrome – a twenty-five years experience. In: Sleep disorders, Dr. Chris Idzikowski, editor. 2012. ISBN: 978-953-51-0293-9.

15. Sutherland K, Vanderveken OM, Tsuda H, Marklund M. Oral appliance treatment for obstructive sleep apnea. A review. J Clin Sleep Med. 2014;10(2):215–27.
16. Pham LV, Schwartz AR. The pathogenesis of obstructive sleep apnea. J Thorac Dis. 2015;7(8):1358–72.
17. Iber C, Ancoli-Israel S, Chesson A, et al. The AASM manual for the scoring of sleep and associated events: rules, terminology and technical specifications. 1st ed. Westchester: American Academy of Sleep Medicine; 2007.
18. Hoekema A, Stegenga B, De Bont L. Efficacy and co-morbidity of oral appliances in the treatment of obstructive sleep apnea-hypopnea: a systematic review. Crit Rev Oral Biol Med. 2004;15(3):137–55.
19. Lim J, et al. Oral appliances for obstructive sleep apnea. Cochrane Database Syst Rev. 2003;(4);CD004435.
20. Bailey D, Attanasio R. Sleep disorders: dentistry's role. Dent Cl N Am. 2001;45(4).
21. Clark G. Mandibular advancement devices and sleep disordered breathing. Sleep Med Rev. 1998;2(3):163–74.
22. Schmidt-Nowara W, Lowe A, Wiegand L, et al. Oral appliances for the treatment of snoring and obstructive sleep apnea: a review. Sleep. 1995;18(6):501–10.
23. Practice parameters for the treatment of snoring and obstructive sleep apnea with oral appliances. Sleep. 1995; 18(6):511–513.
24. Mehta A, Qian J, Petocz P, et al. A randomized, controlled study of a mandibular advancement splint for obstructive sleep apnea. Am J Respir Crit Care Med. 2001;163:1457–61.
25. Marklund M, Sahlin C, Stenlund H, et al. Mandibular advancement device in patients with obstructive sleep apnea. Long- term effects on apnea and sleep. Chest. 2001;120:162–9.
26. Ferguson K, Ono T, Lowe A, et al. A randomized crossover study of an oral appliance vs nasal-continuous positive airway pressure in the treatment of mild-moderate obstructive sleep apnea. Chest. 1996;109:1269–75.
27. Clark G, Blumenfeld I, Yoffe N, et al. A crossover study comparing the efficacy of continuous positive airway pressure with anterior mandibular positioning devices on patients with obstructive sleep apnea. Chest. 1996;109:1477–83.
28. Walker-Engstrom M, Tegelberg Å, Wilhelmsson B, Ringqvist I. 4-Year follow-up of treatment with dental appliance or uvulopalatopharyngoplasty in patients with obstructive sleep apnea. A randomized study. Chest. 2002;121:739–46.
29. Pantin CC, Hillman DR, Tennant M. Dental side effects of an oral device to treat snoring and obstructive sleep apnea. Sleep. 1999;22(2):237–40.
30. Fritsch K, et al. Side effects of mandibular advancement devices for sleep apnea treatment. Am J Respir Care Med. 2001;164(5):813–8.
31. Robertson CJ. Dental and skeletal changes associated with long-term mandibular advancement. Sleep. 2001;24(5):531–7.
32. Bailey DR, Atannasio R. Screening and comprehensive evaluation for sleep related breathing disorders. In sleep medicine and dentistry. Dent Clin N Am. 2012;56:331–42.
33. Atannasio R, Bailey DR. Sleep assessment studies. In: Atannasio R, Bailey DR, editors. Dental management of sleep disorders. Iowa: Blackwell Publishing; 2010.
34. Pliska BT, Almeida F. Effectiveness and outcome of oral appliance therapy. Dent Clin N Am. 2012;56(2):433–44.

Part VI

Temporomandibular Disorders and Occlusal Dysfunction

Temporomandibular Joint Disorders

14

Jeffrey P. Okeson, Cristina Perez, and James R. Fricton

Pearls of Wisdom

- Temporomandibular joint functional disorders are classified into derangements of the condyle-disc complex, structural incompatibility of the articular surfaces, and inflammatory joint disorders.
- Clinical signs and symptoms may range from non-painful signs of joint noises to acute and chronic pain and dysfunction.
- These conditions are prevalent; nevertheless, only some require treatment.
- Diagnostic criteria are described in the AAOP guidelines [1] and diagnostic criteria for TMD [2].
- The clinician should always match the level of complexity of the management program with the complexity of the patient. In complex patients, the use of a pain clinic team to facilitate success is often needed.
- Employing clinical paradigms of self-care, education, and self-responsibility in the patient's care will enhance long-term outcomes and maintain positive relationships between the patient and the clinician.

J.P. Okeson, DMD (✉)
Division of Orofacial Pain, University of Kentucky College of Dentistry,
Lexington, Kentucky 40536-0297, UK
e-mail: okeson@uky.edu

C. Perez, DDS, MS
Division of Pediatric Dentistry, University of Kentucky College of Dentistry,
Lexington, Kentucky 40536-0297, UK
e-mail: cristina.perez@uky.edu

J.R. Fricton, DDS, MS, Dip. ABOP
Division of TMD and Orofacial Pain, University of Minnesota School of Dentistry,
Minneapolis, MN, USA

J.N.A.R. Ferreira et al. (eds.), *Orofacial Disorders*,
DOI 10.1007/978-3-319-51508-3_14

14.1 Introduction

One major category of temporomandibular disorders relates to functional disorders of the temporomandibular joints. They are often called internal derangements, but this term only represents one subcategory. Functional disorders of the TMJ can be classified into three broad categories:

1. Derangements of the condyle-disc complex
2. Structural incompatibility of the articular surfaces
3. Inflammatory joint disorders

The first two categories have been collectively referred to as disc-interference disorders. The term disc-interference disorder was first introduced by Welden Bell [3] to describe a category of functional disorders that arise from problems with the condyle-disc complex. Some of these problems are due to a derangement or alteration of the ligaments that attach the disc to the condyle; others to an incompatibility between the articular surfaces of the condyle, disc, and fossa; and still others to the fact that relatively normal structures have been extended beyond their normal range of movement. Although these broad categories have similar clinical presentations, they are treated quite differently. It is therefore important that they be differentiated.

Inflammatory disorders may arise from any localized response of the tissues that make up the TMJ. They are often the result of chronic and sometimes progressive disc derangement disorders. The two major symptoms associated to functional TMJ disorders are pain and dysfunction.

These three broad categories are described below in detail:

14.1.1 Derangements of the Condyle-Disc Complex

These disorders present as a range of conditions that relate to the functional relationship between the articular disc and the condyle. Under normal conditions the disc is attached to the condyle by the medial and lateral collateral ligaments. These attachments allow the disc to rotate anteriorly and posteriorly on the condyle as the condyle translates out of the fossae (Fig. 14.1).

If the morphology of the disc is altered and/or the discal ligaments become elongated, the disc is then permitted to slide (translate) across the articular surface of the condyle. This type of movement is not present in the healthy joint. When this occurs the disc can become displaced from its normal position and thus this is known as a *disc displacement* [4]. When a disc displacement is present, opening the mouth will bring the condyle forward to a more stable position on the disc, and an unusual movement can occur between the condyle and disc resulting in a joint sound (click). With time and further elongation of the ligaments, the disc can gain more freedom to move (translate) between the condyle and fossae.

Eventually, the disc can be forced through the discal space, collapsing the joint space behind. When this occurs, inter-articular pressure will collapse the discal space, trapping the disc in the forward position. Then, the next full translation of the condyle is inhibited by the anterior and medial positioning of the disc. The person

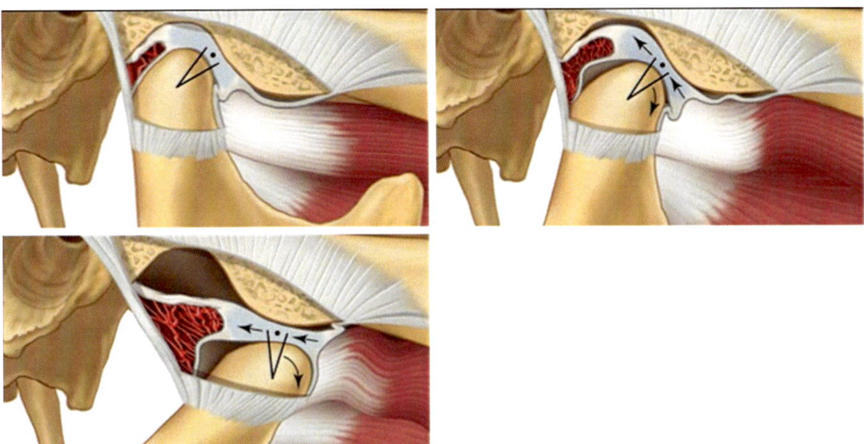

Fig. 14.1 Normal condyle and disc movement during opening of the mouth. Note: The disc always remains between the condyle and fossa, but it also rotates posteriorly on the condyle during the opening movement (From Okeson [15])

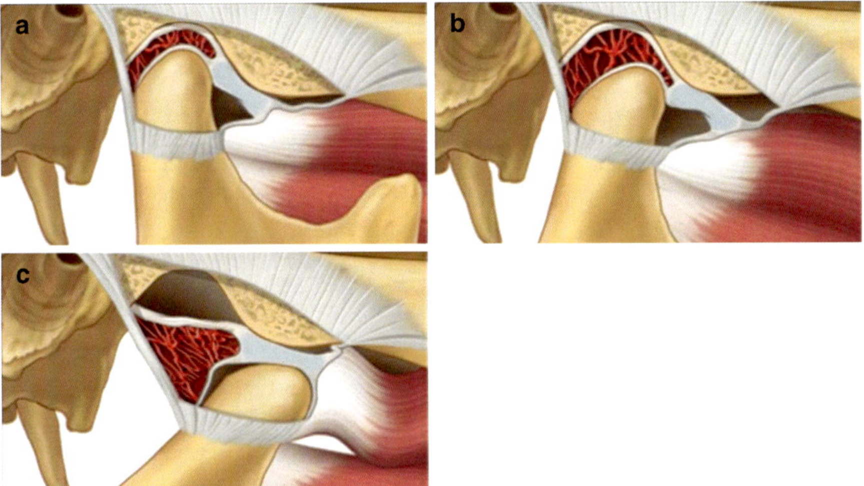

Fig. 14.2 The articular disc is displaced anterior to condyle in the normal closed mouth position (**a**). During opening (**b**) the condyle pushes the disc forward until it is reduced into its normal position (**c**). This condition is called a disc dislocation with reduction (From Okeson [15])

feels the joint being locked in a limited closed position [5]. Since the articular surfaces of the disc have actually been separated from the condyle, this condition is referred to as a *dislocation of the disc.*

Some individuals with dislocation of the disc are able to move the mandible in various lateral or protrusive directions to accommodate the movement of the condyle over the posterior border of the disc, and the locked condition is resolved. If the lock occurs only occasionally and the person can resolve it with no assistance, it is referred to as a *dislocation with reduction* (Fig. 14.2).

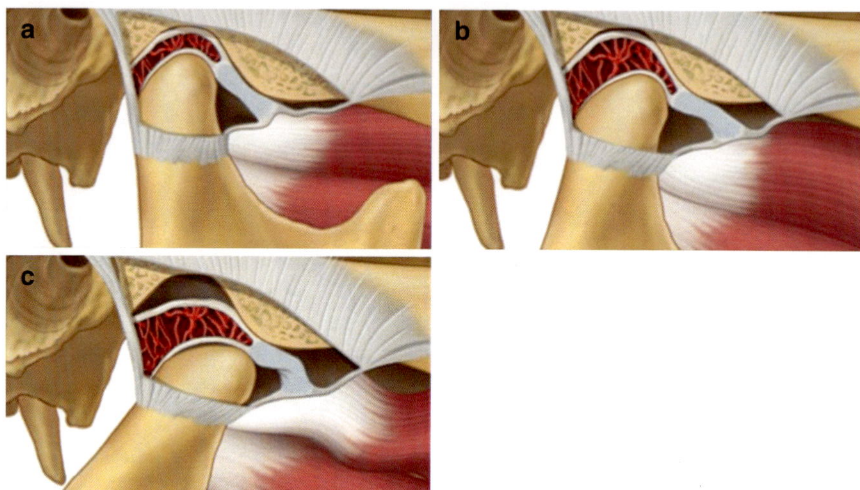

Fig. 14.3 The articular disc is displaced anterior to condyle in the normal closed mouth position (**a**). During opening (**b**) the condyle pushes the disc forward; however, the disc is never reduced into its normal position (**c**). This condition is called as a "disc dislocation without reduction." Since this condition often limits full opening of the mouth, it is often referred to as a "closed lock" (From Okeson [15])

The next stage of disc derangement is known as *disc dislocation without reduction*. This condition occurs when the person is unable to accommodate the condyle to return the dislocated disc to its normal position on the condyle. The mouth cannot be opened maximally because the position of the disc does not allow full translation of the condyle (Fig. 14.3).

14.1.2 Structural Incompatibility of the Articular Surfaces

Some disc derangement disorders result from problems between the articular surfaces of the joints. In a healthy joint, the articular surfaces are firm and smooth and when lubricated with synovial fluid move almost without friction against each other. However, if these surfaces become altered by trauma or inflammation, movement can be impaired. As a result *Adhesions* and *Adherences* can form. *Adherences* are considered to be a temporary sticking of the articular surfaces, while *adhesions* are more permanent. Disc perforations are another form of structural incompatibility [6].

In some individuals, clinical observations of full mouth opening reveals a momentary pause, followed by a sudden jump or leap to the maximally open position. This jump does not produce a clicking sound but instead is accompanied by more of a thud. This condition is called *subluxation* or *hypermobility* [7].

On occasion the mouth is opened beyond its normal limit and the mandible locks. This is called *spontaneous dislocation* or an *open lock*. It should not be confused with the closed lock, which occurs with a functionally dislocated disc without reduction. With spontaneous dislocation the patient cannot close the mouth. This condition is almost always produced by wide opening, for example, an extended yawn or a long dental procedure. Open lock can be produced when the disc and the condyle as a whole translate past the eminence and when trying to return the posterior thicker part of the disc does not permit its return.

14.1.3 Inflammatory Joint Disorders

Inflammatory joint disorders are a group of disorders in which various tissues that make up the joint structure become inflamed as a result of an insult or breakdown. Any or all of the joint structures may be involved. Disorders that form part of this category are synovitis, capsulitis, retrodiscitis, and the arthritides. *Synovitis* and *capsulitis* are characterized by inflammation of the synovial tissues and the joint capsule. These disorders are often mentioned together due to the difficulty in separating them clinically. *Retrodiscitis results from an encroachment of* retrodiscal tissues by the condyle due to an altered forward position of the disc.

Joint *arthritides* represent a group of disorders in which destructive bony changes are seen. One of the most common types of TMJ arthritide is called osteoarthritis (also known as degenerative joint disease). Osteoarthritis represents a destructive process by which the bony articular surfaces of the condyle and fossa become altered. It is generally considered to be the body's response to increased loading of a joint [8]. There are certainly other types of arthritides that can affect the TMJs. Many of these are considered polyarthritides such as traumatic arthritis, infectious arthritis, rheumatoid arthritis, gout, psoriatic arthritis, and ankylosing spondylitis.

14.2 Clinical Presentation

Many of the common joint disorders present as non-painful conditions with clinical symptoms that include joint sounds, deviation of the jaw on opening, or limitation of opening. However, on occasion pain and dysfunction are present in which the following clinical findings are common:

- *Pain*: Common sites of pain in the temporomandibular joint include preauricular pain, earache, jaw pain, facial pain, and temple/parietal headaches. Pain can be acute or chronic and present as a constant steady dull ache that fluctuates in intensity or acutely sharp and only associated to movement. Duration may vary from hours to days.
- *Joint tenderness*: In arthralgia, the tenderness is reported as deep and localized on the lateral or posterior aspects of the joint capsule.
- *Limited or deviation in range of motion*: With disc displacement and disc dislocation with reduction, mandibular deviation may be seen at the point of the joint sound, but normal range of movement is usually achieved. With disc dislocation without reduction, gross limitation of opening is often seen (<30 mm), especially when the disorder is acute.

- *Joint sounds*: Joint sounds alone are not diagnostic of joint pathology. However, specific types of sounds couple with clinical signs, in these cases imaging, may be helpful to make a diagnosis. These may include reciprocal clicking (both opening and closing) associated with disc displacement and disc dislocation with reduction. Non-reproducible opening or closing clicks or fine crepitus may occur with later stages of disc dislocation. Coarse crepitus may occur with osteoarthritis or osteoarthrosis.
- *Other associated signs and symptoms*: These would include occlusal changes such as an anterior open bite with loss of condylar height or posterior open bites associated with anterior condylar displacement with inflammation or tumors. Pain is increased with movement of the joint and occasionally otologic symptoms such as tinnitus, and plugged ears may be present.

14.3 Etiology and Epidemiology

14.3.1 Prevalence

Temporomandibular joint disorders are a common cause of pain and dysfunction in the masticatory system affecting up to 25–30% of the general population with about 5% having symptoms severe enough to warrant treatment [9]. The prevalence of osteoarthritis in the TMJ is significantly less.

14.3.2 Comorbid Conditions and Complicating Factors

- Osteoarthritis, rheumatoid arthritis, and other systemic rheumatological or connective tissue conditions
- Fibromyalgia, myofascial pain, and muscle pain in the jaw and other parts of the body
- Malocclusion and occlusal dysfunction
- If chronic, medication dependencies, disuse, and psychological factors such as emotional difficulties or pain behaviors

14.3.3 Etiologic Factors

- Direct macrotrauma to the joint through direct blow or opening the mouth too wide or for too long a period during activities such as dental visits, eating, yawning, and sexual activity.
- Indirect trauma due to whiplash type of injury in some cases may be an initiating factor.
- Occupational and repetitive strain injury may contribute to joint pain.

- Microtrauma to the TM joint produced by oral parafunctional muscle tension produced by habits such as teeth clenching, jaw thrust, gum chewing, and jaw tensing.
- Poor positioning of the head, neck, or tongue.
- Gross occlusal instability.
- Psychosocial stressors such as relationship conflicts, monetary problems, feeling hurried, over scheduled, and poor pacing skills can play an indirect role in reinforcing chronic pain.

14.4 Pathophysiology and Mechanisms

14.4.1 Biomechanical Strain Hypothesis

The genesis of disc disorders and TMJ arthralgia has been at least partially attributed to abnormal biomechanical forces on the condyle. These alter the shape, form, and function of articular tissues. Friction due to abnormal jaw function and malposition of the disc may exacerbate both jaw displacement and changes to the form and function of the disc. In other cases, a blow to the jaw, inadvertent biting of a hard object, or excessive chewing may be inciting factors. Occasionally, whiplash injury may indirectly contribute to biomechanical trauma.

14.4.2 Molecular and Cellular Hypothesis

Multiple cellular and molecular mechanisms are also involved in initiation and progression of degenerative joint disease because they modify the adaptive capacity of the joint. Trauma and mechanical stresses may release free radicals such as free iron and directly or indirectly damage cellular components and play a role in TMJ adhesion formation through oxidative modification of proteins and the formation of intramolecular and intermolecular cross-linking of fibrinogen and fibronectin [10]. Inflammatory mediators including cytokines, TNF-α, and IL-1 are expressed and produce large amounts of matrix metalloproteinases (MMPs), which in turn degrade extracellular matrix components including collagens and proteoglycans. The increase in arachidonic acid metabolism and extracellular matrix degradation lead to deformation of the disc-condyle apparatus. There are also neurogenic contributions to pain and modulation of cell adhesion in the inflammatory state.

14.5 Diagnostic Criteria

The diagnostic criteria for each TMJ disorder has been described in two documents: the AAOP guidelines [1] and Diagnostic Criteria for Temporomandibular Disorders DCTMD [2]. They are summarized below:

14.5.1 TMJ Disc Displacement/Dislocation with Reduction

1. Reproducible joint noise that occurs usually at variable positions during opening and closing mandibular movements.
2. Soft tissue imaging reveals displaced disc that improves its position during jaw opening, and hard tissue imaging shows an absence of extensive degenerative bone changes.
3. Any of the following may accompany the above:
   - Pain, when present, is precipitated by joint movement.
   - Deviation of the mandible during movement coinciding with a click.
   - No restriction in mandibular movement.
   - Episodic and momentary catching of smooth jaw movement during mouth opening (<35 mm) that self-reduces with voluntary mandibular repositioning.

14.5.2 TMJ Acute Disc Dislocation Without Reduction

1. Persistent marked limited mouth opening (<35 mm) with history of sudden onset.
2. Deflection to the affected side on mouth opening.
3. Marked limited laterotrusion to the contralateral side (if unilateral disorder).
4. Soft tissue imaging reveals displaced disc without reduction, and hard tissue imaging reveals no extensive osteoarthritic changes.
5. Any of the following may accompany the above:
   - Pain precipitated by forced mouth opening
   - History of clicking that ceased with the locking
   - Pain with palpation of the affected joint
   - Ipsilateral hyperocclusion
   - Moderate osteoarthritic changes with hard tissue imaging

14.5.3 Chronic TMJ Disc Dislocation Without Reduction

1. History of sudden onset of limited mouth opening that occurred more than 4 months ago.
2. Soft tissue imaging reveals displaced disc without reduction, and hard tissue imaging reveals no extensive osteoarthritic changes.
3. Any of the following may accompany the above:
   - Pain, when present, is markedly reduced from acute stage and usually presents only as a feeling of stiffness.
   - History of clicking that resolved with sudden onset of the locking.
   - Moderate osteoarthritic changes with imaging of hard tissues.
   - Gradual resolution of limited mouth opening.

14.5.4 Spontaneous Dislocation of the TMJ

1. Inability to close the mouth without a specific manipulative maneuver.
2. Radiographic evidence reveals condyle well beyond the eminence.
3. Pain at time of dislocation with mild residual pain after the episode.

Differential diagnosis: condyle fracture secondary to trauma

14.5.5 Synovitis, Capsulitis, and Retrodiscitis

1. Localized TMJ pain exacerbated by function.
2. Tenderness to superior or posterior joint loading and palpation.
3. No extensive osteoarthritic changes with hard tissue imaging.
4. The following may accompany the above:
   - Limited range of motion secondary to pain.
   - Fluctuating swelling (due to effusion) that decreases ability to occlude on ipsilateral posterior teeth.
   - A hyperintense MRI signal when fluid is present (T2 weighting).
   - Ear or preauricular pain.

Differential diagnosis: osteoarthritis, polyarthritis, ear infection, and neoplasia

14.5.6 TMJ Osteoarthritis

1. TMJ pain at rest and with function.
2. Joint tenderness on palpation.
3. Radiographic evidence of structural bony change (subchondral sclerosis, osteophytic formation, erosion) and joint space narrowing.
4. The following may accompany the above:
   - Limited range of motion, deviation to the affected side
   - Crepitus or multiple joint noises

Differential diagnosis: inflammation, polyarthritis, and neoplasia

14.5.6.1 Diagnostic Tests

1. Imaging studies that may be useful for TMJ functional disorders include:
   - Magnetic resonance imaging (MRI) scans to view disc position
   - CT scans and tomography to view structural joint pathology and degenerative joint disease
   - Panoramic radiographs to view dental, maxillary, and mandibular pathology
2. Lab studies: blood and urine studies are generally normal unless caused by a concomitant disorder.
3. Psychometric tests: the DC/TMD axis II, Beck Depression Inventory, and SCL-90 can help identify specific psychosocial contributing factors.

14.6 Rationale for Treatment

Some general considerations in the management of TMJ disorders are as follows:

- Treatment should be directed toward rehabilitating the joint, improving range of motion, reducing tenderness and inflammation, and reducing contributing factors.
- Treatment should attempt to reduce biomechanical strain to the joint from repetitive straining activities, poor postural activities, and sustained muscle activity, which should encourage healing.
- Treatment should attempt to inhibit peripheral and central neural input through various treatment modalities such as cold, heat, analgesic/anti-inflammatory medications, massage, trigger point injections, and transcutaneous electrical stimulation.
- Treatment should attempt to reduce factors that facilitate continued sustained central and peripheral neural activity such as reduction of clenching, joint trauma, and CNS alterations such as depression.

14.7 Treatment Options

14.7.1 Self-Care

- Most acute symptoms are self-limited and resolve with minimal intervention.
- Initial treatment should be a self-care program to reduce repetitive strain of the masticatory system and encourage relaxation and healing of the joint and muscles.
- This includes jaw exercises, habit change, and gentle use of the jaw.
- Most patients respond well to self-care in 4–6 weeks. If symptoms do not resolve, further assessment and treatment are indicated [11].

14.7.2 Pharmacotherapy

- Nonsteroidal anti-inflammatory drugs (NSAIDs)
- Precaution: gastrointestinal side effects. Gastrointestinal safety of COX-2 inhibitors may be greater than that of nonselective NSAIDs, but recent evidence of increased cardiovascular disease needs to be considered. Examples include:
  - Naproxen, 250–500 mg BID with meals
  - Ibuprofen, 400–800 mg TID with meals
  - Celecoxib, 100–200 mg BID
- Muscle relaxants for muscle spasm, muscle tension, nocturnal bruxism, and improving sleep. Common side effects are sedation, dizziness, dry mouth, and, if allergy, rash.
  - Cyclobenzaprine, 10–20 mg HS
  - Tizanidine, 4 mg HS or BID
  - Methocarbamol, 500–750 mg QID
  - Metaxalone, 400–800 mg TID

- Benzodiazepines are useful to manage anxiety. However, if used daily, dependency is likely to occur. Examples include:
  - Clonazepam, 0.5–1.0 mg HS
  - Diazepam, 5 mg HS or BID

14.7.3 Physical Rehabilitation Medicine Procedures

Certain physical medicine procedures can be efficacious for patients with TMJ restriction and pain as well as for other TMD symptoms.

- Jaw exercise is the primary and often the only physical medicine treatment required:
  - Relaxation
  - Rotation and arthrokinematics
  - Stretching (range of motion)
  - Isometric and strengthening exercise
  - Postural exercise
- Physical modalities can reduce jaw pain and increase range of motion, thereby allowing jaw exercises to more effectively proceed. These can be particularly helpful with muscle spasm and contracture.
  - Thermotherapy
  - Coolant therapy
  - Ultrasound
  - Phonophoresis
  - Iontophoresis
  - Electrogalvanic stimulation therapy
  - Transcutaneous stimulation therapy (TENS)
  - Laser

14.7.4 Orthopedic Intraoral Splints

These appliances can allow protection of the joint and reduce oral habits [12]. There are three major types of splints:

- *Stabilization splint*: to allow passive protection of the jaw and reduction of oral habits. Full arch occlusal contacts on flat surface with mild anterior tooth disocclusion is most scientifically supported. These can be made for the maxillary or mandibular arch.
- *Anterior positioning splint*: can be efficacious for painful TMJ disc displacement or dislocation with reduction associated with reciprocal clicking and/or intermittent jaw locking, especially upon awakening. Recommended for short-term, part-time use, primarily during sleep, because they can cause occlusal changes if worn continuously [14].
- *Partial coverage splint*: may cause occlusal changes in some patients. Splints should cover all of the mandibular or maxillary teeth to prevent supraeruption of unopposed teeth.

14.7.5 Cognitive-Behavioral Therapy (CBT)

- CBT approaches can help change maladaptive habits and behaviors that contribute to strain placed on the joint such as jaw tensing, teeth clenching, and teeth grinding [13].
- Although many simple habits are easily abandoned when the patient becomes aware of them, changing persistent habits requires a structured program that is facilitated by a clinician trained in behavioral strategies. Habits do not change themselves. Patients are responsible for initiating and maintaining behavior changes.
- Habit reversal can be accomplished by (1) becoming more aware of the habit, (2) knowing how to correct it (i.e., what to do with the teeth and tongue), and (3) knowing why to correct it, combined with the patient's commitment to conscientious self-monitoring and a focus upon the goal. Correcting it during the day will help reduce it at night.
- Supplement with additional behavioral strategies such as biofeedback, meditation, stress management, or relaxation techniques.
- Address poor pacing or hurrying related to a day overloaded with commitments.
- Address depression, anxiety, and other emotional problems through psychological therapy and medications.
- Address sleep disorders (e.g., snoring, obstructive sleep apnea – discussed in Chap. 12) with sleep hygiene self-care, medications, and if needed a sleep laboratory evaluation.

14.7.6 TMJ Surgery

- If persistent pain is localized in the TMJ and is associated with specific structural changes in the joint, surgical intervention can be considered if comprehensive nonsurgical care is unsuccessful.
- Muscle pain and associated contributing factors should be addressed and controlled prior to TMJ surgery.
- In general, the less invasive surgeries are as efficacious as those that are more invasive, so the health-care provider should consider an arthrocentesis or arthroscopic procedure before more invasive interventions such as discectomy, discal repair, or complete TM joint replacement.
- Postoperative management includes appropriate medications, physical therapy, splint therapy when indicated, and continued psychological treatment as appropriate.

14.8 Sequence of Care

- Treatment goals include:
  1. Reduce or eliminate pain
  2. Restore normal jaw function
  3. Reduce the need for future health care
  4. Restore normal lifestyle functioning

- Short-term strategy is to restore the joint to normal function, obtaining full range of motion. Jaw exercises can help achieve this goal.
- Long-term strategy includes reducing the symptoms and their negative effects while helping the patient return to normal function without the need for future health care.
- Acute cases of recent onset can often be managed with palliative self-care strategies designed to protect the joint and encourage healing.
- Behavioral and psychosocial evaluation should be conducted on all patients with persistent pain to determine complexity and contributing factors.

References

1. Orofacial pain: guidelines for classification, assessment, and management. In: de Leeuw R, Klasser G, editors. 4th ed. Chicago: Quintessence Publ. Co.; 2013.
2. Schiffman E, Ohrbach R, Truelove E, et al. Diagnostic Criteria for Temporomandibular Disorders (DC/TMD) for clinical and research applications: recommendations of the International RDC/TMD Consortium Network* and Orofacial Pain Special Interest Group. J Oral Facial Pain Headache. 2014;28(1):6–27.
3. Bell WE. Recent concepts in the management of temporomandibular joint dysfunctions. J Oral Surg. 1970;28(8):596–9.
4. Guler N, Yatmaz PI, Ataoglu H, Emlik D, Uckan S. Temporomandibular internal derangement: correlation of MRI findings with clinical symptoms of pain and joint sounds in patients with bruxing behaviour. Dentomaxillofac Radiol. 2003;32(5):304–10.
5. Westesson PL, Bronstein SL, Liedberg J. Internal derangement of the temporomandibular joint: morphologic description with correlation to joint function. Oral Surg Oral Med Oral Pathol. 1985;59(4):323–31.
6. Murakami K, Segami N, Moriya Y, Iizuka T. Correlation between pain and dysfunction and intra-articular adhesions in patients with internal derangement of the temporomandibular joint. J Oral Maxillofac Surg. 1992;50(7):705–8.
7. Bell WE. Temporomandibular disorders. 3rd ed. Chicago: Year Book Medical Publishers; 1990.
8. Stegenga B, de Bont L, Boering G. Osteoarthrosis as the cause of craniomandibular pain and dysfunction: a unifying concept. J Oral Maxillofac Surg. 1989;47(3):249–56.
9. Schiffman EL, Fricton JR, Haley DP, Shapiro BL. The prevalence and treatment needs of subjects with temporomandibular disorders. J Am Dent Assoc. 1990;120(3):295–303.
10. Milam SB, Zardeneta G, Schmitz JP. Oxidative stress and degenerative temporomandibular joint disease: a proposed hypothesis. J Oral Maxillofac Surg. 1998;56(2):214–23.
11. Gray RJ, Quayle AA, Hall CA, Schofield MA. Physiotherapy in the treatment of temporomandibular joint disorders: a comparative study of four treatment methods. Br Dent J. 1994;176(7):257–61.
12. Kurita H, Kurashina K, Kotani A. Clinical effect of full coverage occlusal splint therapy for specific temporomandibular disorder conditions and symptoms. J Prosthet Dent. 1997;78(5):506–10.
13. Oakley ME, McCreary CP, Clark GT, et al. A cognitive-behavioral approach to temporomandibular dysfunction treatment failures: a controlled comparison. J Orofac Pain. 1994;8(4):397–401.
14. Nilner M. Does splint therapy work for temporomandibular pain? Evid Based Dent. 2004;5(3):65–6.
15. Okeson JP. Management of temporomandibular disorders and occlusion. 7th ed. St Louis: Elsevier Publishers; 2013. p. 244.

Temporomandibular Muscle Disorders 15

Edward F. Wright

Pearls of Wisdom

- Diagnosing and treating temporomandibular muscle disorders is a challenging yet very rewarding venture. It requires carefully listening to patients so as to obtain a thorough history and identify potential contributing factors. An in-depth clinical exam confirms or refutes the suspicious structures contributing to the temporomandibular muscle disorder.
- Identifying and reducing the contributing factors is the key to developing the most cost-effective long-term management for patients with temporomandibular muscle disorders.
- With the patients' participation, methodically develop the most cost-effective treatment plan, focusing upon each patient's identified contributors. TMD self-management and education are the foundation for empowering self-reliance and enhancing a positive patient to practitioner relationship.
- Treatment often involves enlisting the help of other practitioners who provide therapies that are outside of the dentist's realm of treatment, e.g., physical therapist and psychologist.
- As treatments are implemented, ensure the patient's temporomandibular muscle pain is sufficiently reduced and the masticatory function is restored.
- Patients are not passive recipients of our therapies but are active partners in obtaining and maintaining their treatment goals.

E.F. Wright, DDS, MS, MAGD
Department of Comprehensive Dentistry, University of Texas Health Science Center – San Antonio, San Antonio, TX, USA
e-mail: WrightE2@uthscsa.edu

J.N.A.R. Ferreira et al. (eds.), *Orofacial Disorders*,
DOI 10.1007/978-3-319-51508-3_15

15.1 Introduction and Diagnostic Subtypes

Temporomandibular muscle disorders (TMD) are the most common cause for patients' temporomandibular pain, and they may coexist with temporomandibular joint disorders (see Chap. 14). They are characterized by pain arising from dysfunctional processes within the masticatory muscles and not from the joint itself. There are a number of muscle disorders that may occur among the masticatory muscles including myalgia, myofascial pain with referral, myositis, and spasm (Tab. 15.1) [1].

Myalgia is the most common masticatory muscle disorder and is diagnosed when the patient's muscle pain is aggravated by mandibular movement, function, or parafunction; and the patient's pain is reproduced by palpating the painful muscle [1].

Myofascial pain with referral is a subcategory of myalgia in which, through central processes (e.g., sensitization and convergence), patients perceive their muscle pain in a distant location. Many dentists have observed patients

Myalgia: repetitive strain
Generally a dull aching pain in the masseter and/or temporalis muscle region that is aggravated by mandibular movement, function, or parafunction; and the patient's pain is reproduced by palpating the painful muscle.

Myofascial pain with referral: muscle pain perceived in a distant location from the source
Generally a dull aching pain in a location where there is no pathology and this pain can be reproduced by firmly palpating a tender region within a muscle at a distant location (e.g., tooth pain caused by referred pain from the masseter muscle).

Spasm: acute onset of contracted muscle
Acute onset of a continuously contracted muscle causing constant muscle pain with a significantly limited range-of-motion. If due to a closure muscle (masseter, temporalis, or medial pterygoid muscle), the patient will have a limited opening. If due to a lateral pterygoid muscle, the patient will have increased pain when trying to occlude into maximum intercuspation and will have a limited ability to translate the ipsilateral condyle causing a limited mandibular movement to the contralateral side. The involved muscle is generally exquisitely tender.

Myositis: acute onset of infection or injury
Acute onset of constant muscle pain with a significantly limited range-of-motion and has clinical characteristics of an infection, or the muscle pain is secondary to trauma to the muscle.

Tab. 15.1 Diagnostic criteria for temporomandibular muscle disorders

complaining of tooth pain when there is no pathology associated with the teeth. This tooth pain may be due to referred pain from a masticatory muscle, suggested by reproduction of the tooth pain by firm palpation of tender regions within a masticatory muscle and ruling out other potential sources (e.g., sinus congestion) [1].

Spasm is an immediate onset of a constant muscle contraction causing pain and limited range of motion [1]. Most of us can relate to this disorder by the spasm that has occurred in our calf muscle that awoke us in the middle of the night. This disorder may develop within any of the masticatory muscles, but it most commonly occurs with the lateral pterygoid muscle or the medial pterygoid muscle following an inferior alveolar injection [2, 3].

Myositis is another acute disorder in which the muscle has clinical characteristics of an infection (e.g., edema, erythema, and/or increased temperature) or inflammation, in addition to meeting the criteria for myalgia. The onset of the patient's symptoms is directly related to an infection or trauma to the muscle [1].

15.2 Clinical Presentation

Patients with temporomandibular muscle disorders generally complain of pain in the masseter and/or temporalis muscle region. This pain is most commonly a constant dull ache with an intensity that generally fluctuates with function (e.g., eating), parafunction (e.g., clenching teeth), activities (e.g., holding tension in muscles and resting chin in one's hand), and stress. The pain may last for minutes, hours, or be constant; this may be an acute or chronic disorder [4, 5].

Patients may also have various associated pain complaints, the most common being tooth pain where there is no dental pathology and neck pain [1, 3]. The tooth pain may be from localized inflammation from heavy clenching activities or referred pain from the masticatory structures (e.g., myofascial pain with referral). The neck pain may be due to a disorder within the cervical structures and/or secondary to the TMD disorder. There are many other potential symptoms that can occur secondary to the TMD disorder, e.g., otologic symptoms (i.e., tinnitus, ear pain, etc.) and neurologic deficits due to nerve entrapment [4, 6].

Palpation of the painful muscles reproduces the patient's pain, and these painful muscles will generally not elongate to their normal length. If this involves a closure muscle (masseter, temporalis, or medial pterygoid muscle), this will manifest as a limited range of motion (less than 40 mm). Myalgia and myofascial pain with referral generally cause a slight limitation (10–20%), while myositis and spasm may cause a gross limitation (50% or more).

15.3 Etiology and Epidemiology

Temporomandibular disorder (affecting muscles and the joint), or TMD, is one of the most prevalent of all musculoskeletal disorders, with approximately 25–33% of the general population having some TMD symptoms and 3.6–7% having it with sufficient severity to desire treatment [1, 7]. Women request TMD treatment more often than do men, and their symptoms are less likely to resolve than for men [7, 8].

These TMD severe muscle symptoms significantly correlate with masticatory muscle tension, tooth clenching, grinding, and other oral parafunctional habits [5, 9]. They are also significantly correlated with an increase in psychosocial factors (e.g., worry, stress, irritation, frustration, and depression), and patients with poor psychosocial adaptation have significantly greater TMD improvement when the dentist's TMD therapy is combined with cognitive-behavioral intervention [7, 8].

15.4 Pathophysiology and Mechanisms

There are no specific anatomical changes within the muscle that account for temporomandibular muscle pain, and there is currently no consensus on the specific pathophysiology for this pain. Some authors speculate the pain is secondary to vasoconstriction of arteries from repetitive muscle strain. This forms an ischemic region that accumulates metabolic waste products, causing the release of algogenic substances, and the muscle pain develops. It is also known that temporomandibular muscle pain is greatly influenced by central mechanisms, e.g., phasic modulation of excitatory and inhibitory tonic muscular input, convergence of multiple afferent inputs, and inhibition or facilitation of central input [4, 10].

15.5 Diagnosis and Diagnostic Criteria

- The diagnosis is based upon the patient's history, symptomatology, and clinical evaluation (see Tab. 15.1). The suspected offending muscle(s) is palpated to ensure aggravation of this muscle can reproduce the patient's pain [3, 7]. These palpations are performed by starting with light force and increasing the force until the patient's pain is aggravated or reproduced, or the force reaches 0.5–1 kg (recommended force varies with the muscle according to the new diagnostic criteria for TMD) [11].
- Blood, urine, and imaging studies are usually normal for these muscle disorders [4].
- A TMD questionnaire is often helpful to identify the contributing factors (e.g., daytime clenching) and rule out other potential contributors (e.g., similar muscle pain throughout the body) [7].

15.6 Rationale for Treatment

- Myalgia is by far the most common cause for temporomandibular muscle pain. Some patients will awake with the muscle pain that resolves within an hour. Other patients will awake without symptoms, and the muscle pain develops as the day progresses, while other patients will have constant pain that generally has some daily variation of the pain intensity.
- The most cost-effective therapy for the long-term management of myalgia is through identifying and satisfactorily reducing the contributing factors [4, 7]. The most common contributing factors are nighttime and/or daytime masticatory parafunctional activity and other masticatory habits (including holding tension in the muscles) [3, 12].
- Nighttime masticatory parafunctional activity and habits predominately contribute to patients' pain upon awaking, and daytime habits predominately contribute to the pain that occurs later in the day. Some treatments are more effective for the various times of the day in which these habits occur, so the daily symptom pattern helps in selecting the most effective therapies for each patient. A way to determine this is to ask patients what is their average pain intensity (on a 0–10 scale, where 0 is no pain, and 10 is the worst pain imaginable) upon awaking and later in the day [7, 12].
- Other pain in the region tends to cause the masticatory muscles to tighten in response to this pain and may cause referred pain to the masticatory muscles. So these potential sources (e.g., sinus, tooth, and cervical pain) for the masticatory muscle pain must be investigated and treated if contributing to the masticatory muscle pain. Heavy snoring or sleep apnea may also cause patients to awake with myalgia, so this disorder should also be considered as a potential cause or contributor for patients' temporomandibular muscle pain.

15.7 Treatment Options

There are great variations in the severity and complexity with which patients present. There are also considerable variations as to which therapies patients are receptive to receiving and the degree of relief they would consider to be sufficient; these are often related to personal finances and insurance coverage.

The recommended treatments for each diagnostic muscle subtypes will vary, but in general, nearly all patients who are diagnosed with a temporomandibular muscle disorder would benefit from the TMD self-management therapies (Tab. 15.2), and this should be one of the first therapies provided.

1. Massage your painful muscles. 2. Apply heat, ice, or a combination to the painful muscles. Use which ever provides the greatest amount of relief; most patients prefer heat. 3. Do not chew gum, eat hard foods (e.g., raw carrots), or eat chewy foods (e.g., caramels, steak, and bagels); and cut large pieces of food into small pieces. 4. Limit daily caffeine consumption to 1 regular cup of coffee, 2 cups of tea, or 1 can of soda. 5. Keep your jaw muscles relaxed throughout the day so your teeth do not touch; do not clench your teeth or hold tension in your jaw muscles. Ask for a coach to help, if one is desired. 6. Eliminate other habits that could put unnecessary strain on your jaw muscles (e.g., tapping your teeth together; resting your jaw on your hand; biting your cheeks, lips, finger nails, cuticles, or any other objects you may put in your mouth; pushing your tongue against your teeth; and holding your jaw in an uncomfortable or tense position). 7. Sleep on your side or your back; do not sleep on your stomach. 8. Restrain from opening your mouth wide (e.g., yawning, yelling, and eating large pieces of food). 9. Use over-the-counter therapies as needed: - Apply topical creams/gels/patches containing NSAIDS over the painful areas - Take tablets/caplets per os: naproxen, ibuprofen, acetaminophen, etc.

Tab. 15.2 TMD self-management therapies

15.7.1 Myalgia

The various contributing factors (e.g., nighttime activity, daytime activity, neck pain, and sinus pain) are identified through patients' history and clinical exam. The recommended myalgia therapies will vary with the contributors, e.g., nighttime activity, daytime activity, or a combination of these; patients with non-masticatory contributors are generally referred to other providers who can best treat them [3, 4].

The therapies that have been suggested to be *effective for awaking TMD symptoms* are as follows: improve sleep position, wear a flat stabilization appliance at night, take medications that decrease nocturnal EMG activity, wear a soft appliance to oppose a hard appliance, and perform a relaxation session just prior to going to sleep (Tab. 15.3). The author treats the nighttime contributors by recommending these therapies to his patients in this order in addition to applicable therapies in Tab. 15.5.

Stomach sleeping tends to aggravate the masticatory and cervical musculoskeletal systems, so recommend patients change their sleep posture to sleeping on one or both of their sides and/or on their back. If this and the rest of the TMD self-management instructions do not provide adequate symptom relief, provide a flat stabilization appliance for the patient to wear at night.

1. Improve sleep positions 2. Wear a flat stabilization appliance at night 3. Take medications that decrease nocturnal EMG activity, e.g., gabapentin, amitripty line, nortriptyline, or cyclobenzaprine 4. Wear a soft appliance to oppose a hard appliance 5. Perform a relaxation session just prior to going to sleep; this may require referring the patient to a psychologist to train the patient how to perform this session. 6. Awaking headache can be present and may be related to snoring or sleep apnea

Tab. 15.3 Therapies primarily for awaking TMD symptoms (provided in this order)

There are a variety of medications that can help reduce the symptoms with which patients awake. A recent study revealed that 200–300 mg of gabapentin taken at bedtime will reduce the nighttime muscle activity similar to a stabilization appliance [13]. Clinically, this has been observed to be effective for the more healthy patients who are not taking a large number of medications.

Other medications that are often prescribed for this contributor are the tricyclic antidepressants (for long-term use) or Flexeril (for short-term use). For the tricyclic antidepressants, the author prescribes either 10 mg tablets of amitriptyline or nortriptyline (causes less drowsiness than amitriptyline) and asks patients to start with one table near bedtime and slowly increase the dose (up to five tablets) and titrate to the dose that provides satisfactory relief with minimal side effects. For short-term interventions, the author generally prescribes 5 mg tablets of Flexeril and asks patients to take one to two tablets at bedtime; many other muscle relaxants appear to provide a similar effect.

If these therapies do not provide adequate symptom improvement, the patient could be provided an opposing soft appliance that occludes with the hard flat stabilization appliance. One study provided patients, who had not obtained adequate improvement from wearing a flat stabilization appliance at night, an opposing soft appliance occluding with the hard appliance. They found that patients obtained a significant decrease in their TMD symptoms; 63% rated it as good TMD symptom improvement and 12% rated it as some improvement [14].

If the patient has not obtained adequate awaking symptom relief, it has been suggested that the patient may find benefit from performing a relaxation session just prior to going to sleep; some patients may need a psychologist to help the patient perform this. Providers must keep in mind that awaking myalgia may be from heavy snoring or sleep apnea, which should have been ruled out during the initial patient evaluation.

The therapies that have been suggested to be *effective for daytime TMD symptoms* are breaking daytime parafunctional and muscle-tensing habits; use relaxation, stress management, and/or biofeedback; wear a flat stabilization appliance

- Break daytime parafunctional and muscle-tensing habits
- Use relaxation, stress management, and/or biofeedback
- Wear a flat stabilization appliance during the day as a temporary crutch until the patient can satisfactorily decrease the daytime habits and/or to facilitate cognitive awareness for breaking the daytime habits
- Take a tricyclic antidepressant that causes minimal drowsiness (e.g., desipramine)

Tab. 15.4 Therapies primarily for daytime TMD symptoms (selection varies with each patient)

- Use medications, i.e., topical or oral NSAIDs, muscle relaxants, tricyclic antidepressants, etc.
- Use physiotherapy (i.e., heat, ice, ultrasound, iontophoresis, etc.); they may be provided by the patient at home or by a physical therapist
- Perform masticatory and/or cervical exercises provided by the dentist and/or physical therapist
- Therapies provided to relieve neck pain

Tab. 15.5 Additional therapies beneficial for both symptom patterns (selection will vary with each patient)

during the day; and take a tricyclic antidepressant that causes minimal drowsiness (Tab. 15.4). The order in which these are provided will vary with the patient's desires; applicable therapies in Tab. 15.5 are also provided.

Symptoms that occur during the day are generally secondary to daytime habits. The TMD self-management therapies requested that patients work to keep their jaw muscles relaxed throughout the day so their teeth do not touch and to not clench their teeth. If patients are unable to satisfactorily relax their masticatory muscles or break this habit on their own, they may desire a "coach" to help them. Some psychologists have training and experience with this and generally use relaxation, stress management, and/or biofeedback to achieve this goal.

Another treatment beneficial for daytime pain is to wear a flat stabilization appliance during the day. Patients prefer wearing mandibular (rather than maxillary) appliances during the day, because they are less visible and patients speak better with them [4]. Patients should use the appliance as a habit-breaking appliance, so whenever their opposing teeth touch the appliance, this should alert them that their muscles are contracted and work at relaxing their muscles. If after 2 months, patients want to continue wearing the appliance, they should limit their daytime wear to 3–5 h. Patients should never wear their appliance while eating [7].

Tricyclic antidepressants have been shown to be beneficial for musculoskeletal pain [15]. Patients generally find 25 mg of desipramine taken in the morning and afternoon helpful and that it does not cause drowsiness.

Additional therapies that are *beneficial for both symptom patterns* include medications, physiotherapy (provided by dentists and/or physical therapists), masticatory and cervical exercises, and therapies to relieve neck pain (Tab. 15.5).

Patients generally find topical and oral NSAIDs beneficial for myalgia. Patients appear to prefer topical NSAID in the gel rather than the liquid formulation, because it is easier to apply to the masticatory region. Most patients who experience gastric upset with oral NSAIDs can tolerate the topical formulations. Oral NSAIDs should not be taken on a continuous basis long term. A low-dose muscle relaxant may be taken during the day, if it does not cause drowsiness.

Physiotherapy (i.e., heat, ice, ultrasound, iontophoresis, etc.) can also benefit both daily patterns. Patients can apply heat, ice, or the combination at home multiple times a day. Patients can be referred to a physical therapist who may use these or other physiotherapy modalities. Patients generally find masticatory and cervical exercises beneficial; these may be given by the dentist or physical therapist.

Cervical pain can cause referred pain to the masticatory region; patients tend to unconsciously clench their teeth in response to cervical pain, and the masticatory muscles often tighten in response to cervical pain. Studies have shown that patients with cervical pain do not respond to TMD therapies as well as those without cervical pain [16]. Hence, patients with cervical pain generally have improvement in their TMD symptoms from cervical therapies.

15.7.2 Myofascial Pain with Referral

Treatment for temporomandibular muscles that are causing referred pain to distant locations is the same as the treatment for the diagnosis of myalgia. As the muscle pain improves, the referred pain pattern will resolve.

15.7.3 Spasm

The most effective treatment for a spasm is to stretch the muscle in spasm. A masticatory muscle spasm does not immediately release once the muscle has been stretched, so patients will need to be taught how to stretch the muscle and perform this stretch numerous times throughout the day. This stretch should be slow, gentle, and held in the restricted range. The stretch should be held for 30–60 s, and the force applied should be determined by patient tolerance while ensuring the muscle is not aggravated. A series of six stretches with 5 s breaks can be performed sequentially [2, 7].

The stretch is more beneficial if patients first warm the region. The masticatory muscles in which a spasm most commonly occurs are the lateral and medial pterygoid muscles. Since these muscle are not superficial muscles, it would appear that superficial heat would not be beneficial, but patients commonly report using a heating pad 15–20 min prior to stretching is helpful [2, 7].

An analgesic (e.g., 800 mg ibuprofen, tid) is commonly provided for patients with a spasm; this appears to enable patients to better tolerate the discomfort and allow patients to provide a better stretch of the muscle. When the disorder is more severe, a muscle relaxant (e.g., 5 mg diazepam, one to two tablets hs or bid) is indicated. These therapies are similarly recommended for spasms of other muscles in the body [2, 7].

Within a day or two, patients should start to show signs of improving. Depending upon the severity of the spasm and patient compliance, full recovery ranges from days to many weeks. If a patient does not begin to respond to this therapy after 2 or 3 days, consider referring the patient to an orofacial pain specialist [2, 7].

15.7.4 Myositis

If the myositis is due to an infection, the infection must be treated to resolve the myositis. If the myositis is due to trauma, treatment involves the patient taking a nonsteroidal anti-inflammatory drug (NSAID), limiting the use of the masticatory muscles (e.g., soft diet and avoiding oral habits), and applying ice over the affected area for the first 24–48 h after the trauma; afterwards apply heat and/or ice as desired [3]. If there is residual muscle pain after these therapies, treat the muscle as described under the myalgia diagnosis.

15.8 Treatment Goals and Sequencing of Care

- The goal of treatment is to satisfactorily reduce the patient's pain and restore masticatory function. The acute disorders are treated as described above and ensure this is not a reoccurring problem for these patients.
- For patients with chronic disorders, the most prominent contributing factors for the temporomandibular muscle disorder must be identified. These may entail the patient's habits, harmful activities, non-masticatory pains, and psychosocial contributors [4, 7].
- Through the patient's history, symptomatology, and clinical evaluation, the practitioner can determine the patient's temporomandibular muscle disorder (Tab. 15.1).
- These contributing factors need to be adequately reduced with a treatment strategy that will be individualized for each patient. Many of these therapies can be provided concurrently, so complex patients are generally best treated with a team of providers (e.g., dentist, physical therapist, and psychologist) simultaneously reducing the various contributing factors within their realm of practice [4].
- TMD self-management therapies (Tab. 15.2) are generally one of the first therapies provided for all of these disorders.
- Myalgia is unquestionably the most common cause for temporomandibular muscle disorders. Numerous therapies are used to treat this disorder, but the most cost-effective long-term management is determined through identifying and reducing the patient's contributing factors.

- Myofascial pain with referral is confusing for both practitioners and patients, because the pain's source is at a different location than where the patient perceives it. Practitioners must first rule out pathology at the location it is perceived and then reproduce the pain by firm palpation of tender regions within the muscle causing this pain. This disorder is a subcategory of myalgia; the muscle is treated as described for myalgia, and as the myalgia disorder improves, the referred pain stops.
- Spasm is best treated by patients gently stretching this muscle into its restricted range numerous times throughout the day. Adjunction therapies of applying heat prior to the stretches, and taking an analgesic and possibly a muscle relaxant, should speed recovery. It generally takes days to many weeks for the patient to obtain full recovery.
- Myositis may be due to an infection or trauma to the muscle. If it is due to an infection, the infection must be treated to resolve the myositis. If it is due to trauma, treat with NSAID, soft diet, limiting oral habits, and applying ice over the affected area for the first 24–48 h after the trauma.

References

1. de Leeuw R, Klasser GD, editors. Orofacial pain: guidelines for assessment, diagnosis and management, vol. 127. 5th ed. Chicago: Quintessence; 2013. p. 146–8.
2. Wright EF. Medial pterygoid trismus (myospasm) following inferior alveolar nerve block: case report and literature review. Gen Dent. 2011;59(1):64–7.
3. Clark GT. Classification, causation and treatment of masticatory myogenous pain and dysfunction. Oral Maxillofac Surg Clin North Am. 2008;20(2):145–57. v
4. Fricton J. Myogenous temporomandibular disorders: diagnostic and management considerations. Dent Clin N Am. 2007;51(1):61–83.
5. Magnusson T, Egermarki I, Carlsson GE. A prospective investigation over two decades on signs and symptoms of temporomandibular disorders and associated variables. A final summary. Acta Odontol Scand. 2005;63(2):99–109.
6. Wright EF. Otologic symptom improvement through TMD therapy. Quintessence Int. 2007; 38(9):E564–71.
7. Wright EF. Manual of temporomandibular disorders. 3rd ed. Ames: Wiley Blackwell; 2014. p. 1–2. 31–70, 97–101, 114–6, 125–9
8. Velly AM, Fricton J. The impact of comorbid conditions on treatment of temporomandibular disorders. J Am Dent Assoc. 2011;142(2):170–2.
9. Carlsson GE, Egermark I, Magnusson T. Predictors of bruxism, other oral parafunctions and tooth wear over a 20-year follow-up period. J Orofac Pain. 2003;17(1):50–7.
10. Okeson JP. Bell's oral and facial pain. 7th ed. Chicago: Quintessence; 2014. p. 287.
11. Schiffman E, Ohrbach R, Truelove E, et al. Diagnostic Criteria for Temporomandibular Disorders (DC/TMD) for clinical and research applications: recommendations of the International RDC/TMD Consortium Network and Orofacial Pain Special Interest Group. J Oral Facial Pain Headache. 2014;28(1):6–27.
12. Blanco Aguilera A, Gonzalez Lopez L, Blanco Aguilera E, De la Hoz Aizpurua JL, Rodriguez Torronteras A, Segura Saint-Gerons R, Blanco HA. Relationship between self-reported sleep bruxism and pain in patients with temporomandibular disorders. J Oral Rehabil. 2014;41(8): 564–72.

13. Madani AS, Abdollahian E, Khiavi HA, Radvar M, Foroughipour M, Asadpour H, Hasanzadeh N. The efficacy of gabapentin versus stabilization splint in management of sleep bruxism. J Prosthodont. 2013;22(2):126–31.
14. Lindfors E, Nilsson H, Helkimo M, Magnusson T. Treatment of temporomandibular disorders with a combination of hard acrylic stabilisation appliance and a soft appliance in the opposing jaw. A retro- and prospective study. Swed Dent J. 2008;32(1):9–16.
15. Haviv Y, Rettman A, Aframian D, Sharav Y, Benoliel R. Myofascial pain: an open study on the pharmacotherapeutic response to stepped treatment with tricyclic antidepressants and gabapentin. J Oral Facial Pain Headache. 2015;29(2):144–51.
16. Raphael KG, Marbach JJ. Widespread pain and the effectiveness of oral splints in myofascial face pain. J Am Dent Assoc. 2001;132(3):305–16.

Orofacial Dystonias and Dyskinesias

16

Gary M. Heir and José L. de la Hoz

Clinical Pearls

- A dentist trained in orofacial pain or oral medicine plays a primary role in the diagnosis and management of orofacial movement disorders. These conditions have the potential to impair jaw function, affect orofacial expressions, facial appearance, and aesthetics, and impact on the quality of life of these patients.
- The aging population is becoming more dentally conscious, reinforcing the importance of adequate knowledge of these clinical entities by the orofacial pain and oral medicine dental provider, as well as the general dentist, in order to deliver appropriate treatment to these patients.
- There is a striking lack of methodologically sound studies to support the various therapeutic options. This reinforces the importance of conservative and noninvasive restorative modalities that assist in the maintenance of an orofacial functional equilibrium.

G.M. Heir, DMD (✉)
Center for Temporomandibular Disorders and Orofacial Pain, Rutgers School of Dental Medicine, Newark, NJ, USA
e-mail: heirgm@sdm.rutgers.edu

J.L. de la Hoz, MD, DDS, MS
Master Program in Temporomandibular Disorders & Orofacial Pain, School of Medicine, CEU San Pablo University, Madrid, Spain

J.N.A.R. Ferreira et al. (eds.), *Orofacial Disorders*,
DOI 10.1007/978-3-319-51508-3_16

16.1 Introduction

Orofacial dyskinesia and orofacial dystonia (OFD) includes involuntary muscle contractions causing slow repetitive movements or abnormal postures. Orofacial dyskinesia is a group of neurological syndromes characterized by excessive, deficient, or aberration of movement of orofacial structures unrelated to muscle weakness or spasticity [1] and includes blepharospasm, uncontrolled mandibular depression, puckering of the lips, spasm of the platysma muscle, and uncontrolled movements of the tongue. It is a neurological condition that is seen in older adults, usually in seventh decade of life [2].

16.1.1 Basic Functional Neuroanatomy Review

The pyramidal system (PS) is a group of motor axons that travel from the precentral gyrus, or primary cerebral motor cortex, where upper motor neurons (UMNs) are located. Neurons from the precentral gyrus supply axial and limb muscles. These axons travel through the brain stem to the anterior horn of the medulla oblongata, through the corticobulbar tract (CBT) or spinal cord corticospinal tract (CST), where approximately 75–90% of the axons decussate or cross the midline within the medulla at a point referred to as the decussation of the pyramids.

The pyramids are the corticospinal tracts as they pass through the medulla. The fibers that decussate innervate the limbs and travel through the lateral corticospinal tract (LCST) to the appropriate spinal cord level where they synapse with lower motor neurons (LMNs) located in the anterior horn of the spinal cord. The remaining axial fibers, approximately 10%, do not decussate at the pyramidal level. They travel through the anterior corticospinal tract (ACST) and decussate within the spinal cord, also synapsing on anterior horn cells with the lower motor neurons (LMNs), which then project to the axial and limb muscles. This explains why the movements of one side of the body are controlled by the opposite side of the brain. The PS contains only motor axons (Fig. 16.1).

The nuclei of the UMN are located in the precentral gyrus in the frontal lobe of the cerebral cortex. This area is also referred to as the "motor strip." UMNs that control facial and oral movements are near the Sylvian or lateral fissure. These axons descend and converge in the cerebral peduncle toward the internal capsule of the midbrain, forming the CBT and CST (Fig. 16.2).

Axons innervating the facial muscles are located medially (in the CBT) and exit at different levels to synapse with motor neurons located in the motor nuclei of the cranial nerves. The axons of the UMN synapse with LMN in the anterior horn of the spinal cord and their axons, which can measure up to 5 feet in length in tall subjects, exit through the ventral root of the spinal cord, and converge with the dorsal sensory tracts to form the spinal nerves that supply the skeletal muscles. Injury of the LMN results in flaccid paralysis.

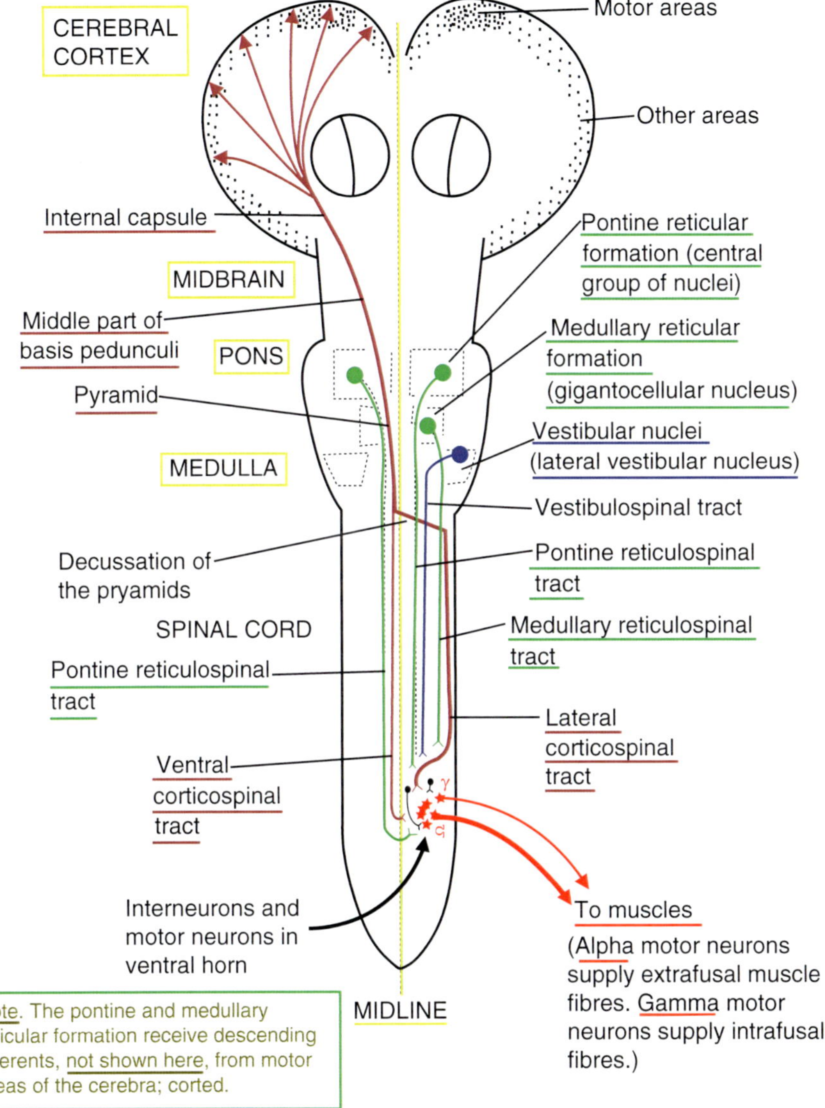

Fig. 16.1 Descending pathways involved in motor control [3]

The CBT includes two motor neurons, the UMN in the primary motor cortex (Brodmann area 4), and the LMN in the motor nuclei of the cranial nerves. The axons of the CBT UMN follow the same path, as does the CST to the medulla, where they synapse with the LMNs. The CBT supplies the nuclei of cranial nerves bilaterally (with contralateral predominance), except for cranial nerves CN-VII and CN-XII, which are both contralateral and unilateral.

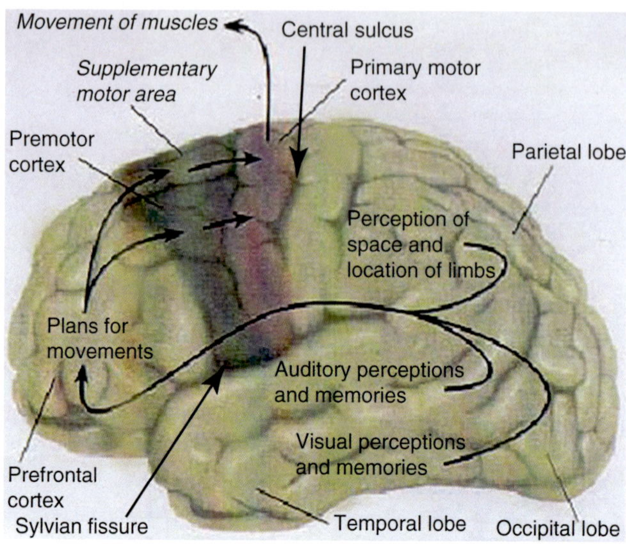

Fig. 16.2 Primary motor cortex, central sulcus, and Sylvian fissure [4]

Cranial nerves with exclusive motor function are CN-IV, CN-VI, CN-XI, and CN-XII. Those exclusively responsible for sensation are CN-I, CN-II, and CN-VIII, and those with mixed (motor, sensation, and vegetative parasympathetic) function CN-III, CN-V, CN-VII, CN-IX, and CN-X.

The extrapyramidal system (ES) is a neural network within the central nervous system (CNS) and is part of the motor system associated with the coordination of movement. It consists of polysynaptic nerve pathways including the basal nuclei (BN) and the subcortical nuclei (SN). This system is called "extrapyramidal" to distinguish it from the tracts of the motor cortex traveling through the pyramids of the medulla.

The tracts of the ES arise mainly from the reticular formation of the pons and the medulla; their target neurons in the medulla and spinal cord are related to reflexes, locomotion, complex movements, and postural control, complementing the PS that is responsible for voluntary movement. These tracts are, in turn, modulated by various areas of the CNS, including the striatum, the basal ganglia, the cerebellum, the vestibular nuclei, and various sensory areas of the cerebral cortex. All of these regulatory components are considered part of the ES, as they modulate motor activity without directly innervating the motor neurons. Neurotransmitters involved in the function of the ES are dopamine, serotonin, acetylcholine, and gamma-aminobutyric acid (GABA).

The basal ganglia (BG) are composed of an accumulation of cell bodies in the telencephalon near the base of the brain. They connect with the cerebral cortex, thalamus, and brain stem. They are associated mainly with unconscious voluntary movements such as those that involve the entire body controlling routine or everyday tasks. The BG are in the corpus striatum.

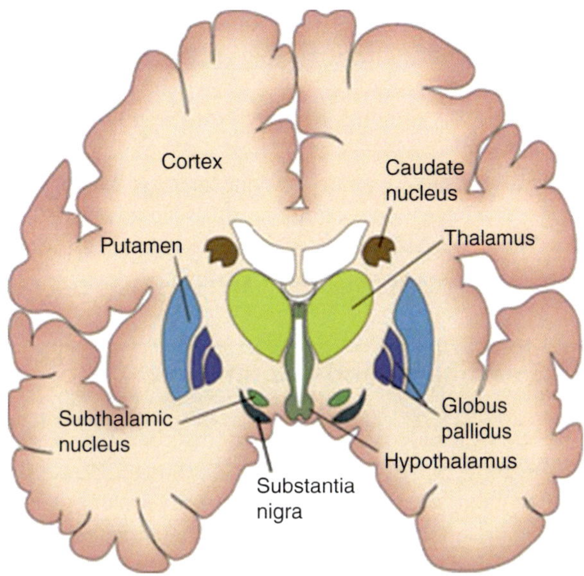

Fig. 16.3 Basal ganglia [5]

The basal ganglia are five prominent nuclei: the caudate nucleus, putamen, globus pallidus, the subthalamic nucleus, and substantia nigra (Fig. 16.3). Functional impairment of the BG is associated with a lack of coordination of bodily movements and results in the clinical presentation of diseases such as Parkinson's disease, ballism, and Huntington's chorea.

Extrapyramidal system functions include:

1. Control of muscle tone
2. Control of body posture
3. Harmonization of motor activity
4. Fine-tuning control of voluntary and involuntary movements

16.2 Clinical Presentation

According to the anatomical clinical presentation, orofacial dystonias and dyskinesias are classified as follows:

- Focal: blepharospasm, torticollis, oromandibular dystonia, spastic dysphonia, writer's cramp, occupational cramp
- Segmental: two or more contiguous parts of body, e.g., cranial + brachial, cranial + axial, cranial + cervical (Meige's syndrome)
- Generalized: involves several regions on both sides of the body, e.g., combination of leg involvement in addition to other body areas

- Multifocal: involves two or more noncontiguous parts of the body
- Hemidystonia: affects one-half of the body – symptomatic rather than primary

The most common forms of dystonia and dyskinesia include blepharospasm or twitching around the eye; cervical dystonia or spasmodic torticollis affecting the neck; segmental cranial dystonia such as Meige's'syndrome affecting the jaw, tongue, and eyes; oromandibular dystonia affecting the jaw, tongue, and lips; spasmodic dysphonia affecting the vocal cords; axial dystonia affecting the trunk; and dystonia of the arm, e.g., writer's cramp.

16.3 Etiology and Epidemiology

The etiology underlying movement disorders can be genetic, primary/idiopathic, or secondary/acquired during adulthood (due to functional overuse, medications, dental treatment, etc.); however, the majority are not well understood.

The prevalence of bruxism (sleep and awake) in the adult population is 20%, with a female predominance [6, 7]. Sleep bruxism (SB) is estimated as present in approximately 8% of the population, making it the most common of the OFDs [8]. The prevalence of SB in children is estimated at 14–20%, 13% in young adults between the age of 18 and 29, 9% in adults aged 30–65 years, and 3% in persons beyond 65 years [9, 10]. Awake bruxism has a prevalence of 22%, 1–31% [11].

The prevalence of oromandibular dystonias is 3–30/100,000 in the US population [12]. It is more common in women between 30 and 70 years [13].

Primary idiopathic dyskinesia typically affects the elderly population. The prevalence ranges between 1% and 38%, being two to three times more common in women, though this difference may be partly due to methodological biases of epidemiological studies [14].

The general prevalence of secondary dyskinesias (also named tardive dyskinesia or TD) in patients treated with neuroleptic medications is approximately 20%, with a variable incidence depending on age and gender. It is more frequent in the elderly and females [15]. No epidemiological data exist regarding the prevalence of TD in various psychiatric disorders nor the duration of exposure or dose-related risk for its occurrence, indicating an individual susceptibility trait. However, the prevalence of tardive dyskinesia seems to be dependent on the type of antipsychotic drugs used.

16.4 Pathophysiology and Mechanisms

The exact pathophysiological mechanisms underlying movement disorders are not completely understood. Normally, the prefrontal cortex gathers information to plan and execute movement by projecting signals to the premotor cortex and supplementary motor area, and then to the primary motor cortex. This, in turn signals the appropriate area of the spinal cord for movement.

The basal ganglia regulate the initiation, grading, and control of the amplitude and direction of movement. At the same time, some movements are facilitated, while others are suppressed, controlling fine, coordinated movements. Movement disorders may arise from biochemical or structural abnormalities in the BG "braking" system which prevents the target structures from generating unwanted motor activity. Many available muscles may be activated at any given time. For example, when altered as in disorders such as Huntington's disease or Wilson disease, unwanted movements such as involuntary jerking movements of an arm or leg or spasmodic movement of facial muscles occur.

There are several hypotheses for dysfunction of this system that include basal ganglia dysfunction and hyperexcitability of interneurons involved in motor signaling [16]; reduced inhibition of spinal cord and brain stem signals coming from supraspinal input; and dysfunction of neurochemical systems involving dopamine, serotonin, and noradrenaline [17].

Other risk factors for developing movement disorders include injury at birth, e.g., lack of oxygen, infection, reactions to medications, heavy metal poisoning, carbon monoxide poisoning, trauma, stroke, and inherited abnormalities of the basal ganglia.

Depending on the location of the pathology, movement disorders include:

1. Lesion of the PS:
    (a) Weakness or paralysis of the muscles responsible for the movements
2. Lesion of the ES:

(a) Altered muscle tone, posture, and coordination of movements

16.5 Diagnosis and Diagnostic Criteria

Orofacial movement disorders can be classified as follows:

1. Deficit of movement:
    (a) Akinesia (lack of movement)
    (b) Hypokinesia (decreased range of motion)
    (c) Bradykinesia (slowness of movement)
2. Excess of movement (hyperkinesias or dyskinesias)
    (a) With jerky movements:
        (i) Myoclonus/tics
        (ii) Chorea (including ballism)
    (b) No jerky movements:
        (i) Dystonia (including athetosis
        (ii) Tremor

Hypokinesia is generally referred to as Parkinsonism and includes:

1. Idiopathic Parkinsonism or Parkinson's disease
2. Secondary Parkinsonism to medications, toxins, drugs, infections
3. Atypical Parkinsonism: syndromes related to Parkinson's disease associated with other degenerative neurological disorders – multiple systemic atrophy, progressive supranuclear palsy, corticobasal ganglionic degeneration, Lewy's body disease

Hyperkinesias/dyskinesias include [18]:

1. With jerky movements:
   (a) Myoclonus/tics
   (b) Chorea (including ballism)
2. No jerky movements:
   (a) Dystonia (including athetosis)
   (b) Tremor
3. Additional classifications include:
   (a) Fast: myoclonus/tics, chorea, ballism
   (b) Slow: dystonia, athetosis
   (c) Rhythmic: tremor

16.5.1 Orofacial Dyskinesias

Orofacial dyskinesias are caused by the functional impairment of cranial nerves V, VII, and XII affecting the masticatory muscles, muscles of facial expression, and the lingual musculature [19]. These result from anomalies in the basal ganglia and/or in their interaction with other areas of the brain and can be divided into dystonias and dyskinesias. Dystonias are brief and recurrent sustained muscle contractions that cause abnormal movements and postures. Dyskinesias are involuntary, repetitive, and uncoordinated muscle movements.

Orofacial dyskinesias may be:

- Primary, idiopathic, or essential
- Secondary or tardive
- "Dental" (to be discussed later in this chapter)
- Orofacial dyskinesias are as follows [20]:
  - Bruxism
  - Oromandibular dystonia
  - Orofacial dyskinesia
- Drug-induced dystonic-type extrapyramidal reactions (DERs)

16.5.2 Bruxism

Bruxism is a repetitive jaw muscle activity characterized by clenching or grinding of the teeth and/or by bracing or thrusting of the mandible. Bruxism has two distinct circadian manifestations: it can occur during sleep (referred to as sleep bruxism) or during wakefulness (referred to as awake bruxism) [21]. For more information on awake bruxism, please review Chap. 12.

Pathophysiology is multifactorial with elements such as genetic predisposition, sleep structure (microarousals), environment, emotional distress, anxiety, and other psychological factors. CNS catecholaminergic imbalance, autonomic nervous system dysfunction, some recreational drugs (ecstasy, alcohol, caffeine, tobacco), and medications (e.g., selective serotonin reuptake inhibitors, and benzodiazepines, dopaminergic drugs) play a significant role [22].

Currently, the etiology of sleep bruxism is considered as a central and autonomic nervous system etiology beginning as oromandibular activity during sleep. Motor activities may increase during sleep and induce rhythmic masticatory muscle activity (RMMA). This represents jaw movements secondary to this muscle activity seen as bruxism [23]. It is further suggested that bruxism secondary to RMMA may be triggered by brief brain stem arousal in the reticular ascending system contributing to an increase in activity of autonomic-cardiac and motor modulatory networks [24].

Clinically, bruxism may result in oral manifestations including abnormal tooth wear, failure of dental restorations or fracturing of teeth, indentations of the lateral borders of the tongue, gingival recessions, linea alba along the biting plane or maxillary/mandibular tori, muscular or articular pain (arthrogenous temporomandibular disorder [25]), and headaches among other symptoms. Contrary to general belief in the dental and medical professions, most chronic bruxers do not present with painful or functional symptomatology related to jaw function [26].

Presently, there is no treatment that effectively or permanently eliminates bruxism [27]. Consequently, the therapeutic management aims to prevent and treat the eventual detrimental effects that bruxism may have on the masticatory system. Conservative multimodal approach by means of muscle relaxants, oral appliances, physical therapy, and psychoemotional counseling is enough, in most cases, to obtain this goal for daytime bruxism [27]. Nocturnal bruxism is considered a movement disorder associated with sleep [28–30]. For those cases in which the conservative approach does not adequately control the bruxing habit, the use of botulinum toxin has offered positive results [31].

16.5.3 Oromandibular Dystonia

Oromandibular dystonia (OMD) is a focal dystonia in which patients present with intermittent, short-lasting, sustained, and recurring muscle contractions of the masticatory, facial, and/or lingual musculature [32]. There may be opening, closing, or deflected movements, usually bilateral, due to a central origin [33]. In some instances, it can significantly compromise the quality of life of the patient affecting speech, mastication, swallowing, and social interaction [34].

Pathophysiology is due to [17]:

- Basal ganglia dysfunction
- Hyperexcitability of interneurons
- Failure (inhibition) of spinal and medullar neuromodulation
- Dopaminergic, serotonergic, and/or adrenergic systems dysfunction

There are of three types of OMD: primary, idiopathic, or essential (±63%). Secondary OMD include trauma, tumor, brain stem injury, systemic conditions (MS, Parkinson, cerebral vascular stroke), and due to medications/drugs (DER).

OMD may occur concomitant to placement of "dental or prosthetics" (to be discussed later in this chapter), in the presence of stress, exposure to glaring lights, driving, reading, talking, praying, fatigue, and chewing, which may act as triggering or aggravating factors [33]. Conversely, OMD may diminish when relaxing, talking, singing, humming, lip biting, tongue posturing, swallowing, chewing gum, and in some instances with the intake of alcohol [35]. In addition, the tactile stimulation of the affected area ("sensory trick" or "geste antagoniste") [36] or the use of certain types of sensory feedback intraoral devices [37] may diminish or temporarily eliminate the dystonic movement. This is more frequent in the OMD.

If OMD presents with blepharospasm (focal dystonia of the orbicularis oculi muscles), it is called Meige's or Brueghel's syndrome [33].

16.5.4 Orofacial Dyskinesia

Orofacial dyskinesia (OD) is defined as involuntary, repetitive, stereotypical movement of the face, tongue, and jaw that may be occasionally painful [38]. It may present as one of these three types:

1. Primary or idiopathic
2. Secondary (a.k.a. tardive dyskinesia)
3. "Dental or prosthetic" (to be discussed later in this chapter)

16.5.4.1 Primary or Idiopathic Dyskinesia

Primary or idiopathic dyskinesia is frequently comorbid, but not secondary to schizophrenia, Alzheimer's disease, dementia, autism, mental retardation, and Rett syndrome. It has been suggested that in these cases, the use of medications to treat these conditions may unmask dysfunctional subcortical circuits and trigger a dyskinesia in a predisposed patient [39]. The clinical presentation is usually milder than that of tardive dyskinesia.

16.5.4.2 Secondary or Tardive Dyskinesia (TD)

The clinical presentation consists of rapid, repetitive, nonrandom, stereotypic movements involving the tongue, lips, and jaw areas secondary to exposure to an offending drug, typically conventional antipsychotic drugs, such as chlorpromazine, haloperidol, and perphenazine [40]. Trunk and muscles of the extremities are also occasionally involved.

TD is a secondary condition that arises in some instances due to the use of certain drugs, mainly neuroleptic medications [40] and occasionally other dopamine receptor-blocking agents, such as atypical antipsychotic drugs, antiemetics, tricyclic antidepressants, and selective serotonin reuptake inhibitors. The clinical presentation consists of rapid, repetitive, nonrandom, stereotypic movements involving the tongue, lips, and jaw areas. They may present in combination with tongue twisting and protrusion, lip smacking and puckering, and chewing movements. Occasionally trunk and extremities are involved. Several activities and other factors may temporarily interrupt or increase the intensity of the dyskinesia.

TD seems to be due to hypersensitivity of basal dopaminergic receptors by chemical denervation due to chronic blockade with these medications. However, this does not explain why TD only appears in ±20% of patients treated pharmacologically. Other pathophysiological hypotheses have been formulated such as an underlying polymorphic genetic susceptibility due to the association between serine and glycine in exon 1 of the gene DRD3 [41]. Other possible anomalies are the presence of alterations in GABAergic pathways, adrenergic and cholinergic production, and O_2 radicals [42].

The diagnosis of TD requires a minimum of 3 months of treatment and persistence of symptoms beyond 3 months after discontinuation of treatment.

Drug-induced extrapyramidal reactions (DERs) are a group of oromotor hyperactivity disorders triggered by the use of certain medications and illegal or stimulant drugs (Table 16.1). In Table 16.2, a list of medications/drugs known to induce drug-induced extrapyramidal reactions (DERs) and subsequent orofacial movement disorders can be viewed.

Table 16.1 Clinical forms of drug-induced extrapyramidal reactions (DERs)

Dystonia (involuntary, tonic contractions of skeletal muscles)
Akathisia (subjective experience of motor restlessness)
Parkinsonism (tremor, rigidity, and akinesia or bradykinesia)

Table 16.2 Medications and drugs related to drug-induced extrapyramidal reactions (DERs)

Common medications prescribed by health-care professionals[a]
Fluoxetine
Fluvoxamine
Paroxetine
Sertraline
Citalopram
Escitalopram
Uncommon stimulant drugs prescribed by health-care professionals or illegal[b]
Methylphenidate
Phentermine
Pemoline
Dextroamphetamine
Amphetamines
Diethylpropion
Illegal stimulant drugs[c]
Methamphetamine
Cocaine
3,4-Methylenedioxymethamphetamine (ecstasy)

Notes:

[a]Prescribed for the treatment of depression and anxiety. Rather than a clenching or grinding bruxing type of masticatory musculature hyperactivity, patients complain of muscle pain, facial tightness, and fatigue due to sustained isometric muscle contraction

[b]Used for the treatment of obesity, attention deficit hyperactivity disorder, and narcolepsy

[c]May cause tooth clenching and grinding, tics, and dystonic reactions

16.5.4.3 "Dental or Prosthetic" Dyskinesias

There are isolated reports in the literature that implicate dental treatment as a factor in the onset of orofacial dyskinesia [43, 44]. It has been suggested that wearing ill-fitting prostheses poses a higher risk factor for oral stereotypes than not wearing prostheses [45]. Several factors, such as ill-fitting and unstable prostheses, oral discomfort, and lack of sensory contacts, have been proposed to explain the pathophysiology of oral dyskinesia in the so-called prosthetic stereotypes, but the exact mechanism remains unclear [46].

16.6 Rationale for Treatment

Providing a correct differential diagnosis of OFD is of upmost importance in order to establish the appropriate therapeutic protocol in which the OFP dentist must be part of the interdisciplinary team. A comprehensive neurological examination including MRI and MR angiography is necessary to rule out the possibility that the motor dysfunction may be due to a central degenerative, demyelinating, space-occupying, or sclerotic lesion of the nervous system. OFDs may be primary or essential, secondary to the use of certain medications (as SSRIs in bruxism or neuroleptics as in tardive dyskinesias) or illegal recreational drugs (amphetamine, cocaine, ecstasy), or comorbid with some hereditary or neurological degenerative disease (Parkinsonism, choreas, tremors, tics, orofacial dyskinesias) or psychiatric diseases [47].

Characteristic clinical features including amelioration by action, augmentation by distraction, partial volitional suppressibility, and lack of subjective distress help differentiate TD from other movement disorders such as resting tremor, Huntington's disease, spontaneous dyskinesias, and abnormal movements accompanying psychiatric illnesses [48].

The dentist is responsible for the examination and diagnosis of possible local pathological causes of the masticatory system (masticatory, perioral/facial, or tongue muscles).

Electromyographic assessment may be indicated to identify specifically which muscles are involved and to assess the patient for a motor or sensory nerve conduction deficit, a peripheral-origin myopathic disease, or motor neuron abnormality.

In severe cases of bruxism, including some forms of myoclonic-type bruxism, it will be necessary to conduct a nocturnal polysomnogram [20].

16.7 Treatment Options

Identification and withdrawal from medications with the propensity toward inducing dyskinesia should be the first objective of treatment. Adjustment of a pharmacological regimen, rather than adding another medication, may be effective, however, not in all cases.

Where dyskinesia or dystonia may be due to neurotransmitter imbalance, certain medications may help to correct these imbalances [49]. They include the following:

Anticholinergics, which are typically the most effective. However, side effects including dry mouth, blurred vision, constipation, and urinary retention must be considered. Narrow-angle glaucoma is a contradiction.

Trihexyphenidyl, typically, the first choice, is a muscarinic acetylcholine receptor antagonist. It is useful for generalized and segmental dystonia [50]. Side effects are dose related and include drowsiness, confusion, difficulty with memory, and hallucination. One of the more prominent side effects is dry mouth. It may also cause nausea. Dental hygiene in medication-induced hyposalivation is important to prevent caries. Other side effects include blurred vision, dizziness, headache, photophobia, lightheadedness, constipation, loss of appetite, trembling of the hands, and vomiting.

Baclofen targets presynaptic GABA receptors. Acting as a GABA agonist, it is effective in treating spasticity. Baclofen may be helpful for oromandibular dystonia. Side effects include dizziness, weakness, drowsiness, tiredness, headache, difficulty with sleep, nausea, constipation, and increased urination. Care must be taken when administering baclofen to diabetics as the blood glucose levels may increase. Discontinuation of baclofen must be gradual.

Benzodiazepines, of which clonazepam is the most commonly prescribed, may be effective for a small percentage of patients [51]. They may be useful for treatment of head tremor [52, 53], cervical dystonia, and blepharospasm [54]. These medications are useful as short-term muscle relaxants for reduction of skeletal muscle tone, and may have some utility for the relief of painful muscle contractions or spasms. The use of benzodiazepines in the elderly should be avoided due to the side effect of dizziness and weakness that may result in falling. Other side effects include sedation, cognitive impairment, and disturbed sleep patterns. Rapid withdrawal may result in seizures.

Dopaminergic medications are inconsistent in the treatment of dystonias supporting the etiological heterogeneity of dystonia and dyskinesia [55]. Treatment with tetrabenazine and reserpine, presynaptic dopamine depleters, has met with some success. Trials of dopamine receptor antagonists have also been met with mixed results [56]. Levodopa is rarely helpful in patients with idiopathic or other types of dystonia. Numerous side effects have been reported with the use of dopaminergic medications including headache, anxiety, nausea, vomiting, and chills. Less frequent side effects reported include chest pain, palpitations, and confusion.

Botulinum toxin injections, directly in the muscles affected by dystonia, can result in their weakening. This may improve symptoms for 3–4 months. This can be effective treatment for focal dystonias such as oromandibular dystonia, blepharospasm, dysphonia, and cervical dystonia.

Surgery to ablate the nerves leading to muscles affected by dystonia or removing the muscles altogether may help reduce dystonic muscle contractions. This technique of selective denervation is mostly indicated for cervical dystonia [57]. Some

Table 16.3 Other potentially useful pharmacologic and nonpharmacological therapies for orofacial dystonias and dyskinesias

Blepharospasm
Clonazepam, lorazepam
Botulinum toxin
Trihexyphenidyl
Orbicularis oculi myectomy
Oromandibular dystonia
Baclofen
Trihexyphenidyl
Botulinum toxin
Jaw closure dystonia
Masseter muscle
Jaw opening dystonia
Submental muscle or lateral pterygoid muscle
Spasmodic dysphonia
Botulinum toxin
Cervical
Trihexyphenidyl
Diazepam, lorazepam, clonazepam
Botulinum toxin
Tetrabenazine
Carbamazepine
Baclofen
Task-specific dystonia (writer's cramp)
Benztropine, trihexyphenidyl
Botulinum toxin
Occupational therapy

success has been reported with deep brain stimulation to reduce symptoms of dystonia [58]. Nonpharmacological or surgical treatment includes physical and supportive therapy, substitute for a "sensory trick," muscle relaxation techniques, and sensory feedback therapy.

Other treatment options are displayed in Table 16.3.

16.8 Treatment Goals and Sequencing of Care

The dental management of orofacial movement disorders is necessary when daily jaw functions are impaired. The restorative dentist plays a primary role in the management of the dental implications of OFD [59]. Unfortunately, there is a significant lack of evidence-based scientific literature to support the possible associations and efficacy of therapeutic dental modalities for these clinical entities. Most publications are dated and empirically based clinical reports [60–62]. It must be emphasized that dental treatment can only assist in the improvement of oral health and masticatory function and accordingly contribute to the maintenance of an adequate nutritional status of the OFP patient but will not provide a definitive solution for these complex multifactorial pathologies.

Several therapeutic modalities are available as adjuvants in the control of the orodental consequences of OFD, such as the prudent and judicious use of correctly adjusted oral appliances to distribute and optimize the occlusal load and prevent the damage to dental structures. In some instances, these appliances may also play the role of a "sensory trick," temporarily alleviating the intensity of the dyskinetic movement.

Fixed, either conventional or implant-supported, prosthodontic restorations are preferable over removable options to facilitate retention and prevent orodental injuries due to uncontrolled movements. These restorations must be carefully planned, designed, and adjusted using the least invasive restorative procedures to facilitate their integration in the already hypersensitive masticatory system of the patient in order to assist in the maintenance of the functional equilibrium and minimize any peripheral input that could act as trigger of the OFD.

A comprehensive clinical examination including mounted study casts, interocclusal records, correct vertical dimension, static and dynamic intermaxillary relations, and restorative material selection is of upmost importance.

Occasionally, dental treatment must be provided under conscious sedation or general anesthesia.

16.9 Conclusion

The primary responsibility of the dental practitioner confronted by a patient with abnormal facial or jaw movements is first to arrive at a differential diagnosis. This may be a difficult task, but depends on a detailed history including a review of systems, physical and psychological disorders, and knowledge of past or current medications. Once recognized as a movement disorder rather than parafunction, the dental practitioner, working with the appropriate health-care providers, plays the important role of maintaining health of the dentition and all intraoral structures to maintain optimal function regarding facial expressions and appearance, and to facilitate adequate nutrition. Care must be taken to provide conservative, or the least invasive treatment and maintenance of the oral cavity, as in many cases the etiology of movement disorders affecting masticatory musculature is unclear.

References

1. National Institute of Neurological Disorders and Stroke. http://www.ninds.nih.gov/disorders/dystonias/detail_dystonias.htm. 2016.
2. From Adams et al. Principles of neurology. 6th ed. McGraw Hill Medical: New York, Chicago, San Francisco. p. 108.
3. http://instruct.uwo.ca/anatomy/530/descmoto.gif.
4. Carlson N. Physiology of behavior. 6th ed. Needham Heights: Allyn and Bacon; 1998.
5. http://humanphysiology.academy/Neurosciences2015/Chapter3/A.3pThalamus.html.
6. Lavigne GJ, Khoury S, Abe S, Yamaguchi T, Raphael K. Bruxism physiology and pathology: an overview for clinicians. J Oral Rehabil. 2008;35:476–94.

7. Goulet JP, Lund JP, Montplaisir JY. Daily clenching, nocturnal bruxism and their association with TMD symptoms [abstract]. J Orofac Pain. 1996;10:120.
8. Lavigne GJ, Montplaisir JY. Restless legs syndrome and sleep bruxism: prevalence and association among Canadians. Sleep. 1994;17:739–43.
9. Hublin C, Kaprio J, Partinen M, Koskenvuo M. Sleep bruxism based on self-report in a nationwide twin cohort. J Sleep Res. 1998;7:61–7.
10. Okeson JP, Phillips BA, Berry DT, Cook Y, Paesani D, Galante J. Nocturnal bruxing events in healthy geriatric subjects. J Oral Rehabil. 1990;17:411–8.
11. Manfredini D, Winocur E, Guarda-Nardini L, Paesani D, Lobbezoo F. Epidemiology of bruxism in adults: a systematic review of the literature. J Orofac Pain. 2013;27:99–1110.
12. Nutt JG, Muenter MD, Aronson A, et al. Epidemiology of focal and generalized dystonia in Rochester, Minnesota. Mov Disord. 1988;3(3):188–94.
13. Brin MF, Comella C, Jankovic J. Dystonia: "etiology, clinical features, and treatment". Philadelphia: Lippincott Williams & Wilkins; 2004.
14. Blowers AJ, Borison RL, Blowers CM, et al. Abnormal involuntary movements in the elderly. Br J Psychiatry. 1981;139:363–4.
15. Kane JM, Woerner M, Lieberman J. Tardive dyskinesia: prevalence, incidence, and risk factors. J Clin Psychopharmacol. 1988;8(Suppl 4):52S–6S.
16. Cardoso F, Jankovic J. Dystonia and dyskinesia. Psychiatr Clin North Am. 1997;20(4):821–38.
17. Richter A, Loscher W. Pathology of idiopathic dystonia: findings from genetic animal models. Prog Neurobiol. 1998;54(6):633–77.
18. Abdo WF, et al. The clinical approach to movement disorders. Nat Rev Neurol. 2010;6:29–37. doi:10.1038/nrneurol.2009.196.
19. Thomas GA. Abnormal movements in the orofacial region. Diagnosis, assessment and control. A guide for the dental clinician. Aust Prothodont J. 1988;2:41–4.
20. Glark GT. Four oral motor disorders: bruxism, dystonia, dyskinesia and drug-induced dystonic extrapyramidal reactions. Dental Clinics Of North America [Dent Clin North Am] 2007;51(1):225-43, viii-ix.
21. Lobbezzoo F, et al. Bruxism defined and graded: an international consensus. J Oral Rehabil. 2012; doi:10.1111/joor.12011.
22. De-La-HozAizpurua JL, Díaz-Alonso E, LaTouche-Arbizu R, Mesa-Jiménez J. Sleep bruxism. Conceptual review and update. Med Oral Patol Oral Cir Bucal. 2011;16(2):e231–8.
23. Klasser GD, Rei N, Lavigne G. Sleep bruxism etiology: the evolution of a changing paradigm. J Can Dent Assoc. 2015;81:f2.
24. Lavigne GL, Huynh N, Kato T, Okura K, Adachi K, Yao D, Sessle B. Genesis of sleep bruxism: motor and autonomic-cardiac interactions. Arch Oral Biol. 2007;52(4):381–4.
25. Schiffman E, Ohrbach R, Truelove E, Look J, Anderson G, Goulet JP, List T, Svensson P, Gonzalez Y, Lobbezoo F, Michelotti A, Brooks SL, Ceusters W, Drangsholt M, Ettlin D, Gaul C, Goldberg LJ, Haythornthwaite JA, Hollender L, Jensen R, John MT, De Laat A, de Leeuw R, Maixner W, van der Meulen M, Murray GM, Nixdorf DR, Palla S, Petersson A, Pionchon P, et al. Diagnostic criteria for temporomandibular disorders (DC/TMD) for clinical and research applications: recommendations of the international RDC/TMD consortium network* and orofacial pain special interest groupdagger. J Oral Facial Pain Headache. 2014;28:6–27J.
26. Benoliel R, Svensson P, Heir GM, Sirois D, Zakrzewska J, Oke-Nwosu J, Torres SR, Greenberg M, Klasser G, Katz J, Eliav E. Persistent orofacial muscle pain. Oral Dis. 2011;17(Suppl 1): 23–41.
27. Huynh NT, Rompré PH, Montplaisir JY, Manzini C, Okura K, Lavigne GJ. Comparison of various treatments for sleep bruxism using determinants of number needed to treat and effect size. Int J Prosthodont. 2006;19:435–41.
28. American Academy of Sleep Medicine. In: International Classification of Sleep Disorders, 3rd ed. Darien: IL American Academy of Sleep Medicine; 2014.
29. Sleep related bruxism. In: International classification of sleep disorders: diagnosis and coding manual. 2nd ed. Westchester: American Academy of Sleep Medicine; 2005. p. 189–92.

30. Lavigne GJ, Manzini C, Kato T. Sleep bruxism. In: Kryger MH, Roth T, Dement WC, editors. Principles and practice of sleep medicine. Philadelphia: Elsevier; 2005. p. 946–59.
31. Long H, Liao Z, Wang Y, Liao L, Lai W. Efficacy of botulinum toxins in bruxism: an evidence-based review. Int Dent J. 2012;62:1–5.
32. Balasubramaniam R, Saravanan R. Orofacial movement disorders. Oral Maxillofac Surg Clin North Am. 2008;20:273–85.
33. Tolosa E, Marti MJ. Blepharospasm-oromandibular dystonia syndrome (Meige's syndrome): clinical aspects. Adv Neurol. 1988;49:73–84.
34. Lee KH. Oromandibular dystonia. Oral Surg Oral Med Oral Pathol Oral Radiol Endod. 2007;104(4):491–6.
35. Sankhla C, Lai EC, Jankovic J. Peripherally induced oromandibular dystonia. J Neurol Neurosurg Psychiatry. 1998;65(5):722–8.
36. Lo SE, Gelb M, Frucht SJ. Geste antagonistes in idiopathic lower cranial dystonia. Mov Disord. 2007;22:7.
37. Verma SP, Sinha UK. Use of an intraoral sensory feedback device in the management of jaw opening dystonia. Otolaryngol Head Neck Surg. 2009;141:142–3.
38. Assael LA. Maxillofacial movement disorders. Quintessence Pub: Hanover Park; 2006.
39. Blanchet PJ, Abdillahi O, Beauvais C, et al. Prevalence of spontaneous oral dyskinesia in the elderly: a reappraisal. Mov Disord. 2004;19(8):892–6.
40. Jankovic J. Tardive syndromes and other drug-induced movement disorders. Clin Neuropharmacol. 1995;18(3):197–214.
41. Steen VM, Lovlie R, MacEwan T, McCreadie RG. Dopamine D3-receptor gene variant and susceptibility to tardive dyskinesia in schizophrenic patients. Mol Psychiatry. 1997;2(2): 139–45.
42. Lohr JB. Oxygen radicals and neuropsychiatric illness – some speculatins. Arch Gen Psychiatry. 1991;48(12):1097–106.
43. Scutcher HD, et al. Orofacial diskinesia: a dental dimension. JAMA. 1971;216(9):1459–63.
44. Koller WC. Edentulous orodyskinesia. Ann Neurol. 1983;13:97–9; Ghika J, et al. Sensory symptoms in cranial dystonia: a potential role in the etiology? J Neurol Sci. 1993;116: 142–47.
45. Blanchet PJ, Rompré PH, Lavigne GJ, Lamarche C. Oral dyskinesia: a clinical overview. Int J Prosthodont. 2005;18(1):10–9.
46. Girard P, Monette C, Normandeau L, et al. Contribution of orodental status to the intensity of orofacial tardive dyskinesia: an interdisciplinary and video-based assessment. J Psychiatr Res. 2012;46(5):684–7.
47. Casey DE. The differential diagnosis of tardive dyskinesia. Acta Psychiatr Scand Suppl. 1981;291:71–87.
48. Cummings JL, Wirshing WC. Recognition and differential diagnosis of tardive dyskinesia. Int J Psychiatry Med. 1990;19(2):133–44.
49. Cloud LJ, Jinnah H. Treatment strategies for dystonia. Expert Opin Pharmacother. 2010;11(1):5–15. doi:10.1517/14656560903426171.
50. Jabbari B, Paul J, Scherokman B, van Dam B. Posttraumatic segmental axial dystonia, movement disorders, published online: 12 Oct 2004.
51. Greene P, Shale H, Fahn S. Analysis of open-label trials in torsion dystonia using high dosages of anticholinergics and other drugs. Mov Disord. 1988;3(1):46–60. [PubMed: 3050472].
52. Hughes AJ, Lees AJ, Marsden CD. Paroxysmal dystonic head tremor. Mov Disord. 1991;6(1):85–6. [PubMed: 2005930].
53. Davis TL, Charles PD, Burns RS. Clonazepam-sensitive intermittent dystonic tremor. South Med J. 1995;88(10):1069–71. [PubMed: 7481966].
54. Jankovic J, Ford J. Blepharospasm and orofacial-cervical dystonia: clinical and pharmacological findings in 100 patients. Ann Neurol. 1983;13(4):402–11. [PubMed: 6838174].
55. Jinnah HA, Hess EJ. Experimental therapeutics for dystonia. Neurotherapeutics. 2008;5:198–209.

56. Greene P, Shale H, Fahn S. Experience with high dosages of anticholinergic and other drugs in the treatment of torsion dystonia. Adv Neurol. 1988;50:547–56.
57. Arce CA. Selective denervation in cervical dystonia. In: Stacey MA, editor. Handbook of dystonia. New York: Informa Healthcare USA; 2007. p. 381–92.
58. Krauss JK. Deep brain stimulation for dystonia in adults. Overview and developments Stereotact Funct Neurosurg. 2002;78(3–4):168–82.
59. Lobbezoo F, Hamburger HL, Naeije M. Movement disorders in the dental office. In: Paesani DA, editor. Bruxism, theory and practice. London: Quintessence Publishing Co. Ltd.; 2010. p. 99–109.
60. Schuter HD, et al. Facial movement disorders: a progress report. Quintessence Int. 1979;10:109–12.
61. Mack PJ. Two part record blocks: a clinical report. J Dent. 1980;8:182–3.
62. Watanabe I, et al. Oral dyskinesia in the aged. II: EMG appearance and dental treatment. Gerodontics. 1988;4:310–4.

Suggested Reading

Oliveira D, Jorge R, Daldas I, Carvalho F, Magalhaes T. Bruxism after 3,4-methylenedioxymetha mphetamine (ecstasy) abuse. Clin Toxicol. 2010;48(8):863–4. 2p. 2.

17 Occlusal Dysesthesia and Dysfunction

Somsak Mitrirattanakul, Tan Hee Hon, and João N.A.R. Ferreira

Pearls of Wisdom

- The majority of the clinical research studies had agreed on one point: any dental procedure (occlusal adjustment, restorative, prosthetic, or orthodontic approaches) that aims to achieve equilibrated occlusal contacts between the maxillary and mandibular teeth (in maximum intercuspation) must be avoided in patients with occlusal dysesthesia (OD).
- Therefore, any dental procedure that interferes with the occlusion of OD patients usually fails to improve the symptoms but could increase the patient's somatosensorial focus on his or her bite.

17.1 Introduction

Occlusal dysesthesia (OD) is characterized as persistent (more than 6 months) uncomfortable or distressing bite sensations which are not affected by any physical alteration related to the occlusion, pulp, periapical tissue, muscles of mastication, or the temporomandibular joint (TMJ). This condition can cause significant functional impairment [4–6]. Other terms for this condition are phantom bite, occlusal neurosis, occlusal mania, positive occlusal awareness, and occlusal hyperawareness.

S. Mitrirattanakul, DDS, PhD (✉)
Department of Masticatory Science, Faculty of Dentistry, Mahidol University, Bangkok, Thailand
e-mail: sammu99@gmail.com

T.H. Hon, BDS, MDS (Prostho)
Endodontics, Operative Dentistry & Prosthodontics, Faculty of Dentistry, National University of Singapore, Singapore, Singapore

J.N.A.R. Ferreira, DDS, MS, PhD, Dip. ABOP
Oral & Maxillofacial Surgery, Faculty of Dentistry, National University of Singapore, Singapore, Singapore

J.N.A.R. Ferreira et al. (eds.), *Orofacial Disorders*,
DOI 10.1007/978-3-319-51508-3_17

17.2 Clinical Presentation

Patients with occlusal dysesthesia may present the following clinical scenarios:

- Sensorial complaint that "bite is off."
- History of unsuccessful dental treatments.
- Unable to define a comfortable bite position.
- Symptoms are exacerbated by dental treatments that focus only on attempting to restore the "ideal" occlusion.

17.3 Etiology and Epidemiology

17.3.1 Epidemiology

OD is generally considered a rare condition [7], although no precise data on its prevalence and incidence in the population have ever been reported [8]. However, in a survey of patients with temporomandibular disorders (TMD), over 30% reported some bite discomfort, and about 10% reported uncomfortable bite almost all of the time [9, 10]. It seems to be differently distributed between the genders with higher female prevalence [1, 3, 11–14], similarly to the higher female prevalence of TMD that sometimes is comorbid with the disease [2, 8, 15, 16]. However, such female preponderance is not reported in all the studies [8, 9]. The age of the patients can vary widely from 20 to 80 years with a mean age of 40–50 years [1, 8, 11, 14]. First, onset of the symptoms occurs at the mean age of 45 years, with mean time of symptoms' duration of 6 years [1]. In a survey by Watanabe et al. [14], among 130 patients over 70% reported that symptoms developed after a dental treatment.

17.3.2 Etiology

There is no consensus on the etiology and characteristics of OD. Current literature proposed that OD etiologies are related to both neurophysiology of the masticatory proprioceptive system and psychological disorders manifested in the orofacial region.

17.4 Pathophysiology and Mechanisms

There are three hypotheses which attempt to explain this unusual condition:

I. *Psychiatric disorders*: various studies based on psychological consultations have associated OD symptoms with somatoform disorders. The symptoms were characterized by obsessive focus on the tooth morphology, dental occlusion, as well as misinterpretation and exacerbation of normal occlusal contact patterns. The patients also presented detailed information of the psychological interaction of heightened threat, health anxiety, and cognition. In addition, the degree of the perceived physical distress could be altered by mood changes.

II. *Phantom phenomenon and neuroplasticity*: this hypothesis is based on the theory that the brain encompasses the self-knowledge of the whole body as an entity. This could be represented as a neuronal network. This brain network could normally be activated and modulated by external stimuli, but it can also be triggered without any peripheral input. It has been assumed that "the knowledge of dental anatomical details comprising the individual's dental occlusion exists in the brain as a coherent unit or "occlusal neurosignature." For vulnerable patients, tooth contact pattern alterations are caused by tooth movement, extraction, or restorative procedures which could be compared as a body part amputation, which in turn could lead to an ambiguous interpretation between the memory of the "loss of bite" and the actual bite within the occlusal neurosignature. The patient could not therefore accept the altered occlusal contact pattern as his own original bite leading to an endless exploration for the "correct bite."

III. *Altered oral proprioceptive inputs and transmission*: this etiologic concept proposed that the main cause of OD is due to a proprioceptive dysfunction, that is, a false peripheral feedback to the central nervous system. The main etiological factor could be caused by the "sensitization" of the periodontal mechanoreceptors of the involved teeth, which could produce an altered peripheral input or hyperawareness signal from the teeth.

17.5 Diagnosis and Diagnostic Criteria

There are several clinical red flags for OD such as complaint of overly disabling bite discomfort, demonstrating substantial obsessive somatic focus and excess emotional distress, exhibiting detailed histories of their problem and of prior treatment failures, expressing anger at their previous dentists and dental procedures, and showing high expectations of the treatment outcome.

Suggested Criteria for the Diagnosis of OD [11]

1. Complaint of uncomfortable bite sensation
2. Significant associated emotional distress
3. The symptoms lasting for more than 6 months
4. History of various bite-altering dental procedure failures
5. Absence of dental occlusal discrepancies or disproportional to the complaint
6. Not attributed to another disorder (dental pathology, muscle, temporomandibular joint, or neurologic disorder)

17.6 Rationale for Treatment

Since OD is not an exclusively physical problem, and the condition is significantly involving some level of psychological disorders, behavioral approach, e.g., patient's education, is the most important treatment tool. In addition, cognitive-behavioral therapy (CBT) had been proposed as a key concept for the management of OD. This treatment concept will focus on four specific areas of intervention: cognition, attention, context, and mood.

The aims of CBT for somatoform disorder are to:

- Reduce physiological arousal and reactivity through relaxation and mindfulness techniques
- Improve activity regulation through increasing exercise and meaningful activities
- Increase awareness of emotions and learn to regulate their emotion and develop tolerance of distress
- Address comorbid mood disturbance
- Modify dysfunctional beliefs through cognitive restructuring

17.7 Treatment Options

In order to improve the symptoms and enhance the quality of the sufferers' lives, OD patients need to understand that there is a need to take control of their symptoms via the application of self-management physical medicine and cognitive-behavioral treatment modalities. However, not all patients are going to respond to therapy. This would be very much dependent on the severity of the disorder and its comorbid physical and psychological conditions.

17.8 Treatment Goals and Sequencing of Care

Based on the biopsychosocial approach model, the following specific treatment strategies for OD are proposed:

1. Do not try to convince the patient that nothing is wrong with their bite.
2. The treatment needs to be structured on time-limited visits with an emphasis on behavior change through self-management modalities. The patient needs to understand that symptom reduction will occur only through their actions and efforts.
3. The CBT and relaxation may need to be introduced before the physical medicine modalities. It may be important to treat the comorbid psychological concerns first before beginning the physical medicine approach.
4. The dentist should not attempt to treat the bite complaint with occlusal adjustments before working with the tight and/or painful muscles. Adjusting the bite

will feed the somatization and shift the patient's attention to their bite and occlusal splint or device.

5. The important role of the dentist in the treatment process is to help the patient to dissociate the bite from their obsessive focus by assisting them to alternatively focus on something that is beneficial for them, such as doing jaw stretching throughout the day and maintaining a jaw posture where the teeth are not touching. Dentist should take the opportunity to educate the patient to use their symptom as a reminder to employ the adaptive coping behaviors.
6. The patient is instructed neither to check their bite nor to allow their teeth to come together. This can be achieved by using mnemonics like "lips together, teeth apart" or "jaw dropped, teeth apart" or "tongue up, teeth apart."
7. The patient should be given positive feedback for their attempts to comply with the recommendations and encouraged to persist if they fall back.

References

1. Baba K, Aridome K, Haketa T, Kino K, Ohyama T. Sensory perceptive and discriminative abilities of patients with occlusal dysesthesia. Nihon Hotetsu Shika Gakkai Zasshi. 2005;49:599–607.
2. Clark G, Simmons M. Occlusal dysesthesia and temporomandibular disorders: is there a link? Alpha Omegan. 2003;96:33–9.
3. Clark GT, Minakuchi H, Lotaif AC. Orofacial pain and sensory disorders in the elderly. Dent Clin N Am. 2005;49:343–62.
4. Hara ES, Matsuka Y, Minakuchi H, Clark GT, Kuboki T. Occlusal dysesthesia: a qualitative systematic review of the epidemiology, aetiology and management. J Oral Rehabil. 2012;39:630–8.
5. Jagger RG, Korszun A. Phantom bite revisited. Br Dent J. 2004;197:241–3.
6. Littler B. Phantom bite revisited. Br Dent J. 2005;198:149.
7. Marbach JJ, Varoscak JR, Blank RT, Lund P. "Phantom bite": classification and treatment. J Prosthet Dent. 1983;49:556–9.
8. Marbach JJ. Phantom bite syndrome. Am J Psychiatry. 1978;135:476–9.
9. Marbach JJ. Phantom bite. Am J Orthod. 1976;70:190–9.
10. Marbach JJ. Psychosocial factors for failure to adapt to dental prostheses. Dent Clin North Am. 1985;29:215–33.
11. Melis M, Zawawi KH. Occlusal dysesthesia: a topical narrative review. J Oral Rehabil. 2015;42:779–85.
12. Mew J. Phantom bite. Br Dent J. 2004;197:660.
13. Reeves JL, Merrill RL. Diagnostic and treatment challenges in occlusal dysesthesia. J Calif Dent Assoc. 2007;35:198–207.
14. Tinastepe N, Kucuk BB, Oral K. Phantom bite: a case report and literature review. Cranio. 2015;33:228–31.
15. Toyofuku A, Kikuta T. Treatment of phantom bite syndrome with milnacipran – a case series. Neuropsychiatr Dis Treat. 2006;2:387–90.
16. Watanabe M, Umezaki Y, Suzuki S, et al. Psychiatric comorbidities and psychopharmacological outcomes of phantom bite syndrome. J Psychosom Res. 2015;78:255–9.

Part VII

Orofacial Pain Disorders

Non-odontogenic "Tooth" Pain

18

Flavia P. Kapos and Donald R. Nixdorf

Pearls of Wisdom

- Non-odontogenic "tooth" pain characteristics are the key to identifying the underlying disorder: a detailed pain history will guide most of the diagnostic process.
- Pain can be referred from local and distant structures, including musculoskeletal, neuropathic, and neurovascular sources.
- Response to provocation tests and administration of local anesthetic may help to rule out or confirm the origin of the pain, as well as determine therapeutic approaches.
- Treatment options vary widely by diagnosis and are directed at the mechanism of the source of pain.
- Missed non-odontogenic "tooth" pain diagnoses may result in unnecessary dental procedures, as well as continued symptomatology.

F.P. Kapos, DDS, MS (✉)
Division of TMD & Orofacial Pain, Department of Diagnostic and Biological Sciences, School of Dentistry, University of Minnesota, Minneapolis, MN, USA

Department of Oral Health Sciences, School of Dentistry, University of Washington, Seattle, WA, USA

Department of Epidemiology, School of Public Health, University of Washington, Seattle, WA, USA
e-mail: kapos@uw.edu

D.R. Nixdorf, DDS, MS
Division of TMD & Orofacial Pain, Department of Diagnostic and Biological Sciences, School of Dentistry, University of Minnesota, Minneapolis, MN, USA

Department of Neurology, Medical School, University of Minnesota, Minneapolis, MN, USA

HealthPartners Institute for Education and Research, Bloomington, MN, USA

J.N.A.R. Ferreira et al. (eds.), *Orofacial Disorders*,
DOI 10.1007/978-3-319-51508-3_18

18.1 Introduction and Diagnostic Subtypes

Pain presenting in the orofacial region, including the teeth, can arise from various local and distant structures. While the most common causes of tooth pain are odontogenic, most other pain-producing orofacial disorders covered elsewhere in this book may also mimic tooth pain. Especially when dental etiologic factors are not evident, or pain does not respond to standard treatment, non-odontogenic causes should be considered in the differential diagnosis.

Non-odontogenic "tooth" pain is referred to as heterotopic pain, meaning that it is felt in a different anatomical location than its actual source. Sources of non-odontogenic "toothache" could be of any one or more of the five following types:

- Musculoskeletal
- Neuropathic
- Neurovascular/headache disorders
- Referred pain from regional or distant pathology

Each of these broad pain categories is generally associated with certain pain characteristics such as onset, timing, duration, quality, intensity, aggravating/alleviating factors, and associated features. Therefore, a thorough pain history may reveal clues about the true origin of the symptoms to the knowledgeable clinician [1].

Common causes of non-odontogenic "tooth" pain include the following disorders:

- Myofascial pain with referral (temporomandibular disorders – TMD)
- Persistent dentoalveolar pain disorder (PDAP)
- Trigeminal neuralgia (TN)
- Headache disorders, such as migraine headaches and trigeminal autonomic cephalalgias

Other regional or distant pathology that may also produce tooth pain-like symptoms:

- Cardiac pain/angina pectoris
- Sinus/paranasal mucosa pain
- Neoplasias of the head and neck

In such instances, for pain relief to occur, treatment must be directed at the underlying pain-producing disorder and its mechanisms and not at the tooth site where the pain is perceived to be [2]. This chapter will focus on the keys for the identification of the most probable causes of non-odontogenic "tooth" pains. Please refer to specific chapters in this publication for a more in-depth discussion on diagnosis and management strategies for each of these disorders.

18.2 Clinical Presentation

As with other pain disorders, the clinical presentation is the most important part in the diagnostic puzzle of non-odontogenic "tooth" pains. Taking time to perform a comprehensive history taking will pay off by avoiding unnecessary diagnostic tests and misdirected attempts at treatment. It will also lead to the true origin of the pain, which is the desired therapeutic target.

Non-odontogenic "tooth" pains will present in a similar way as their underlying pain-producing disorders. For this reason, it is important for dentists to have a sound knowledge of the clinical picture of some of the most common causes of non-odontogenic "toothache." As a general rule, referred or projected pains will not, or will only mildly, be affected by local treatment or provocation tests directed at the pain site (i.e., tooth) but will rather respond more substantially to interventions directed at the source of pain (e.g., myofascial trigger point, headache disorder, cardiac muscle, etc.). Triggers, alleviating and aggravating factors, will also follow the pattern of the specific underlying disorder and will differ from those typical of true tooth pain. For instance, a "tooth" pain of cardiac origin will improve with administration of nitroglycerin and may worsen with physical activity. A "tooth" pain of sinus/nasal origin may be accompanied by a history of purulent nasal discharge and/or subside with intranasal topical anesthetic application. None of these two examples would be expected to respond to a local anesthetic infiltration to the tooth where the patient perceives the pain (Table 18.1).

Table 18.1 Clinical characteristic of four of the most common causes of non-odontogenic "tooth" pain

Pain Characteristics	Myofascial pain	PDAP	Trigeminal neuralgia	Migraine headaches
Onset	Usually associated with history of temporomandibular disorders (TMD)	Spontaneous or associated with potential nerve injury. History often reveals multiple dental procedures that failed to provide sustained pain relief	Often memorable first episode. Sudden onset. May be apparently initiated by a non-noxious event (i.e., wind blow, routine dental procedure)	Usually associated with history of migraine headaches
Location (pain site)	May be felt in one or multiple teeth and change location over time ("migrating tooth pain")	Localized, perceived in the dentoalveolar tissues in or around a tooth (or location of an absent tooth)	Typically unilateral, in the distribution of one trigeminal nerve branch; maxillary (V2) or mandibular (V3)	Ipsilateral to headache presentation, when unilateral
Quality	Dull, ache, pressure, burning. Occasionally sharp with jaw function	Dull, ache, pressure, burning	Sharp, shooting, electric shock	Throbbing, dull, ache, pressure

(continued)

Table 18.1 (continued)

Pain Characteristics	Myofascial pain	PDAP	Trigeminal neuralgia	Migraine headaches
Intensity	Mild to moderate. Occasionally severe with jaw function	Mild to moderate	Severe	Moderate to severe
Frequency/ duration	Continuous or episodic	Continuous (at least 8 h/day, 15 days/month for 3 months)	Paroxysmal (less than a second – up to 2 min). Usually presents multiple attacks per day	Usually episodic, "tooth" pain may last seconds to hours with pain-free periods between migraine episodes
Aggravating factors	Jaw movement, function, parafunction, or muscle provocation tests	Aggravation of other pain conditions (increased pain input to the brain). Pain may or may not be aggravated by local tooth/ gingiva provocation	Attacks may be spontaneous or triggered by non-noxious stimuli (e.g., light touch on ipsilateral skin of the face/gingiva, chewing, vibration)	Physical activity. Triggers may include hormonal cycle for women, as well as dietary and lifestyle factors
Alleviating factors	Jaw rest, heat/ice, or local anesthetic injection of the affected muscle origin	Surgical procedures (surgical root-canal, tooth extractions) typically provide temporary relief of days to weeks before pain returns to its original state or worsens. Local anesthetic infiltration may or may not provide pain relief	Avoiding triggers may provide limited relief	Resting in a dark and quiet room, head/neck cold compress, avoiding migraine triggers
Associated symptoms	Possible jaw pain, headaches	May present altered sensation, such as local hypersensitivity compared to non-affected areas, tingling, numbness-like sensation	Possible ipsilateral autonomic features	Light and/or noise sensitivity, nausea and/ or vomiting. Possible aura (reversible neurologic disturbances, e.g., visual aura) and/or ipsilateral autonomic signs

18.3 Etiology and Epidemiology

The frequency of all-cause persistent pain after root-canal treatment has been reported to be 5% (63/1,267) after 3–5 years. Of those with persistent pain, 62% (39/63) were found to be of non-odontogenic origin [3]. In a study performed in the National Dental Practice-Based Research Network, the differential diagnosis of persistent pain following initial orthograde root-canal treatment was evaluated [2]. Nineteen patients who had persistent pain 6 months after the procedure were examined, and more than half (10/19 = 53%) of them were diagnosed with non-odontogenic causes for their "tooth" symptoms. The source of pain was determined to be myofascial/TMD in nearly all of those cases (8/10 = 80%), and PDAP disorder in the other two cases [4]. Another investigation reported that 44% (44/100) of patients diagnosed with a non-dental orofacial pain at an endodontic practice had previously received root-canal treatment or tooth extractions in a failed attempt to obtain pain relief [5].

A study of 230 patients with TMD performed at a specialty clinic revealed myofascial pain referral patterns to the teeth in 138 occasions, after each patient received a comprehensive masticatory and cervical muscle palpation exam [6]. Different types of headache disorders have also been reported to present as "tooth" pain. A retrospective study of patients at a university-based orofacial pain clinic revealed that 23.5% of patients with headaches reported non-odontogenic "tooth" pain referral [7]. Pain referred to the teeth was reported in 3 of 186 (1.6%) consecutive eligible patients with verified cardiac ischemic episode admitted to cardiology services at three different hospitals [8].

Most orofacial pains affect women more frequently than man (except for cluster headache). Central sensitization is thought to be associated with the occurrence of heterotopic pains. Therefore, chronic pain patients with multiple pain disorders, and/or pain that has been present for longer periods of time, would be at higher risk for development or progression to referred and centralized pains. Psychosocial disorders such as depression, anxiety, somatization, and catastrophizing may be comorbid in orofacial pain patients.

18.4 Pathophysiology and Mechanisms

Many of the different disorders that can present as non-odontogenic "tooth" pain have specific underlying pathophysiologic mechanisms, and some are more comprehended than others. Many times the classification of the phenomena that are thought to allow the most commonly presenting heterotopic "tooth" pains are pain referral and projection [9].

Referred pain is perceived to be in a location innervated by a different branch of the same nerve that innervates the source of pain or by a different nerve altogether. This is thought to be due to central excitatory effects and conversion of neurons in the central nervous system (CNS). Multiple peripheral neurons (primary afferents, or first order neurons) may converge to synapse with a single second-order neuron.

Especially in situations of central sensitization and prolonged deep pain stimuli, the origin of pain may be mistaken when processed by the CNS and perceived to be in a normal structure (site of pain) when reaching the cortex (e.g., myofascial pain or cardiac pain referred to the teeth). Projected pain is perceived to be in the peripheral distribution of the affected nerve branch (e.g., trigeminal neuralgia, nerve impingement/compression).

18.5 Diagnosis, Diagnostic Criteria, and Treatment

18.5.1 Musculoskeletal Pain

18.5.1.1 Myofascial Pain with Referral

Myofascial pain is a musculoskeletal condition characterized by pain that is typically described as dull ache and the presence of localized tender areas (trigger points) that can cause spreading or referred pain to other structures. Referral patterns tend to be consistent across patients, and they have been thoroughly documented [6, 10]. Jaw muscles are known to refer pain to the teeth, and this can be perceived as dental or intraoral pain. Muscle pain felt in the maxillary teeth is most often referred from masseters, as well as from the temporalis and lateral pterygoids. The masseter muscle is also the most common source of referred muscle pain to mandibular teeth, but lateral pterygoids, sternocleidomastoids, and anterior digastric may also be involved.

As with muscle pain felt in the limits of the muscle structure, muscle pain referred to teeth is mostly constant, mild to moderate in intensity, but changes with jaw movement, function, and parafunction, as well as with provocation tests of the offending muscle. Trigger points can be identified by manual palpation, as a taut band or "knot". Sustained firm digital pressure (~1 kg/2 lbs for approximately 5–10 s) over the source tender trigger point can elicit pain that duplicates the patient's "tooth" pain complaint. A graded response to stimuli is expected.

Diagnostic Criteria for Temporomandibular Disorders (DC-TMD) (Schiffman et al. [11])

Myofascial Pain with Referral

History:

1. Pain in the jaw, temple, ear, or in front of the ear
2. Pain modified by jaw movement, function, or parafunction

Exam:

1. Confirmation of the pain location(s) in the temporalis or masseter muscle
2. Report of familiar pain with palpation of the temporalis or masseter muscle
3. Report of pain at a site beyond the boundaries of the muscle being palpated

While anesthetizing the tooth where the pain is perceived is not expected to have a significant effect of the symptoms, performing a local anesthetic injection to the source muscle should greatly reduce the pain. Local anesthetic infiltrations can be used as diagnostic tests but have also been proposed as treatment for the management of trigger points and referred muscle pain. Other treatment alternatives may also include self-care management reducing jaw muscle overuse, physical therapy manual techniques and modalities, dry needling/acupuncture, botulinum toxin injections, and muscle relaxants.

18.5.2 Neuropathic Pain

Pain sensation is usually part of a physiologic process of conveying information from actual or threatened damage to the body through normally functioning neural structures. Conversely, neuropathic pain occurs when the pain sensing system (somatosensory system) itself is affected by a lesion, disease, or dysfunction.

18.5.2.1 Trigeminal Neuralgia (TN)

Trigeminal neuralgia, also known as *tic douloureux*, is a condition affecting the trigeminal nerve and is characterized by episodes of short, severe, sharp, shooting, shock-like pain. This paroxysmal pain is most often unilateral and follows the distribution of one of the three main divisions of the trigeminal nerve: ophtalmic (V1), maxillary (V2), or mandibular (V3). In that sense, it can be felt anywhere within that innervation territory, including teeth, and mimic a toothache [12].

Trigger areas on the skin of the face, oral mucosa, and teeth ipsilateral to the affected trigeminal nerve branch are frequently reported, where harmless stimulation such as teeth brushing, blowing wind, or light touch sets off a painful attack. Independently from the intensity of the stimulus applied, the pain attacks are usually stereotypical and do not present a graded response. Since peripheral input is

International Classification of Headache Disorders (ICHD-3) Beta (IHS [13])
Classical Trigeminal Neuralgia

A. At least three attacks of unilateral facial pain fulfilling criteria B and C
B. Occurring in one or more divisions of the trigeminal nerve, with no radiation beyond the trigeminal distribution
C. Pain has at least three of the following four characteristics:
   1. Recurring in paroxysmal attacks lasting from a fraction of a second to 2 minutes
   2. Severe intensity
   3. Electric shock-like, shooting, stabbing, or sharp in quality
   4. Precipitated by innocuous stimuli to the affected side of the face
D. No clinically evident neurological deficit
E. Not better accounted for by another ICHD-3 diagnosis

associated with the pain episodes, local anesthetic block applied to the trigger zones may reduce symptomatology or triggering. Thus, the clinician should be careful not to mistakenly conclude that the complaint is odontogenic if the pain improves with dental local anesthesia. Pain episodes can also occur spontaneously.

In some cases, when the condition appears in its first stages (*pre-trigeminal neuralgia)*, it can be difficult to diagnose due to the variability of the pain and less classic presentation. Proper diagnostic work-up may include a neurological evaluation and magnetic resonance imaging (MRI) of the brain. For some patients, trigeminal neuralgia is a secondary presentation of an underlying condition such as a brain tumor or multiple sclerosis.

Education, anticonvulsant neuropathic medications (carbamazepine, oxcarbazepine, gabapentin, baclofen, etc.), neurosurgery, and more recently botulinum toxin injections have been used to treat trigeminal neuralgia. It is important to note that due to the severe and disabling characteristic of the condition, patients may request treatment for the teeth, if that is part of their pain presentation. In the absence of identifiable etiology, dental treatment will most likely be ineffective and unnecessary.

18.5.2.2 Persistent Dentoalveolar Pain Disorder (PDAP)

Traditionally, neuropathic orofacial pain follows a known source of injury to the nerves of the face, teeth, or gums, due to facial trauma, surgery, dental procedures, or infection. These can result in pain and possibly other symptoms (e.g., numbness, tingling, hypersensitivity) that persist even after the original injury has healed. There are also cases with a similar clinical presentation to those pains of neuropathic nature, but the onset of pain is seemingly spontaneous, and no initiating event is identified as a possible source of nerve injury [14].

Multiple nomenclatures have been used in the literature to describe persistent orofacial pain that is not otherwise classified in another pain category, such as atypical facial pain, atypical odontalgia, and phantom tooth pain. It is unlikely that these labels represent a single clinical entity, which creates confusion for researchers and clinicians alike. Furthermore, these terms do not provide information on the nature of the disorder, other than its location, and diagnostic criteria are not clear. Despite its still unclear pathophysiologic mechanisms, the more descriptive terminology persistent dentoalveolar pain disorder (PDAP) has been proposed by an expert consensus group, based on ontology, and accompanied by a defined diagnostic criteria:

Diagnostic Criteria for Persistent Dentoalveolar Pain (Nixdorf et al. [14])

A. Persistent[a] pain[b]
B. Localized[c] in the dentoalveolar region(s)
C. Not caused by another disease or disorder[d]

[a]Persistent meaning pain present at least 8 h per day ≥15 days or more per month for ≥3 months during

[b]Pain is defined as per IASP criteria (includes dysesthesia)

[c]Localized meaning the maximum pain defined within an anatomical area

[d]Extent of evaluation nonspecified (dental, neurological examination +/−) imaging, such as intraoral, CT, and/or MRI)

18.5.2.3 Neuritis

Innervation to the mouth and teeth can be irritated by local inflammation, causing what is generally called neuritis [1]. The source of insult could be physical (e.g., compression during implant placement), chemical (e.g., extravasation of endodontic irrigation solution, medicaments, or filling material), or biological (e.g., herpes simplex, herpes zoster [shingles], or bacterial infection). An acute herpes infection or reactivation of dormant virus lodged in the trigeminal ganglion may cause pain in the distribution of the nerve days or weeks prior to outbreak of vesiculobullous lesion on the skin or mucosa. Some cases may not present these lesions, posing a greater diagnostic challenge, but painful trigeminal neuropathy attributed to acute herpes zoster (viral neuritis) should be considered in the differential diagnosis of patients with a history of primary varicella zoster infection (chicken pox).

18.5.2.4 Neuroma

Nerve injury may also result in the development of a traumatic neuroma, a disorganized proliferation of the severed nerve tissue, which can sometimes be painful. In the orofacial region, most cases present in the soft tissues around the mental foramen, lips, and tongue, but intraosseous lesions have also been reported. These have been proposed to be a potential explanation in cases of persistent pain after apparent healing post-extraction or pulpectomy.

International Classification of Headache Disorders (ICHD-3) Beta (IHS [13])

Painful Trigeminal Neuropathy Attributed to Acute Herpes Zoster

A. Unilateral head and/or facial pain lasting >3 months and fulfilling criterion C
B. Either or both of the following:
   1. Herpetic eruption has occurred in the territory of a trigeminal nerve branch or branches.
   2. Varicella zoster virus DNA has been detected in the CSF by polymerase chain reaction.
C. Evidence of causation demonstrated by both of the following:
   1. Pain preceded the herpetic eruption by <7 days.
   2. Pain is located in the distribution of the same trigeminal nerve branch or branches.
D. Not better accounted for by another ICHD-3 diagnosis

Post-herpetic Trigeminal Neuropathy

A. Unilateral head and/or facial pain persisting or recurring for ≥3 months and fulfilling criterion C
B. History of acute herpes zoster affecting a trigeminal nerve branch or branches
C. Evidence of causation demonstrated by both of the following:
   1. Pain developed in temporal relation to the acute herpes zoster.
   2. Pain is located in the distribution of the same trigeminal nerve branch or branches.
D. Not better accounted for by another ICHD-3 diagnosis

When a secondary cause for the pain is present, treatment usually starts by removing or addressing the etiologic agent (nerve decompression, antiviral medication) and can also include anti-inflammatory medications such as corticosteroids. Response to local anesthetic blocks may help to determine the level to which the pain is more peripheral or central, since central pain will not be responsive to a peripheral nerve block. Typically, the longer the pain has been present providing input to the pain processing centers in the brain, the greater is the tendency of central sensitization changes occurring. Oral medications that regulate nerve function (e.g., amitriptyline, gabapentin, pregabalin) are the first-line treatment neuropathic pain, and topical medications may be considered when there is a significant peripheral component.

18.5.2.5 Post-Herpetic Trigeminal Neuropathy

Although less commonly reported as a source of pain presenting in the teeth, post-herpetic neuralgia in the orofacial region, characterized by persistent pain following a herpes zoster reactivation (shingles), may also be a source of non-odontogenic "tooth" pain of neuropathic origin. It is also known as post-herpetic neuralgia, however, the term neuralgia is avoided in this case since it typically refers to paroxysmal pains, while this pain condition tends to present as constant.

18.5.3 Neurovascular Pain

Primary headaches, such as migraines, cluster headaches, and other trigeminal autonomic cephalalgias, have been reported to present as "toothache" [15]. Neurovascular disorders are thought to be associated with transient alterations in the function and sensitization of the trigeminal nerve and vasculature of the head. The pain is referred and felt in somatic structures of the head, such as the forehead, temples, behind the eyes, sinuses, and sometimes the teeth. The episodes of pain can be spontaneous, severe, and throbbing and have periods of remission. Odontogenic toothache can also wax and wane but tends to leave some level of low-grade background pain. In contrast, patients with headaches presenting as "tooth" pain will typically have pain-free periods between episodes. Attention to the timing, duration, and associated features will help to differentiate the underlying disorder. Migraines, affecting approximately 18% of females and 6% of males, are likely the most common headache disorder to present as "tooth" pain.

Trigeminal autonomic cephalalgias such as cluster headache are rare unilateral neurovascular disorders. Pain attacks are accompanied by ipsilateral autonomic features on the face, such as facial erythema, periorbital swelling, eyelid edema, tearing, conjunctival injection, nasal congestion, rhinorrhea, ptosis, or miosis. Treatment differs according to the diagnosis and often includes medications, diet changes, and lifestyle modification.

International Classification of Headache Disorders (ICHD-3) Beta (IHS [13])

Migraine Without Aura

A. At least five attacks fulfilling criteria B–D
B. Headache attacks lasting 4–72 h (untreated or unsuccessfully treated)
C. Headache has at least two of the following four characteristics:
   1. Unilateral location
   2. Pulsating quality
   3. Moderate or severe pain intensity
   4. Aggravation by or causing avoidance of routine physical activity (e.g., walking or climbing stairs)
D. During headache at least one of the following:
   1. Nausea and/or vomiting
   2. Photophobia and phonophobia
E. Not better accounted for by another ICHD-3 diagnosis

Migraine with Aura

A. At least two attacks fulfilling criteria B and C
B. One or more of the following fully reversible aura symptoms:
   1. Visual
   2. Sensory
   3. Speech and/or language
   4. Motor
   5. Brainstem
   6. Retinal
C. At least two of the following four characteristics:
   1. At least one aura symptom spreads gradually over 5 min, and/or two or more symptoms occur in succession.
   2. Each individual aura symptom lasts 5–60 min.
   3. At least one aura symptom is unilateral.
   4. The aura is accompanied, or followed within 60 min, by headache.
D. Not better accounted for by another ICHD-3 diagnosis, and transient ischemic attack has been excluded.

Cluster Headache

A. At least five attacks fulfilling criteria B–D
B. Severe or very severe unilateral orbital, supraorbital, and/or temporal pain lasting 15–180 min (when untreated)
C. Either or both of the following:
   1. At least one of the following symptoms or signs, ipsilateral to the headache:
      (a) Conjunctival injection and/or lacrimation
      (b) Nasal congestion and/or rhinorrhoea
      (c) Eyelid edema
      (d) Forehead and facial sweating

(e) Forehead and facial flushing
(f) Sensation of fullness in the ear
(g) Miosis and/or ptosis
2. A sense of restlessness or agitation

D. Attacks have a frequency between one every other day and eight per day for more than half of the time when the disorder is active.

Paroxysmal Hemicrania

A. At least 20 attacks fulfilling criteria B–E.
B. Severe unilateral orbital, supraorbital, and/or temporal pain lasting 2–30 min.
C. At least one of the following symptoms or signs, ipsilateral to the pain:
    1. Conjunctival injection and/or lacrimation
    2. Nasal congestion and/or rhinorrhoea
    3. Eyelid edema
    4. Forehead and facial sweating
    5. Forehead and facial flushing
    6. Sensation of fullness in the ear
    7. Miosis and/or ptosis
D. Attacks have a frequency above five per day for more than half of the time.
E. Attacks are prevented absolutely by therapeutic doses of indomethacin.
F. Not better accounted for by another ICHD-3 diagnosis.

Short-Lasting Unilateral Neuralgiform Headache Attacks

A. At least 20 attacks fulfilling criteria B–D.
B. Moderate or severe unilateral head pain, with orbital, supraorbital, temporal, and/or other trigeminal distribution, lasting for 1–600 s and occurring as single stabs, series of stabs, or in a sawtooth pattern.
C. At least one of the following cranial autonomic symptoms or signs, ipsilateral to the pain:
    1. Conjunctival injection and/or lacrimation
    2. Nasal congestion and/or rhinorrhoea
    3. Eyelid edema
    4. Forehead and facial sweating
    5. Forehead and facial flushing
    6. Sensation of fullness in the ear
    7. Miosis and/or ptosis
D. Attacks have a frequency of at least one a day for more than half of the time when the disorder is active.
E. Not better accounted for by another ICHD-3 diagnosis.

Hemicrania Continua

A. Unilateral headache fulfilling criteria B–D
B. Present for >3 months, with exacerbations of moderate or greater intensity

C. Either or both of the following:
   1. At least one of the following symptoms or signs, ipsilateral to the headache:
      (a) Conjunctival injection and/or lacrimation
      (b) Nasal congestion and/or rhinorrhoea
      (c) Eyelid edema
      (d) Forehead and facial sweating
      (e) Forehead and facial flushing
      (f) Sensation of fullness in the ear
      (g) Miosis and/or ptosis
   2. A sense of restlessness or agitation or aggravation of the pain by movement

D. Responds absolutely to therapeutic doses of indomethacin

E. Not better accounted for by another ICHD-3 diagnosis

18.5.4 Referred Pain from Regional or Distant Pathology

18.5.4.1 Cardiac Pain

Heart problems such as angina pectoris or acute myocardial infarction refer pain to the shoulder, arm, and even to the jaw or teeth. As in tooth pulp pain which presents in a visceral-like pattern, cardiac "toothache" presents as diffuse and difficult to localize, described as aching or sometimes pulsatile [16]. Although it is usually felt in the lower left jaw, it can also be bilateral. Occasionally, it is associated with chest pain, but it can also present as a sole symptom. When a "toothache" has a cardiac origin, it usually increases with exercise and decreases with cardiac medication such as nitroglycerin tablets, but is not affected by local provocation or local anesthetic blocks of the teeth. After ruling out dental pathology, immediate referral to medical care is needed, and treatment is directed to the underlying heart problem. Other thoracic structures have also been implicated in non-odontogenic "tooth" pain reports, such as in cases of lung cancer and diaphragmatic pain.

18.5.4.2 Sinus/Nasal Pain

Problems in the maxillary sinuses and/or paranasal mucosa can refer pain to the maxillary teeth [17]. The pain is usually felt in several teeth and is described as pressure, fullness, dull, aching, or throbbing. Sometimes, it is associated with pressure below the eyes and can increase with lowering the head, putting pressure over the sinuses, coughing, or sneezing. Tests performed on the teeth such as cold, chewing, and percussion can exacerbate pain from sinus origin. A history of an upper respiratory infection, purulent nasal discharge, nasal congestion, or obstruction should lead to suspicion of a sinus-related "toothache". Further diagnosis and treatment should be provided by an otolaryngologist. Diagnostic tests such as visual nasal exam, sinus X-rays, or MRI may be useful to confirm this condition. While the pain does not subside with dental anesthesia, application of intranasal topical anesthesia to the offending area should eliminate the pain. Treatment options include antihistamines, decongestants, and antibiotics.

18.5.4.3 Pain Related to Neoplasias and Other Lesions in the Head and Neck

Tumors and other space-occupying lesions anywhere near the course of the trigeminal nerve have the potential to cause compression or impingement [18]. And any trigeminally innervated somatic structures can also cause referred pain to the mouth and teeth [19]. The symptom presentation can be highly variable, but trigeminal sensory deficit, paresthesia, or pain in the distribution of the affected branch can be present. When the source disorder is intracranial, headache is a common complaint. Depending on the extent and the location of the lesion, there may be also non-trigeminal neurological deficits.

Due to the highly variable symptom presentation, a comprehensive cranial nerve examination, as well as advanced regional imaging techniques such as computed tomography (CT) or magnetic resonance imaging (MRI), may be needed, especially for patients with a history of cancer. Tumors in the pharyngeal wall, maxillary sinus, and the jaw have been reported to present as "tooth" pain. Vascular disorders, such as carotid artery dissection, aneurisms, and arteritis, have also been involved in cases of non-odontogenic "tooth" pain. The dental symptoms may be accompanied by systemic symptoms, such as weight loss, malaise, or fatigue. Although possible, these problems are very rare and adequate referral for further diagnosis and treatment is indicated.

18.5.5 Pain Disorders Related to Psychological Factors

Psychosensory disturbances in the category of somatoform disorders are characterized by somatic complaints and symptoms that are not explained by a physical cause but could be related to psychological factors. Patients with psychogenic pain, differently than in cases of malingering behavior, do not consciously fabricate symptoms to achieve a certain benefit. However, true psychogenic pain is an extremely rare diagnosis of exclusion when accounting for pains of any kind. To consider that this pain would present in the teeth is even more unlikely. Therefore, this pain category is probably highly overdiagnosed, when the true source of pain has not been yet identified, and psychosocial factor overlay creates a "colorful" symptom presentation.

Pain disorders are often comorbid with mental disorders (i.e., anxiety, depression, catastrophizing, somatization), and those can contribute to the pain experience. Nevertheless, a causal link between psychological factors and "toothaches" of non-dental origin has not been established. A consultation with a health psychologist or psychiatrist may shed light as to possible cognitive-behavioral and/or psychosocial contributing factors to the persistent pain experience.

References

1. Mattscheck D, Law AS, Nixdorf DR. Diagnosis of nonodontogenic toothache. In: Hargreaves KM, Berman LH, Rotstein I, editors. Cohen's pathways of the pulp. 11th ed. St. Louis: Elsevier; 2016. p. 684.
2. Yatani H, Komiyama O, Matsuka Y, et al. Systematic review and recommendations for non-odontogenic toothache. J Oral Rehabil. 2014;41(11):843–52.
3. Vena DA, Collie D, Wu H, et al. Prevalence of persistent pain 3 to 5 years post primary root canal therapy and its impact on oral health-related quality of life: PEARL network findings. J Endod. 2014;40(12):1917–21.
4. Nixdorf DR, Law AS, John MT, et al. Differential diagnoses for persistent pain after root canal treatment: a study in the national dental practice-based research network. J Endod. 2015;41(4):457–63.
5. Linn J, Trantor I, Teo N, Thanigaivel R, Goss AN. The differential diagnosis of toothache from other orofacial pains in clinical practice. Aust Dent J. 2007;52(1 Suppl):S100–4.
6. Wright EF. Referred craniofacial pain patterns in patients with temporomandibular disorder. J Am Dent Assoc. 2000;131(9):1307–15.
7. Molina OF, Huber Simião BR, Yukio Hassumi M, Iuata Rank RC, da Silva J, Félix F, Alves de Carvalho A. Headaches and pain referred to the teeth: frequency and potential neurophysiologic mechanisms. Rev Sul-Brasileira Odontol RSBO. 2015;12(2):151–9.
8. Kreiner M, Okeson JP, Michelis V, Lujambio M, Isberg A. Craniofacial pain as the sole symptom of cardiac ischemia: a prospective multicenter study. J Am Dent Assoc. 2007;138(1):74–9.
9. Okeson JP, editor. Bell's oral and facial pain. 7th ed. Hanover Park: Quintessence Publishing; 2014.
10. Simons DG, Travell JG, Simons LS. Myofascial pain and dysfunction: the trigger point manual. 2nd ed. Baltimore: Williams & Wilkins; 1999.
11. Schiffman E, Ohrbach R, Truelove E, et al. Diagnostic criteria for temporomandibular disorders (DC/TMD) for clinical and research applications: recommendations of the international RDC/TMD consortium network* and orofacial pain special interest groupdagger. J Oral Facial Pain Headache. 2014;28(1):6–27.
12. Law AS, Lilly JP. Trigeminal neuralgia mimicking odontogenic pain. A report of two cases. Oral Surg Oral Med Oral Pathol Oral Radiol Endod. 1995;80(1):96–100.
13. Headache Classification Committee of the International Headache Society (IHS). The international classification of headache disorders, 3rd edition (beta version). Cephalalgia. 2013;33(9):629–808.
14. Nixdorf DR, Drangsholt MT, Ettlin DA, et al. Classifying orofacial pains: a new proposal of taxonomy based on ontology. J Oral Rehabil. 2012;39(3):161–9.
15. Alonso AA, Nixdorf DR. Case series of four different headache types presenting as tooth pain. J Endod. 2006;32(11):1110–3.
16. Kreiner M, Falace D, Michelis V, Okeson JP, Isberg A. Quality difference in craniofacial pain of cardiac vs. dental origin. J Dent Res. 2010;89(9):965–9.
17. Shueb SS, Boyer HC, Nixdorf DR. Nonodontogenic 'tooth pain' of nose and sinus origin. J Am Dent Assoc. 2016;147:457.
18. Uehara M, Tobita T, Inokuchi T. A case report: toothache caused by epidermoid cyst manifested in cerebellopontine angle. J Oral Maxillofac Surg. 2007;65(3):560–1.
19. Wertheimer-Hatch L, Hatch 3rd GF, SKF HB, et al. Tumors of the oral cavity and pharynx. World J Surg. 2000;24(4):395–400.

Trigeminal Neuropathic Pain and Orofacial Neuralgias

19

David A. Sirois and Teekayu P. Jorns

Pearls of Wisdom

- In a suspected trigeminal neuralgia scenario, it is important to rule out intracranial lesions (such as a mass or demyelination) as a source of pain through imaging. Intracranial lesion may be suspected if the patient is young, and there are neurologic deficits (e.g., loss of sensation, numbness) and loss of other sensory function including hearing, sight, or smell.
- Neuropathic orofacial pain is often accompanied by other pain disorders such as myofascial pain or dental pulpitis. Management of any related disorders that contribute to hypersensitivity of the trigeminal nerve may be necessary to obtain improved relief from pharmacological management.
- A multidisciplinary pain team approach is helpful to facilitate success in complex neuropathic pain patients with multiple pain disorders and contributing factors.

D.A. Sirois, DMD, PhD
Department of Oral & Maxillofacial Pathology, Radiology and Medicine, New York University College of Dentistry, New York, USA

Department of Neurology, New York University School of Medicine, New York City, NY, USA

T.P. Jorns, DDS, MDSc, PhD (✉)
Department of Oral Biology, Faculty of Dentistry, Khon Kaen University, Khon Kaen, Thailand
e-mail: teepla@kku.ac.th

J.N.A.R. Ferreira et al. (eds.), *Orofacial Disorders*,
DOI 10.1007/978-3-319-51508-3_19

19.1 Introduction and Diagnostic Subtypes

Trigeminal neuropathic pain disorders refer to chronic orofacial pain conditions maintained primarily by neuropathic mechanisms (due to nervous system injury or dysfunction) and not nociceptive mechanisms (inflammatory). All of the conditions described in this section exhibit varying degrees of nervous system sensitization and hyperexcitability as the primary mechanism for sustained pain. The neuropathic disorders in this category include the classic cranial neuralgias (trigeminal, glossopharyngeal, and post-herpetic), traumatic trigeminal neuropathic pain, trigeminal neuropathic pain of undetermined origin, and primary burning mouth syndrome (stomatodynia). Non-dental tooth pain and burning mouth syndrome are addressed more extensively in Chaps. 18 and 20 of this clinical guidebook, respectively.

These disorders share the common features of chronicity (continuous or intermittent) and loss of typical stimulus-response features seen in nociceptive inflammatory pain. That is, pain may be spontaneous or result from non-painful stimulation and reach magnitudes and qualities inconsistent with a provoking stimulus. It is imperative that the clinician not be misled that the site of the pain is necessarily the source of the pain, leading to misdirected therapy at the site of the pain experience (i.e., endodontia or exodontia).

While a universally accepted disease classification system for trigeminal neuropathic pain has not been established, there is centainly consensus on broad issues of these diagnoses and their treatment. This chapter classifies the disorders according to the diagnostic guidelines of the International Classification of Headache Disorders (ICHD 2013) [1] and the Neuropathic and Orofacial Pain Special Interest groups of the International Association for the Study of Pain [2].

- *Trigeminal Neuralgia (TN)*
  - *Classical Trigeminal Neuralgia (CTN)*
    Unilateral, brief, sharp, lancinating pain in the trigeminal nerve distribution, usually in the second or third division, with severe intensity and pain-free intervals in the absence of any underlying intracranial pathological condition such as a mass or demyelination; often triggered by light (non-painful) touch (i.e., trigger point). Paroxysmal pain is the main compliant, but it may be accompanied by continuous pain. The duration of pain attacks can change over time and become more prolonged as well as severe.
  - *Secondary Trigeminal Neuralgia (STN)*
    Clinical presentation as described for primary trigeminal neuralgia but with an identified intracranial pathological condition such as a mass or demyelination (i.e., multiple sclerosis) or nonneoplastic cysts (i.e., epidermoid or arachnoid cysts). Most of STN patients are younger than expected for cases of TN and develop subtle or frank neurological deficits.
- *Glossopharyngeal Neuralgia (GN)*
  Severe, unilateral, brief, sharp, lacinating pain in the glossopharyngeal nerve distribution (in the ear, base of the tongue, tonsillar fossa, and/or beneath the angle of the jaw) with variable frequency and pain-free intervals in the absence of any underlying intracranial pathological condition such as a mass or demyelination.

Swallowing, talking, and coughing commonly provoke it. Similar to trigeminal neuralgia, glossopharyngeal neuralgia may be primary or secondary in nature, and these two disorders can occur together.

- *Post-herpetic Neuralgia (PHN)*
  Continuous burning pain following a known history of painful skin rashes/blisters (shingles) in the trigeminal nerve distribution after a varicella zoster viral infection (herpes zoster).
- *Painful Traumatic Trigeminal Neuropathy (PTTN)*
  Follows known injury to the trigeminal nerve, such as oral or sinus surgery, or trauma to the orofacial region. Usually presenting as a continuous burning, stinging, or aching pain in the territory of the injured nerve and may additionally have brief paroxysmal sharp pain superimposed on the continuous, background pain. Non-painful symptoms may include pins-and-needles sensation, tingling, or numbness. If the injury involves the lingual nerve, there may be diminished, distorted, or phantom taste and unilateral burning sensation of the tongue on the affected side.
- *Trigeminal Neuropathic Pain of Undetermined Origin (TNPUO)*
  Similar in quality to trigeminal neuropathic pain but without antecedent nerve or tissue injury, and without evidence of related intracranial or local pathology. This is the pain most likely to spread or move to multiple (including bilateral) trigeminal nerve distributions. While this condition has historically been referred to as atypical odontalgia, atypical facial pain, and/or phantom tooth pain, the term trigeminal neuropathic pain of undetermined origin more accurately describes the condition and avoids presumptions of etiology.
- *Primary Burning Mouth Syndrome (BMS) or Stomatodynia*
  Chronic, continuous intraoral burning sensation not associated with an identifiable mucosal abnormality such as candidiasis, trauma, or ulceration and with no underlying contributing systemic illness such as diabetes mellitus or anemia. Burning sensation occasionally may be associated with dysgeusia.

19.2 Clinical Presentation

- *Pain* – while all of the neuropathic face pains run a chronic course, it is important to distinguish the temporal patterns, distribution, quality, and provocation since these characteristics cannot only distinguish neuropathic from nociceptive pain but can also discriminate among the neuropathic pain subtypes. Table 19.1 below summarizes the classical pain characteristics among the neuropathic pain disorders; certainly there can and will be exceptions to these generalizations particularly following invasive treatments or if there is deterioration of the pain condition over many years. Unlike inflammatory, nociceptive pain which will demonstrate consistent hyperalgesia and allodynia (increased pain perception to a painful stimulus or pain perception to a non-painful stimulus, respectively), neuropathic pain may be constant in nature without provocation or paroxysmal in nature without reliable response (i.e., unexplained pain-free intervals). Classical TN lasts for seconds to minutes and has pain free intervals – clearly different from continuous forms of neuropathic pain – and is *not* reliably provoked by touch – clearly different from nociceptive pain.

Table 19.1 Comparison of clinical characteristics of orofacial neuropathic pain

Pain features	Classical cranial neuralgias				Nonclassical neuralgias		
	CTN	STN	GN	PHN	PTTN	TNPUO	BMS
Quality:							
Sharp, shooting, stabbing	+++	+++	+++	+	+	+	
Burning, stinging	+	+	+	+++	++	++	+++
Aching					++	++	
Paresthesia or anesthesia	+	+		+	+		
Trigger:							
Light touch or movement	+++	++	++	+	+	+	
Spontaneous	+	+	+	++	+++	+++	+++
Timing:							
Continuous				+++	+++	+++	+++
Intermittent	+	+	+		+	+	
Paroxysmal	+++	++	+++				
Location:							
Unilateral	+++	++		+++	+++	+	
Multifocal		++			+	+++	+
Neurological deficit		+++			+		
History of trauma or pathogen-related infection				+[a]	+++		

[a]Related to herpes zoster infection. Legend: +++ most likely, ++ less likely, + possible, *PTN* primary trigeminal neuralgia, *STN* secondary trigeminal neuralgia, *GN* glossopharyngeal neuralgia, *PHN* post-herpetic neuralgia, *PTTN* painful traumatic trigeminal neuropathic, *TNPUO* trigeminal neuropathic pain of undetermined origin, *BMS* burning mouth syndrome

- *Neurologic deficits* such as anesthesia, hypesthesia, motor weakness, loss of cranial reflexes (corneal blink, gag), diminished taste, paresthesia, or asymmetry of the face, tongue, or palate may be present following peripheral nerve injury. When focal deficits are present in the absence of an antecedent injury, suspicion is increased for intracranial mass or demyelinating disease. Bilateral facial pain is more common in secondary TN due to multiple sclerosis than in primary trigeminal neuralgia.
- *Muscle tenderness* secondary to myofascial pain can occur in some patients with neuropathic pain, particularly if there is guarding, splinting, or unilateral chewing in an attempt to avoid painful stimuli.
- *Other associated signs and symptoms* may occur including dizziness, tinnitus, and plugged ears, tearing, nasal congestion.

19.3 Etiology and Epidemiology

- *Classical Trigeminal Neuralgia (CTN)* [3]
  - Accounts for the vast majority (>90%) of TN cases (compared to secondary TN)
  - Increased risk with age: most patients over age 50
  - Overall incidence of 5.7 for women and 2.5 for men per 100,000 people
  - Etiology: neurovascular compression of the trigeminal nerve, most frequently by the superior cerebellar artery at the root entry zone

- *Secondary Trigeminal Neuralgia (STN)* [3]
  Can be secondary to:
  - *Multiple sclerosis (MS)* affects approximately 1 in 700 people, with an estimated US prevalence of 250,000–500,000. Approximately 1–2% of patients with MS develop TN (about ten new cases per year and cumulative total of approximately 4,000–5,000 people). Only about 3% of patients with TN have MS.
  - *An intracranial mass* such as a tumor or aneurysm (excluding vascular compression from cerebellar arteries) is accounting for 10–13% of all TN cases.
- *Glossopharyngeal Neuralgia (GN)* [4]
  - Little available data on incidence, though estimated to be <1:100,000.
  - Like trigeminal neuralgia, it affects most often people over age 50.
  - No reliable data on ratio female/male prevalence.
  - Vascular compression may play a role in the primary form of GN, though the data is not as compelling as for primary TN.
  - MS or intracranial mass affecting the GN may lead to hyperexcitability similar to that seen in TN.
- *Post-herpetic Neuralgia (PHN)* [5, 6]
  - Approximately 1,000,000 new cases of varicella zoster virus (shingles) in the United States each year; 20% in the trigeminal distribution and 80% in the spinal distribution.
  - Twenty percent of individuals with shingles go on to develop PHN, and the risk increases with age: 50% of all PHN cases are over age 60, and 75% of all PHN cases are over age 70.
  - Cumulative prevalence of PHN exceeds one million.
  - Viral neuritis leading to axonal degeneration and death, with subsequent altered CNS sensory processing.
- *Painful Traumatic Trigeminal Neuropathy (PTTN)* [7–9]
  - Between 1% and 5% of lower third molar extractions result in nerve injury, of which approximately one-third of injuries are permanent.
  - The estimated incidence of inferior alveolar nerve injury following a mandibular block is 1:25,000–1:50,000 – less than or equal to one event per dentist practice lifetime. In addition to mechanical injury during the injection, local anesthetic neurotoxicity has also been implicated, with prilocaine and articaine having higher risk potential than lidocaine, bupivicaine, or mepivicaine.
  - Three reports have estimated the incidence of post-endodontic neuropathic pain to range from 1% to 3%.
  - Known injury to the trigeminal nerve or tissue in its innervation territory.
  - While most patients recover from therapeutic (i.e., surgical) tissue injury, some do not and instead have a neuropathic response. Indeed, there is emerging data from the human genome project that suggests genetic risk factors for neuropathic pain.
- *Trigeminal Neuropathic Pain of Undetermined Origin*
  - No reliable data on prevalence or incidence, though most authorities agree it is more common than PTTN and that women are affected at least twice as often as men.
  - The average age of onset (age 35) is much earlier than for primary TN (greater than age 50).

- *Primary Burning Mouth Syndrome (Stomatodynia)*
  - Affects 0.7–2% of the population, increasing with age (most patients over age 50).
  - Women are more frequently affected than are men, and the relative proportion is between 3 and 20 females for each male, depending on the study.
  - Excluding burning mouth syndrome secondary to identified local or systemic pathology, primary burning mouth is viewed as a neuropathic pain condition that may result from alterations in the balance of general and special somatic afferent innervation and possible disinhibition (and hyperexcitability) of nociceptive afferents.

19.4 Pathophysiology and Mechanisms

- The pathophysiology of classical trigeminal neuralgia is not known. However, local compression from nearby cerebellar blood vessels at the trigeminal root entry zone is widely held as the underlying cause in most cases. Following whatever initiating event for the pain (demyelination, trauma, compression), the nerve becomes hyperexcitable and results in the paroxysmal pain of CTN [10]. The ignition hypothesis is a provocative explanation recently put forth to explain the unusual behavior of the trigeminal primary afferent in CTN. The model explains how periodic and synchronized spike activity can arise within the nerve and produce the physiological and psychophysical phenomena observed in TN.
- The pathophysiology of PTTN is consistent with known events following nerve injury that lead to CNS sensitization, including decreased response thresholds and increased response magnitudes of affected neurons, expansion of receptive fields, loss of modality properties, and increased spontaneous activity; these pathoophysiological events result in spontaneous and continuous pain as well as the unusual spread and referral of pain [11].
- The understanding of the biophysical events leading to pathological neuronal hyperexcitability and pain is rapidly expanding. The emerging picture of a dynamically maintained neural network that can change phenotypic and functional properties as a result of past events (injury, excitation, etc.) is driving the development of novel classes of analgesics that will focus on reducing the pathological excitability by interacting at key receptor and second messenger system levels. This pharmacologic innovation will lead in the very near future to an expanded inventory of exciting and effective drugs for neuropathic pain.

19.5 Diagnostic Criteria and Diagnostic Tests

The diagnosis of trigeminal neuropathic pain, including TN can be achieved by a careful history taking, i.e., recent history of shingles, trauma, surgery, or medication that may lead to the onset of pain. All of the conditions in this chapter and its diagnostic criteria have been described in the International Classification of Headache Disorders 3rd edition (beta version, 2013) [1]. However, the following are other investigations needed for trigeminal neuropathic pain patients:

- *Hematological and biochemical tests*
  Blood tests are important in patients with burning mouth in order to rule out its primary causes. In TN and other trigeminal neuropathic pain, blood tests are not required for diagnosis but are important in baseline monitoring for patients on future drug therapy.
- *Trigeminal nerve sensory testing*
  May indicate underlying neurological deficits and play a role in differentiating STN from CTN
- *Imaging*
  Neuroimaging is useful to differentiate between CTN and STN.
  When MS plaque, mass, aneurysms, or intracranial vessel compression is suspected, MRI scan of the brain is suggested.
- *Psychosocial assessment*
  The psychological assessment of the patient with chronic pain is essential – not because it is the cause of the patient's pain (this rarely is the case) but because patients with chronic pain will suffer, and demoralization, depression, and disability are not unexpected. Indeed, successful treatment must address these issues, and recent work has indicated that these characteristics of the patient with chronic pain are strong predictors of treatment outcome.

19.6 Rationale for Treatment

Orofacial neuropathies or neuralgias are chronic illnesses with the likelihood for many years of pain of varying intensity and frequency. Therefore, treatment should not only focus on reducing the pain experience but also improving the quality of life by addressing (with the aid as needed of behavioral and physical medicine health providers) any associated psychological distress (e.g., poorly controlled depression and/or anxiety) and disability [12].

19.7 Treatment Options

- *Trigeminal Neuralgia* [13, 14]
  - Carbamazepine is the first-line therapy and is highly efficacious in TN. Recent data implicate the human leukocyte antigen (HLA) allele B*1502 as a marker for carbamazepine-induced Steven-Johnson syndrome and toxic epidermal necrolysis in Asian population, in which this allele is seen in high frequency. The United States Food and Drug Administration (FDA) as well as other public health authorities in Asia have recommended genotyping all Asians for the allele before starting this medication [15]. Alternatively, it's derivative, oxcarbazepine, can also be tried as it is well tolerated with similar efficacy. In refractory cases, gabapentin can also be used [16, 17].
  - Surgical intervention should be considered in medication-resistant cases. The procedural remedies appear to provide significant relief for approximately 75% of patients over a 15 year period. Microvascular decompression (MVD) is recommended as it is the only nondestructive method for the treatment of

TN and involves displacement of the offending cerebellar blood vessel(s) away from the trigeminal root in the cerebellopontine angle. The alternative procedures are all destructive percutaneuous techniques to reduce nerve excitability and pain including radiofrequency thermocoagulation, percutaneous glycerol rhizotomy, and balloon microcompression [18].

- *Painful Traumatic Trigeminal Neuropathy and Pain of Undertermined Origin* [19–21]
  - Tricyclic antidepressants: amitriptyline, nortriptyline
  - Anticonvulsants: gabapentin, pregabalin
  - Topical medications: capsaicin, lidocaine, and doxepin present a challenge when used intraorally (adherence, penetration; enhanced by adhesives and stents) and also present a compliance challenge. An advantage is the lack of systemic side effects and drug interactions.
- *Post-herpetic Neuralgia* [22]
  - Recognizing the significant increased risk for PHN in patients over age 60 who develop shingles is critical and should lead to immediate combination antiviral therapy and a tricyclic antidepressant – this can reduce by 50% the risk for developing PHN. Administration of prednisolone during the acute phase, along with antiviral therapy (famcyclovir, valacyclovir), reduces the neuritis and pain of acute shingles.
  - Tricyclic antidepressants: nortriptyline, amitriptyline, desipramine
  - Anticonvulsants: gabapentin, pregabalin
  - Topical medications: lidocaine 5% transdermal patch
  - Opiods: long-acting, sustained release (oxycodone) proven efficacy
- *Burning Mouth Syndrome* [23, 24]
  - Topical and intraoral medications: lidocaine (topical), clonazepam (in troches or topical)
  - Tricyclic antidepressants: amitriptyline, nortriptyline

Target doses for selected medications for trigeminal neuropathic pain and orofacial neuralgias are provided in Table 19.2. Medications may be prescribed alone but commonly are combined to achieve adequate pain relief. The various combinations and management strategies are beyond the scope of this monograph, and the reader is encouraged to seek consultation with an oral medicine, orofacial pain, or neurologist specialist for complex pain conditions.

19.8 Treatment Goals and Sequencing of Care

- Treatment goals are pain relief, restore patient's function, and improve quality of life. Many of the medications available to treat neuropathic pain have significant adverse and side effects, requiring a thorough understanding of their pharmacology and medical monitoring.
- A stepwise management approach for classical and nonclassical trigeminal neuropathic pains and orofacial neuralgias is summarized below in Fig. 19.1, which includes pharmacological and non-pharmacological therapies.

Table 19.2 Target doses for *selected* medications for neuropathic pains or neuralgias

Generic drug name	Trade name in US	Class	Target dose range[a]
Carbamazepine	Tegretol	Anticonvulsant	200–600 mg PO bid
Carbamazepine XR	Tegretol XR	Anticonvulsant	200–400 mg PO bid
Carbamazepine SR	Carbatrol	Anticonvulsant	200–400 mg PO bid
Oxcarbazepine	Trileptal	Anticonvulsant	300–600 mg PO bid
Gabapentin	Neurontin	Anticonvulsant	300–3600 mg PO tid
Valproate	Valproic acid	Anticonvulsant	250–500 mg PO bid
Lamotrigine	Lamictal	Anticonvulsant	50–200 mg PO bid
Tiagabine	Gabitril	Anticonvulsant	2–4 mg PO bid-qid
Topiramate	Topamax	Anticonvulsant	50–100 mg PO bid
Baclofen	Lioresal	Muscle relaxant	10–20 mg PO tid
Clonazepam	Klonopin	Benzodiazepine	0.5–2 mg PO qhs
Amitriptyline	Elavil	Tricyclic antidepressant	10–75 mg PO qhs
Nortriptyline	Pamelor	Tricyclic antidepressant	10–75 mg PO qhs
Imipramine	Tofranil	Tricyclic antidepressant	10–50 mg PO qhs
Desipramine	Norpramin	Tricyclic antidepressant	10–75 mg PO qhs
Mexiletine	Mexitil	Antiarrhythmics	150–300 mg PO qd
Pregabalin	Lyrica	Anticonvulsants	75–600 mg PO bid

[a]Range going from a initial dose to titrate up and reach therapeutic effect before evaluating outcome. Side effects, adverse effects, and combination strategies are described in selected publications listed in the references section

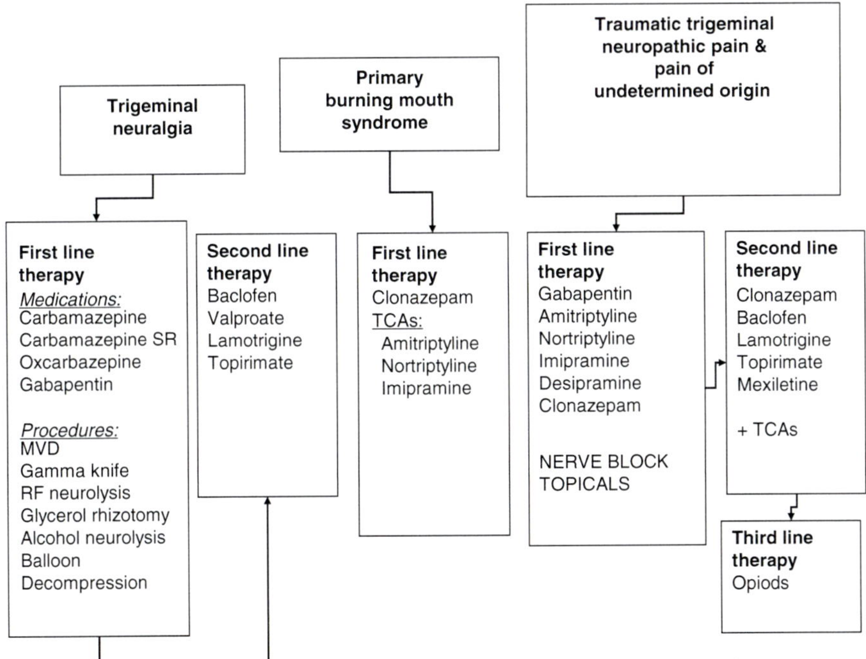

Fig. 19.1 Flow chart with the stepwise management of classical and nonclassical trigeminal neuropathic pains and orofacial neuralgias

References

1. Headache Classification Committee of the International Headache Society (IHS). The international classification of headache disorders, 3rd edition (beta version). Cephalalgia. 2013; 33:629–808.
2. Cruccu G, Finnerup NB, Jensen TS, Scholz J, Sindou M, Svensson P, Treede RD, Zakrzewska JM, Nurmikko T. Trigeminal neuralgia: new classification and diagnostic grading for practice and research. Neurology. 2016;87(2):220–8.
3. Katusic S, Beard CM, Bergstralh E, Kurland LT. Incidence and clinical features of trigeminal neuralgia, Rochester, Minnesota, 1945–1984. Ann Neurol. 1990;27(1):89–95.
4. Katusic S, Williams DB, Beard CM, Bergstralh EJ, Kurland LT. Epidemiology and clinical features of idiopathic trigeminal neuralgia and glossopharyngeal neuralgia: similarities and differences, Rochester, Minnesota, 1945–1984. Neuroepidemiology. 1991;10(5–6):276–81.
5. Dworkin RH. An overview of neuropathic pain: syndromes, symptoms, signs, and several mechanisms. Clin J Pain. 2002;18:343–9.
6. Lipton JA, Ship JA, Larach D. Estimated prevalence of reported orofacial pain in the United States. J Am Dent Assoc. 1993;124:115–21.
7. Merrill RL. Intraoral neuropathy. Curr Pain Headache Rep. 2004;8:341–6.
8. Pogrel MA, Thamby S. Permanent nerve involvement resulting from inferior alveolar nerve blocks. JADA. 2000;131:901–7.
9. Haas DA, Lennon D. A 21 year retrospective study of reports of paresthesia following local anesthetic administration. J Can Dent Assoc. 1995;61(4):319–30.
10. Jensen TS, Baron R. Translation of symptoms and signs into mechanisms in neuropathic pain. Pain. 2003;102:1–8.
11. Lai J, Hunter JC, Porreca F. The role of voltage-gated sodium channels in neuropathic pain. Curr Opin Neurobiol. 2003;13:291–7.
12. Sindrup SH, Jensen TS. Efficacy of pharmacological treatments of neuropathic pain: an update and effect related to mechanism of drug action. Pain. 1999;83:389–400.
13. Jorns TP, Zakrzewska JM. Evidence-based approach to the medical management of trigeminal neuralgia. Br J Neurosurg. 2007;21(3):253–61.
14. Fisher A, Zakrzewska JM, Patsalos PN. Trigeminal neuralgia: current treatments and future developments. Expert Opin Emerg Drugs. 2003;8(1):123–43.
15. Ferrell Jr PB, McLeod HL. Carbamazepine, HLA-B*1502 and risk of Stevens-Johnson syndrome and toxic epidermal necrolysis: US FDA recommendations. Pharmacogenomics. 2008;9(10):1543–6.
16. Reisner L, Pettengill C. The use of anticonvulsants in orofacial pain. Oral Surg Oral Med Oral Pathol Oral Radiol Endod. 2001;91:2–7.
17. Zakrzewska JM. Trigeminal neuralgia. Clin Evid. 2003;9:1490–8.
18. Lopez BC. Hamlyn PJ. Zakrzewska JM. Systematic review of ablative neurosurgical techniques for the treatment of trigeminal neuralgia. Neurosurgery. 2004;54(4):973–82; discussion 982–3.
19. Dworkin R, et al. Advances in neuropathic pain: diagnosis, mechanisms, and treatment recommendations. Arch Neurol. 2003;60:1524–34.
20. Valmaseda-Castellón E, Berini-Aytés L, Gay-Escoda C. Inferior alveolar nerve damage after lower third molar surgical extraction: a prospective study of 1,117 surgical extractions. Oral Surg Oral Med Oral Pathol Oral Radiol Endod. 2001;92:377–83.
21. McQuay HJ, Tramer M, Nye BA, Carroll D, Wiffenband PJ, Moore RA. A systematic review of antidepressants in neuropathic pain. Pain. 1996;68:217–27.
22. Sawynok J. Topical and peripherally acting analgesics. Pharmacol Rev. 2003;55:1–20.
23. Zakrzewska JM, Forssell H, Glenny AM. Interventions for the treatment of burning mouth syndrome: a systematic review. J Orofac Pain. 2003;17(4):293–300.
24. Gremeau-Richard C, Woda A, Navez M, Attal N, Bouhassira D, Gagnieu M, Laluque J, Picard P, Pionchon P, Tubert S. Topical clonazepam in stomatodynia: a randomised placebo-controlled study. Pain. 2004;108:51–7.

Burning Mouth Syndrome 20

Miriam Grushka and Nan Su

Pearls of Wisdom

- Burning mouth syndrome (BMS) is an idiopathic chronic pain condition that remains difficult to both diagnose and treat.
- Various classifications/taxonomy for BMS to date have not led to specific treatments or provided a prognosis for each classification, suggesting that current knowledge are inadequate to properly understand the pathogenesis of BMS for each classification.
- Diagnosis of BMS has been facilitated with blood tests, taste tests, salivary flow collection, and medical imaging studies. Here, we review how to diagnose and treat BMS.

20.1 Introduction

Burning mouth syndrome (BMS) is a chronic pain condition often characterized by burning of the oral mucosa in the absence of clinically notable mucosal changes and affects primarily peri- and postmenopausal women [1]. In the past, it has been referred to as scalded mouth syndrome, stomatodynia, glossodynia, glossalgia, oral dysesthesia, glossopyrosis, and sore tongue, which has led to confusion in diagnosis and treatment [1, 2]. The International Association for Study of Pain (IASP) defines BMS as characterized by "burning oral sensation or pain, unremitting while in the

M. Grushka, MSC, DDS, PhD (✉)
William Osler Health Centre, 974 Eglinton Ave W., Toronto, ON, Canada

Norman Bethune College of Medicine, Jilin University, Changchun, China
e-mail: miriamgrushka@gmail.com

N. Su, BSc, MBBS
Norman Bethune College of Medicine, Jilin University, Changchun, China

J.N.A.R. Ferreira et al. (eds.), *Orofacial Disorders*,
DOI 10.1007/978-3-319-51508-3_20

absence of objective clinical changes in the oral mucosa," and the International Headache Society defined it as "an intraoral burning sensation for which no medical or dental cause can be found" [2].

Several of the classifications of BMS proposed are included:

- Lamey and Lewis (1996) classified BMS into three subtypes based on pain pattern and intensity. In this classification, type 1 was described as daily pain that progresses in intensity over the day, type 2 was described as daily constant pain present throughout the day, and type 3 was described as intermittent burning that presents only on some days and can also affect unusual sites such as the neck [1, 3].
- Scala et al. (2003) classified BMS into two categories depending on etiology: primary (essential/idiopathic) when systemic or local causes cannot be identified and secondary, resulting from local, systemic, or psychological factors [4].
- Jääskeläinen et al. (2012) further classified primary BMS into three subgroups based on pathology. The first subgroup is characterized by focal peripheral small diameter fiber neuropathy; the second subgroup is characterized by subclinical trigeminal neuralgia; and the third subgroup is characterized as having central involvement including hypofunction of dopaminergic neurons [5].

It should be noted that there appear to be no general consensus among researchers and clinicians about which classification system is most useful clinically and none of the classification appear to be a widespread use among patient populations.

20.2 Epidemiology and Etiology

Prevalence findings for BMS have varied widely from 0.7% up to 15% of the population depending on the diagnostic criteria [1, 6]. It has a higher predisposition in females in the fifth to sixth decades of life, with female to male ratio reported at 1:5–1:7 [2, 4, 7]. BMS is rare in patients under 30 and appears to occur infrequently in children and adolescents [1].

BMS is often idiopathic; however, local and systemic factors have been described to be associated with it. Local factors can produce burning via direct irritation of the oral mucosa; these may include dental disease, mechanical or chemical irritation, hypersensitivity reaction, viral or bacterial infection, dry mouth, and oral lesions [2, 8, 9]. Systemic factors include deficiency in vitamin B12, folic acid, iron, and zinc; endocrine disorders such as diabetes; hyposalivation associated with autoimmune disease such as Sjögren's syndrome; medications including angiotensin

-converting enzyme inhibitors (ACEI), benzodiazepines, neuroleptics, antihistamines, and antiretroviral; and taste disorders and reflux disease [2, 10]. Psychological stress and neuropathy have also been suggested [2].

20.3 Clinical Presentation

20.3.1 Burning Symptoms

Burning varies from patient to patient in intensity and location. It can occur in one or multiple locations within the oral cavity and commonly affects the dorsal tongue, palate, lips, and gingival tissue and is often bilateral but can also occur unilaterally [10]. The onset of pain is often spontaneous and can be described by patients as burning, tingling, annoying, tender, or numb and is often constant [1]. Pain intensity varies throughout the day from no pain or mild pain in the morning to moderate to severe pain by late afternoon with the greatest intensity by late evening [6]. Oral stimulation with food or gum and mints often decreases the pain in these patients [10].

20.3.2 Associated Symptoms

The burning sensation is often associated with alteration in taste often reported as bitter, metallic, or sour and with xerostomia or a sensation of oral dryness in approximately two-thirds of patients [1, 10]. Salivary flow studies have demonstrated normal stimulated salivary flow with reduction in resting salivary flow in BMS as well as alterations in the composition of saliva [11–14]. Taste thresholds in BMS have been found to be elevated leading to decreased sensitivity to taste stimuli [15]. Other associated symptoms may include thirst, headache, and temporomandibular joint pain or tenderness [3].

20.3.2.1 Psychosocial

In some cases of BMS, the severe chronic pain can be associated with major depressive disorder, generalized anxiety disorder, hypochondria, cancerphobia, decreased openness, and higher neuroticism [12, 16]. The psychological stress experienced by the patients may lead to poor sleep and decreased quality of life and even to suicidal tendencies [17, 18].

20.4 Pathophysiology and Mechanisms

Although various theories have been described, it is likely that BMS is not the result of a single process. Rather, it is likely that a combination of processes exist in producing the oral burning. Some of the possible processes are described below.

20.4.1 Chorda Tympani Damage

The chorda tympani, which provides taste to the anterior two-thirds of the tongue, has been suggested to be involved in the pathogenesis of BMS. Unilateral chorda tympani damage has been shown to produce altered taste sensation of metallic, bitter, salty, and sore quality, similar to the complaints of BMS patients [19]. It has also been demonstrated that unilateral damage to the chorda tympani can produce increased burning in response to capsaicin contralateral to the side of the damage, a response mediated by the trigeminal nerve [20]. Application of sweet stimuli has also been demonstrated to inhibit oral burning, suggesting that a central loss of inhibition on the trigeminal system from the chorda tympani can lead to oral burning [20]; this finding has been supported by a recent MRI study of the gray matter in both BMS and dysgeusic patients which showed evidence of similarity in the regions affected [21].

20.4.2 Small Fiber Neuropathy

Small fiber neuropathy has been demonstrated with a significant reduction of small fiber density in areas of burning in BMS [22, 23], which has been suggested to relate to changes in immune system function.

It has been noted that burning can be a complaint in autoimmune diseases such as Sjögren's syndrome and oral lichen planus and can also occur as a result of a delayed contact sensitivity reaction [8], suggesting the possibility of a humoral response producing antibody against nerve tissue antigens, leading to small fiber neuropathy [24]. It has also been suggested that nerve growth factor (NGF), found to be elevated in saliva of BMS patients, may interact with mast cells and cause release of inflammatory mediators, which may result in the destruction of small nerve fibers in the oral mucosa [25]. NGF also upregulates expression of transient receptor potential vanilloid channel type 1 (TRPV-1) in tongue papillae and voltage-gated sodium channels 1 and 8 (Na_v 1, 8) in tongue subepithelium; two ion channels associated with nociception in BMS [22, 23, 26], suggesting increased nociceptive activity in the remaining small diameter nerve fiber may contribute to the burning.

20.4.3 Other Theories

Burning pain related to central dopamine deficiency has also been proposed as an etiological factor in BMS in view of the similarities between the BMS and Parkinson patients on nerve conduction tests and the successful treatment of oral burning in some patients with levodopa [27]. Additional support for this mechanism is the demonstration on positron emission tomography (PET) of a reduction in dopamine in the nigrostriatal neurons and the putamen in the basal ganglion [5]. Other suggested pathogenesis includes hormone alterations associated with stress response and menopause and subclinical trigeminal neuralgia [5, 14, 28].

20.5 Diagnosis and Diagnostic Criteria

Burning mouth pain has remained a diagnosis of exclusion despite recent advances in our knowledge of this syndrome and despite awareness of alterations in peripheral and central neural tissues as well as disturbances of taste. Although various classification systems outline different presentation of BMS, they are not especially helpful in determining management or long-term progress (Table 20.1).

Table 20.1 Diagnostic aids for burning pain

Patient complaints
1. Pain quality: burning, constant, mild in the morning, and increase during the day
2. Associated symptoms: dry mouth, metallic taste, sour taste
3. Often have some relief with drinking water, eating, sucking on gum/candy
Physical examination
Examination should include the tongue, buccal mucosa, lips, gingiva, and dentition
Look for striae, vesicles, trauma, and dental erosion to rule out other conditions such as *Candida* infection, lichen planus, herpes, Sjögren's syndrome, head and neck radiation, etc.
Salivary flow [11]
Low unstimulated flow, normal stimulated flow often seen in BMS
Normal unstimulated >1.5 ml/5 min
Normal stimulated >4.5 ml/5 min
Blood tests are done to rule out systemic causes of burning
CBC, ESR, Zinc, B12, folate, ferritin, glucose
Autoimmune panel: Rh, ANA Anti-Ro (SSA), Anti-La (SSB)
Serum hormones
Spatial taste testing [19]
Superthreshold taste solutions [sweet (1 M sucrose), sour (0.032 M citric acid), bitter (0.001 M quinine hydrochloride), and salty (1 M NaCl)] and 50% ethanol (produces pain)
There is often taste deficit in areas of burning
Other studies [1, 3]
Generally, a diagnosis of BMS can be made with a good clinical examination and history; however, other diagnostic test can be performed to exclude other disorders as cause of the burning
Neurological imaging to rule out pathology and degenerative disorder
Patch test to look for presence of allergy
GI assessment to look for reflux
Oral culture to rule out infections include bacterial, viral, and fungal

Table 20.2 Scala et al. (2003) diagnostic criteria of BMS [3]

Fundamental criteria	1. Daily bilateral or unilateral burning of oral mucosa
	2. Pain for at least 4–6 months
	3. Constant and progressively increasing intensity throughout the day
	4. Symptoms improves with eating food or liquid
	5. Pain does not interfere with sleep
Additional criteria	6. Associated symptoms: dysgeusia, xerostomia
	7. Chemosensory changes
	8. Mood disorders

Diagnosis remains complex since patients treated successfully for the physical oral changes may not necessarily improve, suggesting that neural changes may have also occurred as a result of the initial insult including the possibility of changes to taste system which is slow to recover.

Previous studies have shown that even a condition such as geographic tongue which causes transient changes in the architecture of the tongue, including both the filiform and fungiform papillae, can lead to higher risk of developing burning mouth pain [9].

With the possibility that BMS is linked to changes in taste, in addition to other blood tests, determining serum zinc level may also be helpful since zinc has been linked to taste loss, and Cao et al. (2010) have demonstrated that zinc supplementation may be helpful for BMS [29]. Medications which can cause change in taste [30] may be related not only to alteration in taste but also to burning mouth pain secondary to taste changes.

Examination should also include determination of salivary flow rates for evidence of decreased unstimulated salivary flows in the presence of normal stimulated salivary flow [11]. Spatial taste test for deficits in fungiform and circumvallate papillae innervated by the chorda tympani and glossopharyngeal nerve is helpful in determine taste deficit in BMS [19]. Trigeminal testing may also be helpful in determining the sensitivity of the trigeminal system to pain, which may also be a sign of release of inhibition [20].

Rarely, imaging studies may be helpful. However, even with this information, a specific etiological factor for BMS often remains unclear and approach to diagnosis and treatment continues to be by trial and error. See Table 20.2 for proposed diagnosis criteria for BMS [3].

20.6 Rationale for Treatment

In view of the belief that BMS is likely a neuropathic pain, either with no clinical findings or clinical findings which have been successfully addressed without remission of pain, current treatment is directed mostly at pain control and symptom reduction [5]. Medications such as clonazepam (a benzodiazepine), pregabalin, or gabapentin (GABA analogues) are commonly prescribed for BMS because of their ability to enhance inhibitory effect on neurons. Tricyclic antidepressants, such as amitriptyline, which has been used for the treatment of neuropathic pain [31], have also been used in the treatment of BMS. Low-dose benzodiazepine and tricyclic antidepressants are usually too low to affect depression or anxiety and are more likely related to their impact on pain [32], rather than depression or anxiety.

20.7 Treatment Options

Treatment of an underlying cause in secondary BMS may sometimes, but not always, alleviate the symptoms of burning pain with residual symptom treated in the same way as primary BMS. Listed below are some agents that have been trialed in the treatment of idiopathic BMS with varying results for most medications, other than clonazepam which has been shown in multiple studies to have a good effect on relief of symptoms in BMS [33, 34].

20.7.1 Topical Treatment

Topical treatment is aimed at symptom control to reduce the burning pain. Suggested topical treatments include:

- Sucking on 1 mg tablet of clonazepam three times per day for 14 days [1].
- 0.15% benzydamine hydrochloride three times per day [1, 3].
- Local anesthetics such as lidocaine; however, the short duration of activity has rendered them ineffective in pain control [1].
- Salivary substitutes [3].
- Topical antifungals [3].
- Topical aloe vera 0.5 mL gel 70% three times a day together with a tongue protector have been suggested in burning associated with parafunctional activity [1].
- Topical capsaicin (0.025% cream) or rinsing with Tabasco sauce and water (1:2 solution) or hot pepper and water (1:1 solution), although some patient may not be able to tolerate the burning of capsaicin initially [1, 34].

20.7.2 Systemic Treatment

Suggested systemic treatments includes:

- Alpha lipoic acid (ALA) 600 mg/d for 2 months. [1, 34].
- Antipsychotics: amisulpride, levosulpiride, 50 mg/d for 24 weeks [1].
- Antihistamines [3].
- Capsaicin (systemic) 0.25% capsule, three times a day for 1 month may cause gastric pain [1, 34].
- Clonazepam 0.5 mg/d before bed [32, 34].
- Gabapentin 100–300 mg up to three times per day.

- Hormone replacement therapy: premarin (conjugated estrogen) 0.625 mg/d for 21 days and Farlutal (medroxyprogesterone acetate) 10 mg/d from day 12–21 for three cycles in peri- and postmenopausal women [1].
- Pregabalin 25–75 mg up to three times per day.
- Serotonin reuptake inhibitor (SSRIs): sertraline 50 mg/d, paroxetine 20 mg/d for 8 weeks, duloxetine 30–60 mg/d. Dual action serotonin-norepinephrine reuptake inhibitor (SNRIs) appears to have better results [1].
- Supplements in those with abnormal levels on blood tests; B complex, vitamin B12, folic acid, iron, and zinc [1].
- Zinc gluconate 140 mg daily [35].
- Tricyclic antidepressant (TCA) 5–10 mg/d and gradually increase to 50 mg/d, although these medication must be used with care in elderly patients due to adverse effects including sedation, anticholinergic effects, hypotension, etc. [1].

20.7.3 Complementary and Alternative Medicine Therapies

There has been some suggestion that natural remedies may offer some pain relief but there is little evidence of its efficacy. *Hypericum perforatum* for mild to moderate depression, anxiety, and pain has not shown improvement in BMS [34]. Catuama, an herbal product of Brazilian origin, has been shown to have antinociceptive, antidepressant, and vasorelaxing properties and was reported to be effective in reducing the burning in one double-blind clinical trial [34].

Acupuncture in BMS has been studied, although only within China. Despite positive reported results, its efficacy is questionable [34].

20.7.4 Cognitive Therapy

Cognitive therapy, alone or in combination, has been reported to provide significant improvement in some BMS patients [1]. The latest Cochrane review (2005) suggests the best evidence for alpha lipoic acid, clonazepam, and cognitive behavior therapy in symptom reduction in BMS [36].

20.8 Treatment Goal and Sequencing of Care

Ultimately, the goal of BMS treatment is to reduce burning and associated symptoms in patients with the aim of complete resolution of these symptoms. Other important BMS management considerations to make:

- Clinical history and clinical examination are often the key to diagnosis of BMS, in patient with a history of oral burning or oral pain, metallic/bitter taste, or dry mouth in the presence of adequate saliva. If clinical examination or lab work does show changes or a cause of the burning, initial treatment can address the underlying cause. If the burning persists, then treatment should be then aimed at symptom control secondarily to the "usual" treatment for BMS.

- Patients should be followed after several weeks after the initial consultation to determine the impact of treatment and then followed over the next year for reassessment and treatment modification if needed.
- Without treatment, approximately 28% of patients will show moderate improvement, approximately half will have change to their symptoms, and approximately 19% will have worsening in symptoms [3]. It has been suggested in some study the spontaneous remission of BMS rarely occurs [3], so that it is especially important that patient receive excellent clinical care.

References

1. Aravindhan R, Vidyalakshmi S, Kumar MS, Satheesh C, Balasubramanium AM, Prasad VS. Burning mouth syndrome: a review on its diagnostic and therapeutic approach. J Pharm Bioallied Sci. 2014;6(Suppl 1):S21–5.
2. Coculescu EC, Tovaru S, Coculescu BI. Epidemiological and etiological aspects of burning mouth syndrome. J Med Life. 2014;7(3):305–9.
3. Coculescu EC, Radu A, Coculescu BI. Burning mouth syndrome: a review on diagnosis and treatment. J Med Life. 2014;7(4):512–5.
4. Jimson S, Rajesh E, Krupaa RJ, Kasthuri M. Burning mouth syndrome. J Pharm Bioallied Sci. 2015;7(Suppl 1):S194–6.
5. Jaaskelainen SK. Pathophysiology of primary burning mouth syndrome. Clin Neurophysiol. 2012;123(1):71–7.
6. Grushka M, Epstein JB, Gorsky M. Burning mouth syndrome. Am Fam Physician. 2002;65(4):615–20.
7. Kohorst JJ, Bruce AJ, Torgerson RR, Schenck LA, Davis MD. The prevalence of burning mouth syndrome: a population-based study. Br J Dermatol. 2014;172:1654–6.
8. Lynde CB, Grushka M, Walsh SR. Burning mouth syndrome: patch test results from a large case series. J Cutan Med Surg. 2014;18(3):174–9.
9. Ching V, Grushka M, Darling M, Su N. Increased prevalence of geographic tongue in burning mouth complaints: a retrospective study. Oral Surg Oral Med Oral Pathol Oral Radiol. 2012;114(4):444–8.
10. Grushka M, Ching V, Epstein J. Burning mouth syndrome. Adv Otorhinolaryngol. 2006;63:278–87.
11. Poon R, Su N, Ching V, Darling M, Grushka M. Reduction in unstimulated salivary flow rate in burning mouth syndrome. Br Dent J. 2014;217(7):E14.
12. de Souza FT, Kummer A, Silva ML, Amaral TM, Abdo EN, Abreu MH, et al. The association of openness personality trait with stress-related salivary biomarkers in burning mouth syndrome. Neuroimmunomodulation. 2015;22(4):250–5.
13. Lopez-Jornet P, Juan H, Alvaro PF. Mineral and trace element analysis of saliva from patients with BMS: a cross-sectional prospective controlled clinical study. J Oral Pathol Med. 2014;43(2):111–6.
14. Kim HI, Kim YY, Chang JY, Ko JY, Kho HS. Salivary cortisol, 17beta-estradiol, progesterone, dehydroepiandrosterone, and alpha-amylase in patients with burning mouth syndrome. Oral Dis. 2012;18(6):613–20.
15. Eliav E, Kamran B, Schaham R, Czerninski R, Gracely RH, Benoliel R. Evidence of chorda tympani dysfunction in patients with burning mouth syndrome. J Am Dent Assoc. 2007;138(5):628–33.

16. de Souza FT, Teixeira AL, Amaral TM, dos Santos TP, Abreu MH, Silva TA, et al. Psychiatric disorders in burning mouth syndrome. J Psychosom Res. 2012;72(2):142–6.
17. Lopez-Jornet P, Lucero-Berdugo M, Castillo-Felipe C, Zamora Lavella C, Ferrandez-Pujante A, Pons-Fuster A. Assessment of self-reported sleep disturbance and psychological status in patients with burning mouth syndrome. J Eur Acad Dermatol Venereol. 2015;29(7):1285–90.
18. Kontoangelos K, Koukia E, Papanikolaou V, Chrysovergis A, Maillis A, Papadimitriou GN. Suicidal behavior in a patient with burning mouth syndrome. Case Rep Psychiatry. 2014;2014:405106.
19. Bartoshuk LM, Catalanotto F, Hoffman H, Logan H, Snyder DJ. Taste damage (otitis media, tonsillectomy and head and neck cancer), oral sensations and BMI. Physiol Behav. 2012;107(4):516–26.
20. Schobel N, Kyereme J, Minovi A, Dazert S, Bartoshuk L, Hatt H. Sweet taste and chorda tympani transection alter capsaicin-induced lingual pain perception in adult human subjects. Physiol Behav. 2012;107(3):368–73.
21. Sinding C, Gransjoen AM, Schlumberger G, Grushka M, Frasnelli J, Singh PB. Grey matter changes of the pain matrix in patients with burning mouth syndrome. Eur J Neurosci. 2016;43:997–1005.
22. de Tommaso M, Lavolpe V, Di Venere D, Corsalini M, Vecchio E, Favia G, et al. A case of unilateral burning mouth syndrome of neuropathic origin. Headache. 2011;51(3):441–4.
23. Yilmaz Z, Renton T, Yiangou Y, Zakrzewska J, Chessell IP, Bountra C, et al. Burning mouth syndrome as a trigeminal small fibre neuropathy: increased heat and capsaicin receptor TRPV1 in nerve fibres correlates with pain score. J Clin Neurosci. 2007;14(9):864–71.
24. Pavlakis PP, Alexopoulos H, Kosmidis ML, Mamali I, Moutsopoulos HM, Tzioufas AG, et al. Peripheral neuropathies in Sjogren's syndrome: a critical update on clinical features and pathogenetic mechanisms. J Autoimmun. 2012;39(1–2):27–33.
25. Borelli V, Marchioli A, Di Taranto R, Romano M, Chiandussi S, Di Lenarda R, et al. Neuropeptides in saliva of subjects with burning mouth syndrome: a pilot study. Oral Dis. 2010;16(4):365–74.
26. Borsani E, Majorana A, Cocchi MA, Conti G, Bonadeo S, Padovani A, et al. Epithelial expression of vanilloid and cannabinoid receptors: a potential role in burning mouth syndrome pathogenesis. Histol Histopathol. 2014;29(4):523–33.
27. Prakash S, Ahuja S, Rathod C. Dopa responsive burning mouth syndrome: restless mouth syndrome or oral variant of restless legs syndrome? J Neurol Sci. 2012;320(1–2):156–60.
28. Kolkka-Palomaa M, Jaaskelainen SK, Laine MA, Teerijoki-Oksa T, Sandell M, Forssell H. Pathophysiology of primary burning mouth syndrome with special focus on taste dysfunction: a review. Oral Dis. 2015;21:937–48.
29. Cho GS, Han MW, Lee B, Roh JL, Choi SH, Cho KJ, et al. Zinc deficiency may be a cause of burning mouth syndrome as zinc replacement therapy has therapeutic effects. J Oral Pathol Med. 2010;39(9):722–7.
30. Naik BS, Shetty N, Maben EV. Drug-induced taste disorders. Eur J Intern Med. 2010;21(3):240–3.
31. Seltzer Z, Tal M, Sharav Y. Autotomy behavior in rats following peripheral differentiation is suppressed by daily injections of amitriptyline, diazepam and saline. Pain. 1989;37(2):245–50.
32. Grushka M, Epstein J, Mott A. An open-label, dose escalation pilot study of the effect of clonazepam in burning mouth syndrome. Oral Surg Oral Med Oral Pathol Oral Radiol Endod. 1998;86(5):557–61.
33. Zakrzewska J, Buchanan JA. Burning mouth syndrome. BMJ Clin Evid. 2016; pii:1301.
34. Miziara I, Chagury A, Vargas C, Freitas L, Mahmoud A. Therapeutic options in idiopathic burning mouth syndrome: literature review. Int Arch Otorhinolaryngol. 2015;19(1):86–9.
35. Heckmann SM, Hujoel P, Habiger S, Friess W, Wichmann M, Heckmann JG, et al. Zinc gluconate in the treatment of dysgeusia – a randomized clinical trial. J Dent Res. 2005;84(1):35–8.
36. Zakrzewska JM, Forssell H, Glenny AM. Interventions for the treatment of burning mouth syndrome. Cochrane Database Syst Rev. 2005;(1):CD002779.

Part VIII

Headaches

Chronic Daily Headache 21

Roger K. Cady and Kathleen Farmer

Pearls of Wisdom

- Chronic daily headache (CDH) is a descriptive term encompassing many different headache conditions.
- It is easier to prevent CDH than to treat it. Prevention includes:
  - Establish a clear diagnosis early in the natural history of the headache pattern.
  - Set measurable goals of treatment and outcome.
  - Provide limits for acute medication usage.
  - Start preventive medications earlier rather than later.
  - Encourage patients to participate as partners in their headache care.
  - Follow the patient's progress over time.
- In evaluating patients with CDH, look for various mechanisms that may be involved in driving the headache process.
- Address the patient with an interdisciplinary comprehensive approach rather than a linear approach when appropriate.
- Non-pharmacological interventions are the foundation of treatment, not an afterthought when the patient is not compliant with medications.
- Most CDH patients have a good prognosis and are rewarding to treat.

R.K. Cady, MD (✉)
Director, Headache Care Center, Springfield, MO, USA
e-mail: rcady@banyangroupinc.com

K. Farmer, PsyD
Headache Care Center, Springfield, MO, USA

J.N.A.R. Ferreira et al. (eds.), *Orofacial Disorders*,
DOI 10.1007/978-3-319-51508-3_21

21.1 Introduction

Chronic daily headache (CDH) is a diagnostic umbrella that includes many different and often divergent headache diagnoses. Generally, it implies that a person is experiencing headache on more days than not over a specified time period. CDH includes both primary and secondary headaches, and effort should be made to establish a more specific diagnosis whenever possible.

21.2 Clinical Presentation

The current classification of the International Headache Society (IHS) first divides headaches and facial pain disorders into primary and secondary. This differentiation is based on whether or not headaches or facial pain is the result of underlying pathology:

- Common primary headaches include migraine, tension-type headache, cluster headaches, and trigeminal autonomic cephalalgias.
- Secondary headache can result from numerous underlying diseases such as infection, tumor, medication, and trauma.

21.2.1 Primary Headaches

For migraine and tension-type headache, the diagnosis of chronic is based on a frequency of 15 days of headache per month for at least three consecutive months. For cluster headache the assignment of episodic and chronic is based on the duration of a cluster period. When the cluster period lasts more than 1 year without remission more than 1 month, the diagnosis of chronic cluster can be made.

21.2.1.1 Migraine

Migraine is first classified based on the presence or absence of aura into migraine with aura and migraine without aura. An occurrence of two or more auras in a lifetime associated with a headache fulfilling criteria for migraine constitutes the diagnosis of migraine with aura. Aura may occur in as many as 25% of migraine attacks. Many patients experience both migraine with and without aura over their lifetime.

The second division of migraine is based on frequency and is the basis for the diagnosis of episodic and chronic migraine. Episodic migraine is diagnosed when there is less than 15 days of headache per month and constitutes those attacks of migraine with or without aura (see Table 21.1). Attacks not fulfilling these criteria should be another diagnosis. Chronic migraine is diagnosed when there are 15 or greater days with primary headache and eight or more fulfill criteria for migraine or are treated early with migraine-specific medication for a headache believed would be migraine if treated later in its course. Migraine headaches and migraine variants are discussed in detail on Chaps. 22 and 24, respectively.

Table 21.1 Comparison of clinical characteristics between migraine, tension-type headache, and cluster headache

Chronic migraine	Tension-type headache	Cluster headache
Frequency: 15 days or more/month for more than 3 months Pain features (2 of 4): Unilateral location Pulsating quality Moderate or severe pain intensity Aggravation by or causing avoidance of routine physical activity In addition (1 of 2) Nausea and/or vomiting Photophobia and phonophobia	Frequency: 30 min to 7 days Pain features (2 of 4): Bilateral Pressing/tightening Mild to moderate Not aggravated by activity In addition: No nausea Photophobia or phonophobia	Frequency: more than 1 year w/o remission or with remission lasting less than 1 month Pain features: Severe or very severe unilateral orbital Supraorbital and/or temporal pain lasting 15–180 min if untreated Pain (1 of 6) Ipsilateral conjunctival injection and/or lacrimation Ipsilateral nasal congestion and/or rhinorrhea Ipsilateral eyelid edema Ipsilateral forehead and facial sweating Ipsilateral miosis and/or ptosis A sense of restlessness or agitation. Attacks from one every other day to 8 per day

21.2.1.2 Tension-Type Headache

Episodic tension-type headache is diagnosed when there are less than 15 days of headache that is mild to moderate in intensity but otherwise lacking migraine features. Chronic tension-type headache is when there are greater than 15 days of mild to moderate headache. A single associated feature of nausea, photophobia, or phonophobia can be present.

21.2.1.3 Cluster Headache

Cluster headache is a short duration (<3 h) unilateral severe headache associated with autonomic features on the ipsilateral side as the headache such as lacrimation, rhinorrhea, nasal stuffiness, sweating, or miosis with or without ptosis. Cluster attacks occur up to several times a day. It is episodic if the cluster period in less than 1 year and chronic if it persists beyond a year without greater than a month of cluster free time. These are discussed in more detail on Chap. 23.

21.2.1.4 Trigeminal Autonomic Cephalalgias

Other short duration headaches occur but are rare and are differentiated from cluster based primarily on frequency of attacks. These fall into the broad category of autonomic trigeminal cephalalgias. A variety of other uncommon primary headaches such as hypnic headache, chronic hemicrania continua, and chronic paroxysmal hemicranias have also been defined. These are discussed in detail on Chap. 23.

21.2.2 Secondary Headaches

Secondary headaches are the consequence of an underlying disease or pathology. Ideally when the underlying disease resolves, the headache resolves. Etiologies are varied and may include infections, trauma, neoplasm, inflammatory disease, medication, toxic exposures, vascular disease, and psychological disease.

21.3 Etiology and Epidemiology

Worldwide, it has been estimated that prevalence among adults with headache disorder (defined as headache that is symptomatic at least once within the last year) is about 50%. Up to three quarters of adults aged 18–65 years in the world have had headache in the last year. Chronic headache (15 or more days every month) affects 1.7–4% of the adult population globally. Despite country-to-country or regional variations, headache disorders are a worldwide concern, affecting people of all ages, races, income levels, and geographical areas.

The long-term effort of coping with a chronic headache disorder may also predispose the individual to other illnesses. For example, anxiety and depression are significantly more common in people with chronic migraine than in healthy individuals.

Chronic migraine is more common in women, usually by a factor of about 2:1, because of hormonal influences. This type of headache may be related to the activation of a mechanism deep in the brain that leads to release of pain-producing inflammatory substances around the nerves and blood vessels of the head.

Chronic tension-type headache (CTTH) affects 1–3% of adults. It often begins during the teenage years, with a female gender to male ratio of 3:2. Etiological factors of CTTH may be stress-related or associated with musculoskeletal conditions.

21.4 Pathophysiology and Mechanisms

The convergence hypothesis [1] was proposed as a clinical model of headache pathophysiology and suggests that most primary headache disorders arise from a common pathophysiological process. Underpinning this model is that migraine is a process that evolves through multiple phases: prodrome (premonitory), aura, mild, moderate, and severe headache, and postdrome. Not all headaches evolve through all these phases, and this headache process can, under appropriate circumstances, be terminated at any stage in its evolution. Symptoms observed during each of these phases provide the overall observed symptomatology expressed by patients during a primary headache, but only a small subset is actually used in formal diagnostic criteria (Fig. 21.1).

The convergence model predicts multiple clinical expressions of primary headache disorders based on neurological disruption of the central nervous system, peripheral sensitization, central sensitization, and the various sensory inputs into the trigeminal nucleus caudalis and assists in understanding the relationship of cervical, sinus, and temporomandibular factors involved in headache.

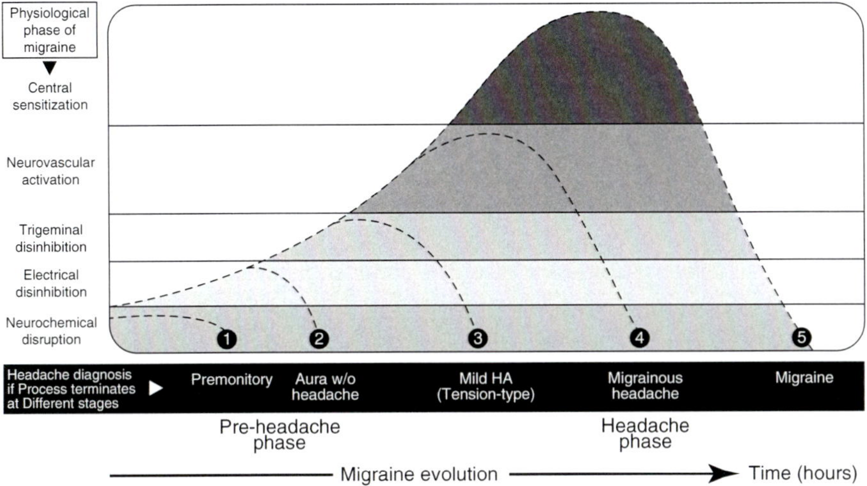

Fig. 21.1 Physiological phases of migraine headache

Over time the frequency of primary headaches can increase, eventually becoming chronic. Many factors can cause transformation of episodic to CDH including head injury, infections such as meningitis, overuse of pain medication, ineffective acute treatment, allergies, asthma, hypothyroidism, and hypertension. As the patient evolves toward a chronic headache pattern, numerous comorbidities are observed such as sleep disruption, affective disease, gastrointestinal symptoms, and myofascial pain [2]. In addition, with the evolution of chronic headache, there is frequently an observed overreliance on symptomatic medications. The overuse of acute symptomatic medication is considered an etiological factor in many chronic headache patients [3].

Risk factors for CDH include genetic factors, trauma (both psychological and physical), physiological factors such as age and hormonal status, obesity, caffeine, medications, and snoring [4]. Recently, it has been observed that patients with suboptimal response to acute medication are also at significant risk of developing chronic migraine [5].

21.5 Diagnosis and Diagnostic Criteria

21.5.1 Diagnosing the Headache Patient

Arguably the most important element of obtaining an accurate headache diagnosis is to establish rapport with the patient. This is best accomplished by beginning the interview with open-ended questions that allow patients to "tell their story." Important areas to define during a headache history include the "5 Ps": pattern, phenotype, patient (comorbidities), pharmacology (all medication usage and its effectiveness), and precipitants [6].

21.5.2 Diagnostic Criteria/Taxonomy

In 1988, the International Headache Society (IHS) established an elaborate taxonomy for the diagnosis of headache and facial pain disorders [7]. This was revised in 2004 and again in 2013 [8]. In the revised edition chronic migraine was recognized for the first time, and thus the taxonomy becomes consistent in defining a chronic form of migraine, tension-type, and cluster headache. These criteria are listed in Table 21.1. Criteria for cervicogenic headache, posttraumatic headache, neuralgias, sinusitis, and temporomandibular disorders and trigeminal autonomic cephalalgias (TAC) have been also defined. For more detailed description, see Chaps. 14 and 15 for TMD, Chap. 19 for neuralgias, Chap. 22 for migraine, Chap. 23 for cluster headaches and TAC, and Chap. 24 for migraine variants.

In clinical reality, primary chronic headache often appears as a complex blending of several diagnostic groupings of the IHS taxonomy. For example, most patients with chronic migraine have some headaches that diagnostically appear to be tension headache. Additionally, most patients with IHS migraine believe they have multiple types of headache [9] most commonly migraine, tension, and sinus, and indeed multiple studies support the idea that patients experience headaches with a wide array of vascular, muscular, and nasal/autonomic symptomatology [10]. This is particularly apparent as headache patterns become more chronic.

21.6 Rationale for Treatment

Evaluation of the patient with CDH requires a holistic approach and a willingness on the part of the medical provider to work as a partner with the patient. It also often requires providers to depart from a linear cause and effect model of disease to a model where multiple factors influence the etiology, outcome, and treatment. Conceptually, an individual patient may have multiple factors influencing their chronic headache, and each component needs to be dissected out, evaluated, and treated. For example, a patient with a traumatic injury to the cervical spine may quickly evolve into a daily headache pattern. However years of unresolved pain can be complicated by depression, disability, and medication overuse. Without addressing the complexity of all factors involved, the treatment outcome of such a patient is compromised. Consequently, many patients with CDH are best treated in interdisciplinary treatment models.

Most patients seeking medical care with chronic daily headache patterns require significant education, behavioral modification, a treatment plan that includes pharmacological and non-pharmacological approaches, and long-term follow-up and follow through. Common complicating factors to chronic daily headache include:

- Comorbid conditions including sinus disorders, temporomandibular disorders, and cervical injury

- Depression and anxiety
- Disability
- Inactivity and lack of exercise
- Medication overuse
- Dietary triggers including caffeine
- Oral parafunctional habits
- Postural habits

21.7 Treatment Options

Treatment needs to be directed at the underlying pain mechanisms whenever possible. The following treatment options should be considered:

1. Education that focuses on engaging the patient as a partner in management is critical to success. Each treatment plan should include behavioral therapies and lifestyle modification such as:
   - Exercise to improve posture, relaxation, and conditioning
   - Relaxation to reduce reaction to stressors and relax musculature
   - Positive self-talk to improve compliance and motivation for lifestyle modification
   - Regular healthy meals to reduce low glucose and other diet triggers
   - Oral habit reversal such as reduced clenching and bruxism
   - Caffeine reduction should be considered if a problem
   - The use of diary records to track medication use, triggering events or factors, compliance, and goals
2. Employing a treatment team is essential in more complicated cases. Members of an interdisciplinary team may often include:
   - Physician for medication management
   - Psychologist for implementing a cognitive behavioral program
   - Dentist to address masticatory dysfunction and temporomandibular disorders
   - Physical therapist to implement an exercise and postural program
   - Massage therapist to address muscular trigger points and relax muscles
   - Other medical or dental specialists to address specific patient needs
3. Pharmacologically, the emphasis is on prophylaxis rather than acute abortive interventions. However, this is not to imply that acute interventions are unnecessary or unimportant. A list of medications used for primary headaches is displayed in (Table 21.2). The choice of prophylactic medication is based largely on the presence of comorbid disorders and avoidance of adverse reactions. For example:
   - Patients with depression and terminal sleep disturbance may do best with a tricyclic antidepressant such as amitriptyline, 50 mg, or nortriptyline, 50 mg QHS.
   - Patients with mood swings may improve with a neuromodulator such as topiramate (100–200 mg/day), valproate sodium (800–1,500 mg/day), or gabapentin (1,000–2,500 mg per day).
   - Patients with obesity or concern about weight gain should avoid steroids and certain antidepressant medications.

Table 21.2 List of medications used for migraine, chronic daily headache, and migraine variants, variants

Anticonvulsants
Gabapentin (Neurontin)
Divalproex (Depakote)
Topiramate (Topamax)[a]
Valproate sodium (Depacon)[a]
Zonisamide (Zonegran)[a]
Triptans
Almotriptan (Axert)
Eletriptan (Relpax)
Frovatriptan (Frova)
Naratriptan (Amerge)
Rizatriptan (Maxalt, Maxalt-MLT)
Sumatriptan (Imitrex)
Zolmitriptan (Zomig, Zomig-ZMT)
Combination drugs
Acetaminophen/aspirin/caffeine (Excedrin Migraine, Excedrin Extra Strength tablets, capsules)
Acetaminophen/caffeine/butalbital
Aspirin/caffeine/butalbital (Fiorinal)
Dichloralphenazone/acetaminophen/ isometheptene (Duradin, Midrin, Migratine)
Ergotamine/caffeine
Other classes
Tricyclics such as Amitriptyline (Elavil, Endep)[a]
Aspirin
OnabotulinumtoxinA (Botox)
RimabotulinumtoxinB (Myobloc)[a]
Candesartan (Atacand)[a]
Coenzyme Q10[a]
Dihydroergotamine (DHE 45)
Ibuprofen (Advil Migraine, Motrin Migraine)
Naproxen sodium
Propranolol (Inderal)
Riboflavin[a]
Timolol (Blockadren)
Tizanidine (Zanaflex)[a]

[a]Unlabeled use

- Patients with morning sedation should avoid amitriptyline or other sedating tricyclics.

4. The need for acute therapy to quickly improve the condition is often paramount in the patient's mind, and it is essential to address directly. To do so, a clinician needs to take into consideration the following:
   - Overuse of analgesic and acute symptomatic medication as an etiological component of the headache pattern. Though somewhat controversial preventative medication may be started before discontinuing the offending acute medication but not in place of stopping it.

- When acute medication is prescribed, it is important to regularly assess its effectiveness and consistency over time. Providing appropriate formulations of abortive medications is also critical given the likelihood of GI impairment associated with chronic headache disorders.
- Prescribing acute therapy from a different pharmacological class is often necessary to disrupt the pharmacologically maintained headache cycle. For example, use bridge therapy to protect the patient through the period of analgesic withdrawal. Though not FDA approved for this indication, commonly used treatments include repeated doses of dihydroergotamine (DHE, 0.5–1 mg/dose IV, IM, SC, or intranasal), a rapid tapering schedule of dexamethasone (12 mg; 8 mg; 4 mg on successive mornings or a Depo Medrol Dosepak), or several consecutive days of a long-acting triptan such as naratriptan (1–2.5 mg/dose po) or frovatriptan (1–2.5 mg/dose po).
- Patients need to be followed regularly and given access to medical advice and prescription refills in order to avoid visits to the emergency departments or unscheduled visits to other providers during this time.
- Use of procedures such as occipital nerve blocks, trigger point injections, or sphenopalatine nerve blocks can also be useful for selected patients.
- OnabotulinumtoxinA can be used in chronic migraine and possibly chronic posttraumatic migraine when the headache has a migraine phenotype.

21.8 Treatment Goals and Sequencing of Care

The goal of treatment is to manage headache, not to cure it. It is important to define the specific goals and timetable with the patient. The following are important considerations in headache management:

- The most common primary management goals include preserve and restore function and establish a treatable episodic headache pattern.
- Tailor the goals whenever possible to ensure that patients participate in their implementation.
- Establishing a timetable to accomplish the goals in stages so that they are obtainable is essential. For example, reduce headaches to a mild headache a few times per week over the next 3 months.
- Patients with CDH often have long established histories of treatment failure. Typically, they have been managed in a linear treatment model where one thing is tried and observed over time to assess what the next step will be.
- Diagnostic workup should be completed quickly so that the therapeutic issues can be addressed without underlying fear that problems are being overlooked.
- Engage the patient in an interdisciplinary model where multiple facets of their headache are addressed simultaneously.
- Include daily behavioral changes for triggering or complicating factors.
- Maintain diaries with written goals that can be assessed regularly to motivate patients.
- With time, the prognosis for most patients is reasonably good.

References

1. Cady R, Schreiber C, Farmer K, Sheftell F. Primary headaches: a convergence hypothesis. Headache. 2002;42:204–16.
2. Cady RK, Schreiber CP, Farmer KU. Understanding the migraine patient: the evolution from episodic headache to chronic neurological disease. Headache J Head Face Pain. 2004;44:426–35.
3. Bigal ME, Rapoport AM, Sheftell FD, Tepper SJ, Lipton RB. Transformed migraine and medication overuse in a tertiary headache centre clinical characteristics and treatment outcomes. Cephalalgia. 2004;24(6):483–90.
4. Scher AI, Stewart WF, Ricci JA, Lipton RB. Factors associated with the onset and remission of chronic daily headache in a population-based study. Pain. 2003;106:81–9.
5. Lipton RB, Fanning KM, Serrano D, Reed ML, Cady R, Buse DC. Ineffective acute treatment of episodic migraine is associated with new-onset chronic migraine. Neurology. 2015;84:688–95.
6. Cady RK, Lipton RB, Rothrock JF. Chronic migraine: a patient-centered guide to effective management. Hamilton: Baxter Publishing; 2013.
7. International headache Society. Classification and diagnostic criteria for headache disorders, cranial neuralgias and facial pain. Cephalalgia. 1988;8(Suppl 7):1–96.
8. Headache Classification Subcommittee of the International Headache Society. The international classification of headache disorders. 2nd edition. Cephalalgia. 2004;24(suppl 1):1–160.
9. Diamond ML. The role of concomitant headache types and non-headache co-morbidities in the underdiagnosis of migraine. Neurology. 2002;58:S3–9.
10. Schreiber CP, Hutchinson S, Webster C, et al. Prevalence of migraine in patients with a history of self-reported or physician-diagnosed "sinus" headache. Arch Intern Med. 2004;164:1769–72.

Migraine

22

Steven B. Graff-Radford†

Pearls of Wisdom

- Migraine is typically a very disabling primary headache disorder that unfortunately remains underdiagnosed and untreated.
- There is no cure for migraine; nevertheless there are numerous interventions that may help restore an improve life for sufferers. These measures should consider the patient in as broad an aspect as possible.
- Triggering factors, neurogenic inflammation, vascular changes, and pain transmission should all be addressed aggressively.
- Individualizing treatment and use of multiple modalities is essential.

22.1 Introduction and Diagnostic Subtypes

Migraine is one of the most common primary headache disorders with high levels of personal disability [1, 2]. It may be very disabling secondary to the pain and associated symptoms including nausea, vomiting, visual aura, and photo- and phonophobia. Missed work and lost productivity secondary to migraine create a significant public burden at great cost. Nevertheless, migraine still remains largely undertreated and underdiagnosed [3]. Less than half the sufferers are diagnosed by their physicians. Migraine must be differentiated from secondary headache disorders. The International Headache Society has put forward specific criteria for headache classification in 1988 [4]. These are currently being revised in a 3rd edition (Beta version) [5]." Please keep the reference intact.

†Author was deceased at the time of publication.

S.B. Graff-Radford, DDS
The Pain Center, UCLA School of Dentistry, Los Angeles, CA, USA
e-mail: denjnarf@nus.edu.sg

J.N.A.R. Ferreira et al. (eds.), *Orofacial Disorders*,
DOI 10.1007/978-3-319-51508-3_22

Table 22.1 Migraine headache subcategories

1. Migraine without aura
2. Migraine with aura
3. Childhood periodic syndromes that are commonly precursors of migraine
3.1. Cyclical vomiting
3.2. Abdominal migraine
3.3. Benign paroxysmal vertigo of childhood
4. Retinal migraine
5. Complications of migraine
5.1. Chronic migraine
5.2 Status migrainosus
5.3. Persistent aura without infarction
5.4. Migraine infarction
5.5. Migraine-triggered seizure
6. Probable migraine

Part I: The primary headaches.
Part II: The secondary headaches.
Part III: Cranial neuralgias, central and primary facial pain, and other headaches. Despite the fact that all pain in the head and face is conducted by the trigeminal nerve, the classification allows for clinical symptoms to be subclassified. This enables each classified entity to be studied, helping determine the pathophysiology and ultimately the treatment.

The subcategories of migraine are listed in Table 22.1.

22.2 Clinical Presentation

Migraine may be very disabling secondary to the pain and associated symptoms including:

- Throbbing headache
- Unilateral location
- Moderate to severe in intensity
- Aggravated by routine physical activity
- Nausea and vomiting
- Photophobia and phonophobia

Aura occurs in approximately 10% of migraine sufferers about 10% of the time. The aura is characterized by recurrent attack of reversible focal neurological symptoms that develop over 5–20 min and last less than 60 min. Migraine presents itself in four clinical stages:

- Stage 1 – Premonitory stage. Patients during this phase complain of tiredness and a craving for sweet or salty foods; they are more moody and don't function as well as normal.
- Stage 2 – Aura. Aura symptoms are described as visual disturbances such as flashing lights (scotoma), a zigzag pattern (fortification spectra), or other visual or sensory changes. The aura usually starts in the middle of the visual field and progresses outward until it disappears. The aura is thought to be caused by an electrical cortical spread described as similar to the spreading depression of Leao. This cortical depolarization is followed by a decrease in cortical blood flow. Aura occurs in 10–20% of migraine patients about 10% of the time.
- Stage 3 – Headache. The pain is started by a change in the brain, known as the migraine generator. This area as seen in sophisticated imaging studies is located in the brainstem and is likely a lack of central inhibition. It results in an inflammation around the brain blood vessels and results in pain messages perceived as throbbing headache.
- Stage 4 – Recovery. During this phase there is normalization and functional restoration.

22.2.1 Etiology and Epidemiology

Migraine generally begins in childhood to early adulthood. While migraines can first occur in an individual beyond the age of 50, advancing age makes other types of headaches more likely. Evaluation for secondary headache should nevertheless be considered if it is a new onset headache below age 5 or over age 50. According to the Global Burden of Disease Survey 2010, migraine was ranked as the third most prevalent disorder and seventh-highest specific cause of disability globally [6].

A family history is usually present, suggesting a genetic predisposition in migraine sufferers. In addition to diagnosing migraine from the clinical presentation, there should be an accompanying normal examination.

Patients with the first headache ever, worst headache ever, or where there is a significant change in headache or the presence of neurological symptoms like visual or hearing or sensory loss may require additional tests. The tests may include blood testing, brain scanning (either CT or MRI), and a spinal tap. Migraine occurs more frequently in females than males. Waters' data indicates the prevalence of migraine as approximately 30% of women and 17% of men in the third decade, 26% vs. 16% in the fourth decade, 17% vs. 13% in the fifth, and 10% vs. 5% after age 75 [7]. A genetic factor or familial history is present in most migraineurs. The migraine occurs commonly in the first four life decades, then the frequency decreases [8]. A small group of migraineurs transforms into chronic daily headache now classified as chronic migraine (ICHD classification 1.5). Chronic migraine requires headache more than 15 days per month, at least eight fulfilling criteria for migraine and headache should last more than 4 h.

22.3 Pathophysiology and Mechanisms

Migraine pathophysiology is best discussed using the various clinical stages as a guide. The migraine problem has four stages referred to as the premonitory stage, the aura stage, and the headache and the recovery stages [9].

Stage 1 – Premonitory stage. The clinical presentation associated with alteration in mood is attributed to changes occurring in the hypothalamus [9]. Little is known as to how this is initiated, but it is postulated that migraine sufferers are genetically predisposed and that emotional, hormonal, or other triggering factors spark the cascade leading to pain.

Stage 2 – Aura. The aura is associated with a brain neural depolarization beginning in the occipital cortex and resultant spreading oligemia (reduction in cerebral blood flow). Woods and colleagues reported changes in regional blood flow in a migraine volunteer using a PET study [10]. This patient did not have an aura, only transient visual disturbance, suggesting the blood flow changes occur in migraine with and without aura. Migraine with aura may be associated with a state of neuronal hyperexcitability linked to N-methyl-D-aspartate (NMDA) [11]. This requires the presence of low magnesium levels and glutamate. It is unlikely the headache is due to the blood flow reduction followed by reflex vasodilatation as the pain develops while the reduction in flow is present. Most clinicians believe the aura symptoms are due to neuronal dysfunction and not ischemia [9].

Stage 3 – Headache. Moskowitz has proposed that the pain perceived in migraine is due to trigeminal neuronal activation surrounding cephalic blood vessels [12]. This system may be activated through (a) biomechanical modulation (hormones, mast cell constituents, alcohol and drugs, platelet contents, foods), (b) mechanical modulation (stretch), (c) ionic modulation (spreading depression), (d) neural modulation (opiate containing fibers, sympathetic and parasympathetic), and (e) central modulation (periaqueductal gray, special senses such as light and sound, altered physiologic states such as sleep and stress). Serotonin and unstable serotonergic neurotransmission have been implicated in the migraine hypothesis [13]. Although there is compelling evidence for serotonin having some role, the exact mechanism has not been identified but may involve effects on the raphe nuclei, platelets, and other sites where serotonin receptors are present. Serotonin agonists such as ergots and the triptans (sumatriptan, naratriptan, zolmitriptan, rizatriptan, and eletriptan) support the serotonergic system role in migraine [9]. There needs to be an altered state of neural excitability causing a change in neurochemistry and neurophysiology. Signals are sent from the "migraine generator" located in the dorsal raphae nucleus and in the dorsal pons [14]. These signals arrive at peripheral perivascular nerve terminals causing release of vasodilators and nerve sensitizing peptides, substance P, calcitonin gene-related peptide (CGRP), and neurokinin A [12]. This plasma extravasation may be produced by nitric oxide [15]. The ensuing vasodilatation and neurogenic inflammation causes nociceptive activation of trigeminal sensory pathways (c fibers). Thus, the pain message is relayed to the trigeminal nucleus, thalamus, and cortex. Recently Burstein has demonstrated the understanding that the peripheral neuronal sensitization can be significantly attenuated by the triptans providing they are used before central sensitization occurs. Clinically this sensitization is seen as an ipsilateral allodynia, which can progress to an extracephalic allodynia if thalamic sensitization occurs [16–18].

Stage 4 – Recovery. During this phase there is a renormalization of brain hyperexcitability and functional restoration.

22.4 Diagnosis and Diagnostic Criteria

While diagnosis is made primarily through history and the ruling out of secondary headache, it is suggested that if patients present with intermittent recurrent headache, asking three questions about three characteristic symptoms can provide a very high probability of making a migraine diagnosis:

1. About nausea: Are you nauseated or sick to your stomach when you have headache?
2. About disability: Has a headache limited your activities for a day or more in the last 3 months?
3. About photophobia: Does light bother you when you have a headache?

As a result, if two out of these three symptoms above are present, then there will be a 93% positive predictive value; if three out of three symptoms, a 98% positive predictive value [19].

22.5 Rationale for Treatment

Treatment can be acute, preemptive, or preventive. *Acute* treatment is initiated during an attack to relieve pain and disability and to stop progression of the attack. *Preemptive* treatment is used when a known headache trigger exists, such as exercise or sexual activity, and for patients experiencing a time-limited exposure to a trigger, such as ascent to a high altitude or menstruation. *Preventive* treatment is maintained for months or even years to reduce attack frequency, severity, and duration. Patients taking preventive medication can also use acute and preemptive medication [20–22].

One of the important parts in managing patients with migraine is to help them learn how to manage their own illness. This includes educating them about the cascade of events that occurs with each attack. Understanding that early treatment will improve response to therapy is an important component to also realizing that this approach will lead to less medication use and less disability. Learning how to recognize migraine vs. other headache types (e.g., tension-type headache) will also help the patient to know when to take a migraine-specific medication or other analgesic. Preliminary studies have been done that assess the efficacy of giving triptans during an aura. When given during an aura, triptans do not show consistent efficacy in aborting or preventing the migraine. Therefore, until further studies are done, it is also helpful to educate the patient to not take their triptan during the aura phase but rather early in the pain phase of the attack.

22.6 Treatment Options

22.6.1 Pharmacological Therapy

A number of medications are available to treat migraine, and choice depends on the severity and frequency of headaches (see Table 22.2). These categories of medications include nonspecific and specific treatments:

Table 22.2 Pharmacological agents used in migraine management

Acute therapies
A. NSAIDs as initial therapy
Aspirin, 325–975 mg/dose po
Ibuprofen, 400–800 mg/dose po
Naproxen sodium, 375–550 mg/dose po
Combination of acetaminophen/aspirin/caffeine, 2 tablets po
B. Migraine-specific agents when NSAIDs are ineffective
Dihydroergotamine, 0.5–1 mg/dose intranasally or parentally
Naratriptan, 1–2.5 mg/dose po
Sumatriptan, 50–100 mg/dose po or 6 mg/dose SC
Combination sumatriptan 85 mg/naproxen sodium 500 mg po
Rizatriptan, 5–10 mg/dose po
Zolmitriptan, 2.5–5 mg/dose po
Eletriptan, 20–40 mg po
Diclofenac powder 50 mg po (dissolved in water)
Preventive therapies
Amitriptyline, 25–150 mg/day[a]
Nortriptyline 10–100 mg/day
Venlafaxine 37.5–150 mg/day[a]
Divalproex sodium, 500–1,500 mg/day
Gabapentin 500–2,000 mg/day[a]
Topiramate 100–200 mg/day
Propranolol, 80–240 mg/day
Timolol, 20–30 mg/day
Atenolol 25–150 mg/day
Nadolol 10–20 mg/day
Candesartan 4–16 mg/day[a]
Verapamil 40–240 mg/day[a]
Methylergonovine 0.2–1.2 mg/day[a]
Memantine 5–20 mg/day[a]
Magnesium 400 mg/day[a]
Riboflavin 400 mg/day[a]
Petadolex 50–75 mg/day[a]
Preventative therapy for Chronic migraine
Onabotulinum toxin (Botox) 155 units

[a]Unlabeled use

A. Nonspecific therapeutic treatments are those effective for any pain disorder and include:
   - Nonsteroidal anti-inflammatory drugs (NSAIDs)
   - Combination analgesics
   - Opioids
   - Neuroleptics/antiemetics
   - Corticosteroids
B. Specific therapeutic agents are those specifically effective for migraine and related disorders [23] and include:
   - Ergotamine-containing compounds
   - DHE
   - Triptans

For patients with early or significant nausea or vomiting, select a non-oral route of administration. Use of transcutaneous and nasal spray on subcutaneous administration may be beneficial.

22.6.1.1 Acute Therapy

Triptans, as a class, represent a significant advancement in the therapeutic management of migraine. These agents have been described as receptor-specific agonists toward serotonin or 5-HT receptors. Specifically, they are selective 5-HT1B/1D agonists having the greatest affinity for these receptors. Blockade of 5-HT1 receptors has been shown to result in acute migraine relief.

- Triptans, relative to nonspecific therapies, including analgesics and NSAIDs, provide rapid onset of action (between 15 min and 1 h, depending on the formulation), are highly effective in relieving migraine pain symptoms, and have a favorable side effect profile.
- All agents in this class have proven therapeutic efficacy (see Table 22.1).
- In the majority of patients, the intensity of adverse effects is mild and of short duration. Adverse effects can include chest pressure, flushing, dizziness, drowsiness, and nausea. Patients who are at risk for coronary heart disease, diabetes, obesity, severe uncontrolled hypertension, or hypercholesterolemia should be screened prior to administration of triptans [9, 24].

22.6.1.2 Preventive Therapy

The major medication groups for preventive migraine treatment include anticonvulsants, ß-adrenergic blockers and calcium channel antagonists, NSAIDs, serotonin antagonists, and others (including riboflavin, minerals, herbs). Preventive medications are taken whether or not headache is present in an attempt to reduce the frequency and perhaps the severity and duration of anticipated attacks. Onabotulinum toxin is the only agent approved for prevention of chronic migraine [25].

A preventive migraine drug could raise the threshold to activation of the migraine process either centrally or peripherally. Drugs conceivably can decrease activation of the migraine generator, enhance central antinociception, raise the threshold for spreading depression, and stabilize the more sensitive migrainous nervous system by changing sympathetic or serotonergic tone.

Preventive drugs most likely work by more than one mechanism. The drugs could, in part, have a peripheral mechanism of action similar to specific acute medications [24, 26–28].

If preventive medication is indicated, the agent preferentially should be chosen from one of the first-line categories, based on the drug's side effect profile and the patient's coexistent and comorbid conditions.

- Preventative therapy should be initiated with the lowest effective dose of the chosen pharmacologic agent.
- Increase the dose slowly until clinical benefits are achieved in the absence of adverse events or until limited by adverse events. Give each treatment an adequate trial. Avoid interfering medications (i.e., overuse of certain acute medications, such as ergotamine and caffeine).
- Monitor compliance. A clinical benefit may take as long as 2–3 months to become apparent. Patients commonly take new treatments for 1–2 weeks without seeing an effect and then discontinue prematurely, with both the physician and patient believing the medication was not effective. Long-acting formulations may improve compliance.
- Maximize compliance by discussing the following with the patient:
  - Rationale for the particular treatment.
  - When and how to use the treatment.
  - Adverse effects that may be likely.
  - Address and establish patient expectations: Discuss the expected benefits of therapy and how long it will take to achieve them, and create a formal management plan based on patient preferences.
- Use daily diary – Monitor the patient's headache by having them keep a user-friendly diary to measure attack frequency, severity, duration, disability, response to type of treatment, and adverse medication effects.
- After a period of stability, consider tapering or discontinuing treatment [24, 26, 27].

22.6.1.3 Considering Coexisting Diseases

Some comorbid conditions are more common in persons with migraine. These conditions include stroke, myocardial infarction, Raynaud's phenomenon, epilepsy, affective disorders, and anxiety disorders. Coexisting diseases present both treatment opportunities and limitations.

- Once the coexistent condition has been identified, select a pharmacologic agent that will treat both disorders.
- Establish that the coexistent disease is not a contraindication for the selected migraine therapies (e.g., β-blockers are contraindicated in patients with asthma).

- Ensure that treatments being used for coexistent conditions do not exacerbate migraine.
- Beware of interactions between pharmacologic agents used for migraine and those used for other conditions. Special attention should be directed to women who are pregnant or want to become pregnant. Preventive migraine medications may have teratogenic effects. If treatment is absolutely necessary, select a treatment with the lowest risk of adverse effects to the fetus [27] or select non-pharmacologic interventions.

22.6.2 Non-pharmacological Therapy

Non-pharmacological, behavioral, and physical techniques should be emphasized in the management of headache particularly with those occurring in pregnant women. These methods should be considered for use with all migraine sufferers as part of a rehabilitation team approach. Even if they are incompletely effective, they may provide important augmentative benefits to pharmacological therapy. Strategies that are found to be useful in migraine management include:

- Biofeedback including both temperature and electromyography control.
- Physical therapy including stretching, aerobic, and postural exercise.
- Relaxation techniques of many varieties. In one study, pregnant patients treated with physical therapy, relaxation, and biofeedback had an 81.2% reduction in headache compared to a 32.7% reduction in a control population. Third party payers that generally do not provide coverage for these methods of treatment will often approve exceptions for pregnant patients, in an effort to avoid medication use.
- Trigger point injections – In women with identifiable trigger points, local anesthetic infiltration can be safely performed during pregnancy.
- "Avoidance therapy," involving the identification and elimination of headache trigger factors such as excess caffeine, lack of sleep, or skipping meals, should also be emphasized.
- A temporary reduction in work hours or a medical leave of absence from work may also be useful in avoiding the need for pharmacologic treatment of headaches.

22.7 Treatment Goals and Sequencing of Care

22.7.1 Goals

The goals of treatment are to:

1. Relieve or prevent the pain and associated symptoms of migraine
2. Optimize the patient's ability to function normally

22.7.2 Stratified Approach

With use of pharmacological agents, a stratification approach, in which definitive successful treatment is used early in the course of the disease and early in the evolution of each attack, as opposed to the step-care approach, in which less powerful or nonselective drugs are tried first and if not working progress to more potent agents. Not only are lower potency agents may be less efficacious in some patients, but if they do not work, the patient often does not return to the office. Patients with less severe migraine may obtain adequate relief from an NSAID. Patients with moderate to severe migraine benefit from using a triptan as a first-line agent.

22.7.3 Evaluating Therapy

It is important to give sufficient trial to the initial acute medication agent. Treat at least two or three attacks before judging the effectiveness of the therapeutic choice. If treatment is not working, consider the following:

- *Reconsider diagnosis*: Secondary headaches, although not as common, may present with clinical signs and symptoms that resemble migraine.
- *Treat early*: Recent studies, both prospective and retrospective, support improved response to triptan therapy when patients treat early in the course of an attack. This is especially pertinent in those who are at risk of developing cutaneous allodynia. Triptans have been shown to be less effective in patients who develop cutaneous allodynia in association with their migraine (summarized below).
- *Dose and route of administration*: If the patient is experiencing some relief from the current medication, would a higher dose be more efficacious? If the patient requires more rapid onset of pain relief, would a nasal spray or an injectable formulation of the present medication suffice?
- *Choice of drug*: If a nonspecific agent, such as a combination analgesic, is being used, would another nonspecific medication, such as an opioid, or a specific medication, such as a triptan, be more effective?
- *Adverse drug interactions*: Investigate the use of interfering medications, including other over-the-counter analgesics and medications for depression and heart disease.
- *Adjunctive therapy*: Patients experiencing nausea and vomiting may benefit from the addition of adjunctive antiemetics.
- *Additionally*, be sure there are no other medications that may be exacerbating or triggering migraine (e.g., caffeine, herbal preparations, oral contraceptives, among others) [21].

References

1. Vos T, et al. Years lived with disability (YLDs) for 1160 sequelae of 289 diseases and injuries 1990-2010: a systematic analysis for the Global Burden of Disease Study 2010. Lancet. 2012;380(9859):2163–96.
2. Lipton RB, Stewart WF, Diamond S, et al. Prevalence and burden of migraine in the United States: data from the American Migraine Study II. Headache. 2001;41(7):646–57.
3. Lipton RB, Scher AI, Kolodner K, et al. Migraine in the United States: epidemiology and patterns of health care use. Neurology. 2002;58(6):885–94.
4. Headache Classification Subcommittee of the International Headache Society. The international classification of headache disorders. Cephalalgia. 1988;8(Suppl 7):1–96.
5. Headache Classification Subcommittee of the International Headache Society. The international classification of headache disorders. Cephalalgia. 2004;24(Suppl 1):160. Headache Classification Subcommittee of the International Headache Society. The international classification of headache disorders, 3rd edition (beta version). Cephalalgia. 2013:33:629–808.
6. GBD 2015 Disease and Injury Incidence and Prevalence Collaborators. Global, regional, and national incidence, prevalence, and years lived with disability for 310 diseases and injuries, 1990-2015: a systematic analysis for the Global Burden of Disease Study 2015. Lancet. 2016;388(10053):1545–1602.
7. Waters WE. Headache (series in clinical epidemiology). London: Croom Helm; 1986.
8. Selby G, Lance JW. Observations on 500 cases of migraine and allied vascular headache. J Neurol Neurosurg Psychiatry. 1960;47:23–32.
9. Silberstein SD, Lipton RB, Goadsby PJ. Headache in clinical practice. Oxford: ISIS Medical Media; 1998.
10. Woods RP, Iacoboni M, Maziotta JC. Bilateral spreading cerebral hypoperfusion during spontaneous migraine headache. N Engl J Med. 1994;331:1689–92.
11. Moskowitz MA, Henrikson BM, Markowitz S, Saito K. Intra- and extravascular nociceptive mechanisms and the pathogenesis of head pain. In: Olsen J, Edvinsson L, editors. Basic mechanisms of headache. Amsterdam: Elsevier; 1988. p. 429.
12. Moskowitz MA, Cutrer FM. Sumatriptan: a receptor-targeted treatment for migraine. Annu Rev Med. 1993;44:145–54.
13. Peroutka SJ. The pharmacology of current antimigraine drugs. Headache. 1990;30(Suppl 1):5–11.
14. Weiller C, May A, Limmeroth, et al. Brain stem activation in spontaneous human migraine attacks. Nat Med. 1995;1:658–60.
15. Strassman AM, Raymond SA, Burstein R. Sensitization of meningeal sensory neurons and the origin of headaches. Nature. 1996;384:560–3.
16. Burstein R. Deconstructing migraine headache into peripheral and central sensitization. Pain. 2000;89:107–10.
17. Burstein R, Yarnitsky D, Goor-Aryeh I, et al. An association between migraine and cutaneous allodynia. Ann Neurol. 2000;47:614–24.
18. Burstein R, Jukubowski M, Burstein R. Analgesic Triptan action in animal model of intracranial pain: a race against the development of central sensitization. Ann Neurol. 2004;55: 27–36.
19. Lipton RB, Dodick D, Sadosvsky R, Kolodner K, Endicott J, Hettiarachchi J, Harrison W. A self-administered screener for migraine in primary care: the ID MigraineTM validation study. Neurology. 2003;61:375–82.
20. Silberstein SD. Preventive treatment of migraine: an overview. Cephalalgia. 1997;17(2):67–72.
21. Silberstein SD, Saper JR, Freitag FG. Migraine diagnosis and treatment. In: Silberstein SD, Lipton RB, Dalessio DE, editors. Wolff's headache and other head pain. 7th ed. Oxford: Oxford University Press; 2001. p. 121–237.

22. Silberstein SD, Goadsby PJ. Migraine: preventive treatment. Cephalalgia. 2002;22(7):491–512.
23. Diener HC, Kaube H, Limmroth V. A practical guide to the management and prevention of migraine. Drugs. 1998;56(5):811–24.
24. Silberstein SD. Practice parameter: evidence-based guidelines for migraine headache (an evidence-based review): report of the Quality Standards Subcommittee of the American Academy of Neurology. Neurology. 2000a;55(6):754–62.
25. Dodick DW, Turkel CC, DeGryse RE, Aurora SK, Silberstein SD, Lipton RB, Diener H-C, Brin MF. OnabotulinumtoxinA for treatment of chronic migraine: pooled results from the double-blind, randomized, placebo-controlled phases of the PREEMPT clinical program. Headache J Head Face Pain. 2010;50(6):921–36.
26. Gray RN, Goslin RE, McCrory DC, et al. Drug treatments for the prevention of migraine headache. technical review 2.3. Duke University: US Dept of Health and Human Services, Agency for Health Care Policy and Research; February 1999. NTIS Accession No. PB99–127953. Available at: http://www.clinpol.mc.duke.edu/.
27. Ramadan NM, Silberstein SD, Freitag FG, Gilbert TT, Frishberg BM. Evidence-based guidelines for migraine headache in prevention of migraine. Neurology [serial online]. Available at: http://www.neurology.org. Accessed 25 Apr 2000.
28. Snow V, Weiss K, Wall E, et al. Pharmacologic management of acute attacks of migraine and prevention of migraine headache. Ann Intern Med. 2002;137:840–9.

Cluster and Facial Headache

23

Robert G. Kaniecki

Pearls of Wisdom

- Trigeminal autonomic cephalalgias (TACs) are primary headache disorders characterized by unilateral head pain of varying duration associated with ipsilateral cranial autonomic features.
- TACs differ primarily in episode duration, frequency, and periodicity.
- Cluster headache and short-lasting unilateral neuralgiform headache with conjunctival injection and tearing (SUNCT) are more common among men, while chronic paroxysmal hemicrania (CPH) and hemicrania continua (HC) among women.
- The duration of headache attacks (15–180 min) helps differentiate cluster headache from the other TACs and also from migraine headache (4–72 h).
- SUNCT is best differentiated from trigeminal neuralgia (TN) by location of pain (V1 versus V2–V3 for TN) and the prominent ipsilateral autonomic features (rare in TN).
- Cerebral blood flow studies reveal hyperactivation of the hypothalamus ipsilateral to the pain in cluster headache, contralateral to the pain in CPH and HC, and bilateral in SUNCT.
- Oxygen therapy and subcutaneous sumatriptan are the agents of choice for the treatment of acute attacks of cluster headache.
- Prevention of cluster headache is most frequently accomplished with short-term corticosteroids and long-term verapamil. Electrocardiographic monitoring is necessary for those patients with cluster headache requiring verapamil doses greater than 240 mg.

R.G. Kaniecki, MD
Department of Neurology, University of Pittsburgh, Pittsburgh, PA, USA
e-mail: kanieckirg@upmc.edu

J.N.A.R. Ferreira et al. (eds.), *Orofacial Disorders*,
DOI 10.1007/978-3-319-51508-3_23

- Paroxysmal hemicrania and hemicrania continua are prevented absolutely by therapeutic doses of indomethacin. Co-administration of a proton pump inhibitor may improve the tolerability of long-term indomethacin dosing.
- SUNCT is the most brief, least common, and most refractory TAC. Lamotrigine is the treatment of choice.

23.1 Introduction and Diagnostic Subtypes

Although occasionally seen after an isolated incident, most patients with head or facial pain will present with patterns of recurrent or chronic discomfort. The vast majority will present with a primary headache disorder arising from a biological disorder of the brain. Formal criteria for the diagnosis of primary and secondary headache disorders were recently updated in the International Classification of Headache Disorders, third edition, beta version (ICHD-3 beta). Among the four primary headache categories, migraine headaches and tension-type headaches are much more common than the trigeminal autonomic cephalalgias (TACs). These conditions share in common attacks of head pain localized mainly in the distribution of the ophthalmic branch of the trigeminal nerve accompanied by one or more ipsilateral cranial autonomic symptoms (Tables 23.1–23.4).

Cluster headache is the most common and well-recognized form of trigeminal autonomic cephalalgia. Previously known as Horton's headache or Sluder's

Table 23.1 ICHD-3 diagnostic criteria for cluster headache

A. At least five attacks fulfilling criteria B–D
B. Severe or very severe unilateral orbital, supraorbital, and/or temporal pain lasting 15–180 min (when untreated)
C. Either or both of the following:
1. At least one of the following symptoms or signs, ipsilateral to the headache:
(a) Conjunctival injection and/or lacrimation
(b) Nasal congestion and/or rhinorrhea
(c) Eyelid edema
(d) Forehead and facial sweating
(e) Forehead and facial flushing
(f) Sensation of fullness in the ear
(g) Miosis and/or ptosis
2. A sense of restlessness or agitation
D. Attack frequency from one every other day to eight per day when the disorder is active
E. Not better accounted for by another ICHD-3 diagnosis

Adapted with permission from Headache Classification Subcommittee of the International Headache Society [7]

ICHD-3 International Classification of Headache Disorders, third edition

Table 23.2 ICHD-3 diagnostic criteria for paroxysmal hemicrania

A. At least 20 attacks fulfilling criteria B–E
B. Severe unilateral orbital, supraorbital, and/or temporal pain lasting 2–30 min
C. At least one of the following symptoms or signs, ipsilateral to the pain:
1. Conjunctival injection and/or lacrimation
2. Nasal congestion and/or rhinorrhea
3. Eyelid edema
4. Forehead and facial sweating
5. Forehead and facial flushing
6. Sensation of fullness in the ear
7. Miosis and/or ptosis
D. Attacks have a frequency above five per day for more than half the time
E. Attacks are prevented absolutely by therapeutic doses of indomethacin
F. Not better accounted for by another ICHD-3 diagnosis

Adapted with permission from Headache Classification Subcommittee of the International Headache Society [7]
ICHD-3 International Classification of Headache Disorders, third edition

Table 23.3 ICHD-3 diagnostic criteria for short-lasting unilateral neuralgiform headache

A. At least 20 attacks fulfilling criteria B-D
B. Moderate or severe unilateral head pain, with orbital, supraorbital, temporal, and/or trigeminal distribution, lasting for 1–600 s and occurring as single stabs, series of stabs, or in a sawtooth pattern
C. At least one of the following symptoms or signs, ipsilateral to the pain:
1. Conjunctival injection and/or lacrimation
2. Nasal congestion and/or rhinorrhea
3. Eyelid edema
4. Forehead and facial sweating
5. Forehead and facial flushing
6. Sensation of fullness in the ear
7. Miosis and/or ptosis
D. Attacks have a frequency of at least once a day for more than half of the time when the disorder is active
E. Not better accounted for by another ICHD-3 diagnosis

Adapted with permission from Headache Classification Subcommittee of the International Headache Society [7]
ICHD-3 International Classification of Headache Disorders, third edition

neuralgia, cluster headache is characterized by unilateral short-duration attacks of severe head pain associated with prominent ipsilateral autonomic symptoms. Episodic cluster typically occurs in periods lasting from 1–12 weeks, separated by pain-free periods lasting at least 1 month. When headache attacks occur for more than 1 year without remission, or when remission periods last less than 1 month, the term chronic cluster is applied. Less common are the other trigeminal autonomic cephalalgias: paroxysmal hemicranias (PH), also divided into episodic (EPH) and chronic (CPH) forms by criteria identical to that for cluster; short-lasting unilateral neuralgiform headache with conjunctival injection and

Table 23.4 ICHD-3 diagnostic criteria for hemicrania continua

A. Unilateral headache fulfilling criteria B–D
B. Present for >3 months with exacerbations of moderate or greater intensity
C. Either or both of the following:
1. At least one of the following symptoms or signs, ipsilateral to the headache:
(a) Conjunctival injection and/or lacrimation
(b) Nasal congestion and/or rhinorrhea
(c) Eyelid edema
(d) Forehead and facial sweating
(e) Forehead and facial flushing
(f) Sensation of fullness in the ear
(g) Miosis and/or ptosis
2. A sense of restlessness or agitation or aggravation of the pain by movement
D. Responds absolutely to therapeutic doses of indomethacin
E. Not better accounted for by another ICHD-3 diagnosis

Adapted with permission from Headache Classification Subcommittee of the International Headache Society [7]
ICHD-3 International Classification of Headache Disorders, third edition

tearing (SUNCT) and the related short-lasting unilateral neuralgiform headache with cranial autonomic features (SUNA); and hemicrania continua (HC). PH and SUNCT/SUNA appear phenotypically similar to cluster headache but are shorter in duration and typically recur at a higher frequency [14]. It is crucial to distinguish among the various TAC subtypes since management strategies differ significantly. Unlike the other TACs, hemicrania continua is characterized by baseline constant or nearly continuous unilateral head discomfort. It was recently reclassified as a TAC with the rationale that the pain is typically strictly unilateral and accompanied by ipsilateral cranial autonomic symptoms [2].

23.2 Clinical Presentation

The location and description of pain and variety of autonomic symptoms are similar among the TACs [12]. The most intense area of pain typically is centered near the temple and orbit, with occasional patients reporting facial, more widespread hemicranial, or occipital radiation. The discomfort is nearly always intense and often described as stabbing, searing, boring, or throbbing. Accompanying the pain is any combination of the following cranial autonomic features: conjunctival injection or lacrimation, nasal congestion or rhinorrhea, eyelid edema, forehead or facial flushing or sweating, miosis, ptosis, or a sense of ear fullness. A sense of restlessness or agitation also is frequently reported. In HC the autonomic features may only be seen during moderate-to-severe exacerbations of the underlying chronic head pain, at which point migraine-like symptoms may also be described. Unlike the other TACs, hemicrania continua patients may describe aggravation of pain with physical activity. A foreign body sensation in the ipsilateral eye, similar in feeling to a grain of sand, is not listed among the criteria for HC but is quite common.

The TACs will differ significantly in episode duration, frequency, and periodicity [6]. Cluster may last 15–180 min and recur one to eight times daily over a span of weeks to months. PH attacks last 2–30 min and recur up to 40 times per day, while SUNCT/SUNA attacks last 1–600 s and may recur more than 100 times daily. Both PH and SUNCT/SUNA possess temporal profiles extending over months to years and sometimes decades. SUNA differs from SUNCT in that it is diagnosed when only one cranial autonomic symptom, conjunctival injection or tearing, is present [3]. Also, the duration of SUNA attacks seems a bit longer, sometimes extending toward 10 min. Paroxysms of the chronic pain in HC may last 30 min to 3 days and often are accompanied by features suggestive of migraine. Precipitating factors also are varied among the TACs. Alcohol only appears to be a trigger for cluster and PH, neck movement only for PH and SUNCT/SUNA, and local cutaneous stimulation only for SUNCT/SUNA. There are no reliable exacerbating factors in HC. By definition, PH and HC are completely responsive to therapeutic doses of indomethacin. Consequently, most guidelines recommend a therapeutic challenge of indomethacin to any patient presenting with a persistently side-locked hemicranial headache disorder.

Migraine is the most common headache disorder seen by physicians, and unilateral pain is typical, while autonomic symptoms may be seen in up to half of patients. Cluster headache may be occasionally misdiagnosed as episodic migraine and hemicrania continua as chronic migraine. Duration of pain (migraine attacks 4–72 h) and the presence of bilateral autonomic complaints when present (more typical of migraine) should aid in the distinction.

23.3 Etiology and Epidemiology

- Cluster headache is the most common TAC, annually affecting 0.1% (124/100,000) of the general population. It preferentially affects males in a ratio of approximately 3:1. Age of onset is typically in the second to fourth decade of life. A slight genetic predisposition may exist, with 5–10% of patients reporting an affected first-degree relative. Tobacco use is a risk factor for cluster headache development.
- PH is significantly less common with an annual prevalence of 2/100,000.
- CPH is seen more commonly in women with a 2:1 ratio versus men, while EPH is evenly distributed between the sexes. No additional risk factors, including any genetic contribution, have been linked to PH.
- SUNCT/SUNA patients are even rarer, with an estimated population prevalence of 1/100,000. SUNCT is seen slightly more frequently in men at a ratio of 1.5:1, and the age of onset of near 50 years is later than either cluster or PH. No genetic links or environmental risk factors have been identified. The incidence and prevalence of HC have not been well established, but the condition appears to be more common than PH and SUNCT/SUNA but less common than cluster. There is a slight female preponderance of 2:1, and mean age of onset seems to be in the 30s. There are no known genetic or environmental risks.

23.4 Pathophysiology and Mechanisms

Pain-sensitive intracranial structures including the dura and extracerebral vessels receive their innervations primarily from the ophthalmic branch of the trigeminal nerve. Until recently, little was known how this nociceptive circuit was activated in the TACs. Findings from functional neuroimaging studies, specifically positron emission tomography (PET) and functional MRI (fMRI), have provided significant insights into the pathophysiologic underpinnings of the trigeminal autonomic cephalalgias. Hyperactivation of the hypothalamus has been documented to occur ipsilateral to the pain in cluster headache, contralateral in PH and HC, and bilateral in SUNCT. Hypothalamic involvement may explain the circadian, circannual, and seasonal periodicity noted by many with cluster headache. Hypothalamic connections to structures along the trigeminovascular nociceptive network may modify nociceptive signal processing in a facilitatory manner. Activation of areas in the pain matrix and central opioid circuits has also been identified in these patients through similar functional imaging techniques. Parasympathetic outflow responsible for the cranial autonomic features arises in the hypothalamus, connects in the superior salivatory nucleus, and then synapses in the sphenopalatine ganglion. Postganglionic fibers then continue to the lacrimal ducts and nasal mucosa with responses of tearing, nasal congestion, and eventual nasal drainage. Parasympathetic control of cerebrovascular tone is also under some hypothalamic control, with activation resulting in vasodilation, plasma protein extravasation, and local release of inflammatory mediators.

23.5 Diagnosis and Diagnostic Criteria

Clinical criteria are used to diagnose cluster headache or any of the TACs. Cluster headache may be divided into episodic (90% of cases) and chronic subtypes. Episodic cluster involves at least two cycles of headache attacks occurring over periods of between 7 days and 1 year, separated by pain-free intervals of remission lasting at least 1 month. Chronic cluster involves attacks occurring without remission, or with remission periods <1 month, for at least 1 year. These same temporal criteria are used to subclassify episodic and chronic paroxysmal hemicranias, although in the case of PH the chronic subtype is much more common.

A detailed history focused on the frequency and duration of pain with a search for associated non-painful features of the headache disorder is crucial. Neurological examination with attention to papillary response, fundoscopic appearance, and visual field assessment should be performed. Typically the physical examination is normal, although occasionally a Horner's syndrome may be noted ipsilateral to the head pain. Imbedded in the formal diagnostic criteria is the requirement that secondary headache disorders be excluded. Headaches symptomatically similar to TACs may be seen with pathological lesions in and around the hypothalamus and pituitary gland. Contrasted brain MRI with attention to the pituitary area must be examined [9]. Although migraine headache is occasionally confused with cluster headache due to some symptomatic overlap, the cyclic pattern of cluster and its shorter attack duration (< 3 h versus 4–72 h for migraine) should aid in the distinction. Although other primary headaches such as primary stabbing and hypnic headache may present with similar short-duration head pain, these generally lack the autonomic component. Similarly trigeminal neuralgia may present with brief episodes of unilateral pain, but unlike the TACs the pain is typically along the second and third branches of the trigeminal nerve and absent cranial autonomic features. Trigeminal neuralgia also displays a refractory period following a series of triggered attacks, while SUNCT and the other TACs do not.

23.6 Rationale for Treatment

Those patients found to have intracranial mass lesions during the work-up of a trigeminal autonomic cephalalgia might require surgery or other procedures in order to reduce morbidity and possibly mortality. Those with primary headaches such as cluster, PH, SUNCT/SUNA, and HC should be treated to reduce morbidity and improve overall quality of life. These disorders are characterized by excruciating, unbearable pain that is often challenging to both diagnose and treat. Diagnosis does provide some measure of reassurance, but rapid introduction of effective management is required to reduce the overall burden of pain. There is a risk of mortality with these headache conditions as well, since those with uncontrolled cluster headache are known to describe suicidal ideations and a small percentage attempt suicide.

All TACs should be managed with preventive medications, which aim to substantially shorten the duration of symptomatic periods or reduce overall attack frequency and intensity [15]. Although the episodes of cluster headache may be of sufficient duration to warrant acute or abortive therapies, attacks of paroxysmal hemicranias and SUNCT/SUNA are too brief to address acutely. With acute therapies, parenteral and intranasal medication delivery is optimal since oral medication typically is not rapid enough to suit the needs of the patient. Hemicrania continua is managed with daily medication, and occasionally acute medication is administered during painful exacerbations of the underlying continuous discomfort. None of the treatment options to be discussed were developed to address any specific trigeminal autonomic cephalalgia. The uncertainty surrounding the true pathogenesis of these headaches renders it difficult to direct therapeutic research toward a specific target. Each treatment was developed for other conditions but was found to be helpful in one or more of these primary headache disorders.

23.7 Treatment Options

Cluster headache may be managed with both acute and preventive approaches [5]. Following the completion of several clinical trials over the past 10–15 years, a number of national and international organizations have published evidence-based treatment guidelines [10, 13].

The most effective treatment options for treatment of an attack of acute cluster headache are subcutaneous sumatriptan and oxygen inhalation (both level A advice). Pure oxygen is delivered through a non-rebreather face mask at 100% concentration and 6–15 l per minute over 10–20 min [4]. Up to 70–75% of patients may respond, although some describe rapid headache recurrence. Subcutaneous sumatriptan at a dose of 6 mg is the drug of choice with onset of action as early as 5 min into the attack. The maximum daily dose of sumatriptan is 12 mg, so many patients may prefer to use 3 mg or 4 mg dosing per attack. Prefilled devices are available in 4 mg and 6 mg strengths, but lower doses may be drawn from a 6 mg vial. Although the onset is not as rapid, there is level A advice supporting the use of zolmitriptan nasal spray at a dose of 5 mg (maximum daily dose 10 mg). Level B advice is available for sumatriptan 20 mg nasal spray (maximum daily dose 40 mg) and zolmitriptan 5 mg tablets (maximum daily dose 10 mg). All triptans are contraindicated in the presence of coronary, cerebral, or peripheral vascular disease, uncontrolled hypertension, or vasospastic angina. Side effects common to the class are chest pressure, throat or jaw tightness, and flushing. Subcutaneous sumatripan is the most likely formulation to generate these adverse events while it also may cause local site reactions, while the nasal spray preparations are often associated with an unpleasant taste. The only medication other than subcutaneous sumatriptan to have an FDA indication for acute cluster is parenteral dihydroergotamine, which generally is delivered intravenously (1 mg three times daily over 3 days) in the attempt at truncating a cycle of cluster headache. Nausea is a common side effect and generally necessitates co-administration with prochlorperazine 10 mg or metoclopramide 10 mg intravenously. Chest or abdominal pain and muscle cramping are other adverse events. Intranasal lidocaine (4–10% via drops or spray) is a less efficacious alternative to oxygen or triptan therapy and may be used multiple times per day. The best results are achieved when the treatment is administered in the supine position with the neck extended, the head turned toward the side of pain, and the medication placed in the nostril ipsilateral to the pain. Nasal stuffiness, throat numbness, and hoarseness are sometimes noted.

Prevention of cluster headache may be divided into short-term and long-term categories. Short-term measures are more rapidly effective and may be used as primary prevention in cases where patients report cycles lasting less than 1 month. In most cases, patients have cycles lasting 6–12 weeks, and short-term preventive measures are considered a bridge to long-term prophylaxis. Corticosteroids are the most common measures used in the short term. Prednisone may be initiated at 80 mg per day and tapered by 10–20 mg every 2–3 days to provide coverage over 10–14 days. Sometimes the course may be repeated if the headache cycle ceases but immediately returns. Dexamethasone at 12 mg per am, tapered by 4 mg every 3–4 days over a similar duration, is an alternative. Methylprednisolone at 250–500 mg daily over 3–5 days can be more effective than prednisone. Insomnia, moodiness, and increased appetite may be seen with short-term steroid administration, while hiccups are occasionally noted. Greater occipital nerve blockade with a local anesthetic (lidocaine or bupivacaine) mixed with corticosteroid (betamethasone, dexamethasone) has been shown to be effective in truncating a cluster cycle (level B advice) [17]. Local pain, bruising, and scalp numbness may be reported following the injections, but most patients tolerate these procedures quite well. The duration of response far outlasts the predicted therapeutic response of the agents delivered, with effective results lasting weeks to months. The injections may be repeated every 1–2 weeks initially if necessary. Prior to the development of the triptans, patients were treated with scheduled ergotamine (1–3 mg daily) over a maximum period of 4–6 weeks, but this eliminates the option of using any triptan for acute attacks. Nausea, abdominal or chest pain, and muscle cramping are common with the ergot derivatives. The agent of choice for long-term prevention is verapamil (level C advice). The immediate-release version may be started at 80 mg twice daily and advanced over 1–2 weeks toward 240–480 mg total daily dosing [11]. The sustained-release option is less bioavailable and may be started at 180 mg and advanced over 1–2 weeks toward doses of 240–720 mg. Doses greater than 240 mg require electrocardiographic monitoring for possible heart block. Common side effects are constipation, hypotension, and pedal edema. Other options for long-term prevention of cluster headache achieving level C advice are lithium carbonate at a dose of 900 mg and melatonin at a nightly dose of 10 mg. The lithium requires monitoring of serum drug levels (best at 0.4–0.8 nmol/L) and renal functions. Side effects include tremor, metallic taste, and hypothyroidism. In refractory cases, topiramate in the range of 100–200 mg has been shown to be effective in open-label trials. Paresthesias, cognitive impairment, mood changes, and appetite suppression are the most frequently reported adverse events.

The diagnosis and management of paroxysmal hemicrania and hemicrania continua are intertwined since included among the formal ICHD criteria for both is the requirement for a complete response to indomethacin. Typically dosing begins with 25 mg tid for 1 week, then advancing to 50 mg tid, and then 75 mg tid weekly until a response is achieved. Due to side effects of nausea or dyspepsia, most dose indomethacin with meals, and many prescribe proton pump inhibitors for those patients on long-term therapy. Monitoring for renal impairment or gastrointestinal bleeding should be undertaken periodically, initially after a treatment period of 3 months and eventually every 6–12 months while on stable dosing. Additional adverse events include tinnitus, dizziness, diarrhea, and development of a different headache. The prevention of SUNCT/SUNA is significantly more challenging. Given the rarity of the disorder, no randomized controlled clinical trials have been performed. Lamotrigine may occasionally be of benefit, beginning at 25 mg daily and gradually raising the dose over the first month toward 100–150 mg. More rapid escalation may increase the risk of serious rash complications. If such doses are unhelpful, further titration toward 200–400 mg daily over the second month may be indicated. Tolerability issues aside from rash include dizziness, fatigue, and moodiness. There is no available abortive treatment for the acute attacks of SUNCT/SUNA.

The use of opioids in the management of TACs should be avoided. There is no data to document benefit over the list of available therapies outlined above. Since many of these disorders are chronic, there are clear risks of opioid dependence and underlying headache aggravation through a potential medication overuse or "rebound" element. Only in rare cases of failure or contraindication to existing therapies should opioids be prescribed.

23.8 Treatment Goals and Sequencing of Care

The management goals of episodic cluster headache are to shorten the duration of headache cycles, lower the frequency of attacks during the cycle, and effectively treat those acute episodes breaking through preventive measures. In the case of the first cycle, the patient should be evaluated in the office and undergo diagnostic work-up. In cases of recurrent cluster headache cycles, treatment should be initiated immediately. Once the cycle has started, the corticosteroid is prescribed and dosed in the morning, while the melatonin is started at night. For those with cycles previously lasting greater than 4 weeks, verapamil is co-administered with these agents in a twice-daily dosing schedule. A baseline electrocardiogram is arranged and repeated 2 weeks following each dose escalation beyond 240 mg per day. Unless prior therapeutic failure has been documented, arrangements for an oxygen tank with non-breather mask are made. In the absence of contraindications, subcutaneous sumatriptan at a dose of either 4 mg or 6 mg is prescribed. If the patient has significant cardiovascular disease risk factors, a functional cardiac evaluation will be required prior to any triptan prescription. Such a process would involve work-up similar to a preoperative evaluation, and should that return unremarkable, many providers may elect to deliver the first dose in the office. Since most health plans restrict the quantity of triptan doses allowable per month, a prior authorization for quantity limit exception should be pursued. If subcutaneous sumatriptan is ineffective or poorly tolerated, nasal administration of sumatriptan, zolmitriptan, or lidocaine are subsequent options for acute attacks. Should the cycle persist, short-term options include repeating the corticosteroid course and/or delivering ipsilateral greater occipital nerve blocks. At that time, the long-term prevention with verapamil should be escalated toward 360–720 mg as necessary and tolerated [18]. In cases of partial response, lithium may be added to verapamil, while in cases of nonresponse, the verapamil should be tapered and discontinued. Topiramate is typically used if both verapamil and lithium fail. Subsequent medical options without clear evidence of benefit include valproate, gabapentin, amlodipine, and diltiazem.

By definition, all patients with the paroxysmal hemicranias or hemicrania continua should respond to adequate doses of indomethacin. Patients should expect to take indomethacin for years, and in many cases, the treatment is lifelong. Sustained efficacy of indomethacin without tachyphylaxis is to be expected. Approximately half of patients will be able to reduce their indomethacin dosing by 50% over time, so attempts to lower dosing should be made every 6–12 months. Other measures may be necessary in those that fail to tolerate the indomethacin despite dosing with meals and coverage with proton pump inhibitors or in those with medical conditions (renal insufficiency, significant gastrointestinal conditions, treatment with anticoagulation) which prohibit its use. Additional treatment options with occasional reported partial benefit include aspirin, celecoxib, naproxen, melatonin, topiramate, acetazolamide, and verapamil. Occipital nerve blocks may also be attempted. In cases of SUNCT/SUNA refractory to lamotrigine, possible options include topiramate, gabapentin, or hospital admission for intravenous phenytoin (250 mg one to three times daily) or lidocaine (1–4 mg/kg/h).

In the past, surgical ablative procedures were performed in cases of refractory cluster headache and also occasionally in cases of SUNCT/SUNA [8]. These procedures had targeted the first branch of the trigeminal nerve or locations along the parasympathetic pathway such as the sphenopalatine ganglion, greater superficial petrosal nerve, or the nervus intermedius. Results were almost universally disappointing, and complications such as corneal ulceration and anesthesia dolorosa were often problematic. Potential new therapies are arising in the field of neuromodulation. Most of the data has been accumulated in patients with refractory chronic cluster headache. Occipital nerve stimulators, vagal nerve stimulators, and more recently sphenopalatine ganglion stimulators all have data to support significant responses in greater than half of treated subjects [1, 16]. A number of studies investigating these options are in process. Deep brain stimulation of the posterior hypothalamus has been shown to be helpful in cases of refractory cluster, but major adverse events including potential mortality have limited its usefulness (Tables 23.1, 23.2, 23.3 and 23.4).

References

1. Burns B, Watkins L, Goadsby P. Treatment of intractable cluster headache by occipital nerve stimulation in 14 patients. Neurology. 2009;72:341–5.
2. Cittadini E, Goadsby P. Update on hemicrania continua. Curr Pain Headache Rep. 2011;15:51–6.
3. Cohen A. Short-lasting unilateral neuralgiform headache attacks with conjunctival injection and tearing. Cephalalgia. 2007;27:824–32.
4. Cohen A, Burns B, Goadsby P. High-flow oxygen for treatment of cluster headache. JAMA. 2009;302:2451–7.
5. Francis G, Becker W, Pringsheim T. Acute and preventive pharmacologic treatment of cluster headache. Neurology. 2010;75:463–73.
6. Goadsby P, Lipton R. A review of paroxysmal hemicranias, SUNCT syndrome and other short-lasting headaches with autonomic features, including new cases. Brain. 1997;120:193–209.
7. Headache Classification Committee of the International Headache Society. The international classification of headache disorders, 3rd edition (beta version). Cephalalgia. 2013;33(9):629–808.
8. Hong RD. The surgical treatment of headache. Headache. 2014;54:409–29.
9. Iacovelli E, Coppola G, Tinelli E, et al. Neuroimaging in cluster headache and other trigeminal autonomic cephalalgias. J Headache Pain. 2012;13:11–20.
10. Lademann V, Jansen J-P, Evers S, et al. Evaluation of guideline-adherent treatment in cluster headache. Cephalalgia 2016;36:760–64.
11. Leone M, D'Amico D, Frediani F, et al. Verapamil in the prophylaxis of episodic cluster headache: a double-blind study versus placebo. Neurology. 2000;54:1382–5.
12. May A. Diagnosis and clinical features of trigemino-autonomic headaches. Headache. 2013;53:1470–8.
13. May A, Leone M, Afra J, et al. EFNS guidelines on the treatment of cluster headache and other trigeminal-autonomic cephalalgias. Eur J Neurol. 2006;13:1066–77.
14. Pareja J, Sjaastad O. SUNCT syndrome. A clinical review. Headache. 1997;47:195–202.
15. Pareja J, Alvarez M. The usual treatment of trigeminal autonomic cephalalgias. Headache. 2013;53:1401–14.
16. Pedersen J, Barloese M, Jensen R. Neurostimulation in cluster headache: a review of current progress. Cephalalgia. 2013;33:1179–93.
17. Peres M, Stiles M, Siow H, et al. Greater occipital nerve block for cluster headache. Cephalalgia. 2002;22:520–2.
18. Tfelt-Hansen P, Tfelt-Hansen J. Verapamil for cluster headache: clinical pharmacology and possible mode of action. Headache. 2009;49:117–25.

Migraine Variants

24

Robert L. Merrill

Pearls of Wisdom

- Migraine variants represent a group of headache disorders that have migrainous characteristics and also which are accompanied by neurological symptoms that are not recognized as "classic" migraine symptoms.
- While it is generally recognized that these conditions represent primary headache disorders, the clinician should go beyond the diagnostic workup accepted for the primary headache disorders, because the potential for these headaches being secondary to central organic causes is greater.
- Migraine variants can be classified into:
  - Late-life migraine
  - Basilar-type migraine
  - Ophthalmoplegic migraine
  - Hemiplegic migraine
  - Retinal migraine
  - Progressive migraine
  - Primary stabbing headache
  - Exertional migraine
  - Vestibular migraine
- Patients are living longer and are often on multiple medications that are not being managed appropriately. This is leading to an increase in late-life migraine sufferers in our pain clinics.

R.L. Merrill, DDS, MS
UCLA School of Dentistry, Los Angeles, CA, USA
e-mail: rmerrill@ucla.edu

J.N.A.R. Ferreira et al. (eds.), *Orofacial Disorders*,
DOI 10.1007/978-3-319-51508-3_24

24.1 Introduction

The discipline of orofacial was recognized as a dental specialty by the Commission on Dental Accreditation in 2010, and the first programs were accredited in 2011. The specialty of orofacial pain bridges the gap between medicine and dentistry and serves a population of patients who have pain problems that neither discipline has been effective in diagnosing or treating.

The practitioners of orofacial pain are at the cutting edge of both dentistry and medicine because they are able to diagnose and successfully treat disorders that have long been and generally still remain a puzzle to both professions. Dentistry is slowly making inroads into the field of headache through the training that is being provided in the various orofacial pain programs. Graduates of these programs add credibility to the important role that dentistry needs to play in addressing head and neck pain. Unfortunately, some dentists advocate unscientific diagnostic and treatment procedures claiming they can cure a migraine headache without being able to perform a neurological examination or being able to actually make an accurate diagnosis of the various headache conditions that may be seen in an orofacial pain practice. This tends to diminish the regard of dentistry in the medical community. This is a very dangerous situation that needs to be remedied by recognizing that practitioners of orofacial pain should be board certified and trained to medically assess and treat headaches. As we gain better understanding of the neuroanatomy, neurophysiology, and neurobiology of pain, we are able to include more orofacial pain conditions in the general nosology of pain and provide explanations for many previously enigmatic orofacial pain conditions. This is certainly the case with orofacial neuropathies.

Neurovascular disorders are an important part of orofacial pain, because the prevalence of headache is high (64% in the UCLA OFP clinic) in OFP patient population, and the headache is a significant part of their chronic pain problems [1]. Temporomandibular disorders are often associated with concomitant headaches. Many referrals to Temporomandibular Joint (TMJ) clinics come from physicians who have been treating the headache without success and refer the patient to the dentist on the assumption that the patient has a "TMJ headache." In addition, dentists treating TM disorders are often blindsided by patients who have a headache disorder such as chronic migraine or "facial migraine" and find that focusing only on the TM symptoms does not relieve their patient's pain. Treating one disorder without recognizing and addressing the other usually results in suboptimal outcomes for the suffering patient. Additionally, the general dentists may not be aware that the pain/headache condition could be the result of a CNS lesion that has not been recognized. This paper will address the "migraine variants" that the orofacial pain specialist should be aware of and consider as he/she delves into the mystery of chronic orofacial pain.

For the most part, the diagnosis of migraine variants is a diagnosis of exclusion. Although most of these conditions are primary disorders, they could be secondary to a more serious and/or life-threatening condition. Therefore, it is important for the orofacial pain specialist to recognize and do an appropriate workup or make an appropriate referral to specialist who can take care of the patient. Migraine variants may be characterized by the following symptoms:

- Confusion
- Dysarthria
- Atypical sensory, motor, or visual aura
- Focal neurologic deficits
- Paroxysmal episodes of prolonged visual auras
- Gastrointestinal (GI) manifestations
- Other constitutional symptoms, with or without a headache

The International Headache Society (IHS) published *The International Classification of Headache Disorders* (ICHD-II) in 2004. This document updated and refined the first classification system published in 1988 [2]. Subsequently, the IHS has published the ICHD-III beta version that has made significant changes to the 2004 version. The changes primarily were informed by research, and some of the disorders classified in the ICHD-II have been reassigned, recategorized, or dropped [3]. This does not mean, however, that the disorders do not exist but that there is not enough evidence to support including them in the updated classification system at this time. In the 28 years since the first publication, great strides have been made in refining the understanding of headache nosology, pathophysiology, and management.

Migraine variants represent a group of headache disorders that have migrainous characteristics but also which are accompanied by neurological symptoms that are not recognized as "classic" migraine accompaniments. While it is generally recognized that these conditions represent primary headache disorders, the clinician should go beyond the diagnostic workup accepted for the primary headache disorders because the potential for these headaches being secondary to central organic causes is greater. Silberstein and Saper in the first and second editions of their *Handbook of Headache Management* listed and discussed their choice of migraine variants [4]. The list on their handbook included:

- Late-life migraine
- Basilar-type migraine (migraine with brain stem aura)
- Ophthalmoplegic migraine (recurrent painful ophthalmoplegic neuropathy)
- Hemiplegic migraine
- Retinal migraine
- Progressive migraine
- Primary stabbing headache (icepick pain)
- Exertional migraine
- Vestibular migraine

Some of these conditions have been reclassified in the ICHD-III beta and will be discussed in more detail below in relation to the ICHD-III beta classification system.

24.2 Etiology, Epidemiology, Diagnostic Criteria, and Treatment of Migraine Variants

24.2.1 Late-Life Migraine

The average age of the population in the orofacial pain clinic is getting older, and the likelihood of seeing elderly patients with headache is significantly increased. Our patients are living longer and are often on multiple medications that are not being managed appropriately. Epidemiological studies have shown that the prevalence of migraine decreases in the above 50 years of age group. Females who suffered from migraine through their productive year will usually see a decline in migraine after menopause, but male migraineurs also see a decline in migraine episodes, as they get older.

A major complication in migraine in the elderly is the fact that elderly patients may be taking medications or combinations of medications that may cause headache. The clinician should be aware of all medications taken by an elderly patient whose presenting complaints may include headache because the medications may be responsible for the pain they are experiencing. This may be due to sensitivity to a medication, misuse of a medication, or medication interactions. The elderly may experience toxic side effects from "appropriately dosed" medications due to their body's decreased ability to metabolize the medications. Often, the elderly have to be given lower doses of a given medication to avoid toxicity or untoward side effects.

New-onset or persistent headache is always a red flag in the elderly, and the workup needs to include neuroimaging since the likelihood of the headache being secondary to a structural lesion is significantly higher for the elderly than for the young. Headache due to disease is more common in the elderly than in the young. The onset of a new headache condition in the elderly patient is certainly a red flag that needs to be pursued in depth and other potential causes of the headache excluded.

Fisher in 1980 [5] described the phenomenon of late-life migraine as attacks of migraine-associated neurological symptoms without the development of headache. He proposed that the symptoms were due to the same neurological process as migraine but without pain. He noted that the attacks would last up to 72 h (similar to migraine) and may also be accompanied by the various manifestations of aura, including visual scotomas, paresthesias, or other sensory and motor symptoms that accompany migraine. These symptoms could also occur in patients who did not have a prior history of migraine.

As indicated at the first of this paper, most of the headaches in this section are diagnosed by exclusion, and this is certainly the case with late-life migraine.

The *differential diagnoses* should include:

- Stroke
- Clotting disorders
- Central lesion
- Medications or substances

The *workup* must include:

1. Neurological assessment
2. Head and neck physical assessment
3. Review of all medications and pattern of use
4. CT and/or MRI/MRA

24.2.2 Migraine with Brain Stem Aura [3] (Formerly Basilar-Type Migraine or Basilar Migraine)

Bickerstaff was one of the first to write about basilar migraine, and the condition has been known as Bickerstaff syndrome [6]. In his paper, he noted that all of the patients were under 35 years of age and most were women. He also noted that the attacks were generally infrequent and that the patient also could have headache with normal non-brain stem aura. The aura phenomena described by Bickerstaff included visual disturbances in both fields of vision (compare with retinal migraine below), diplopia, bilateral limb paresthesia, perioral tingling, dysarthria, vertigo, tinnitus, and ataxia. These symptoms would last 20–30 min and would be relieved by sleep.

Migraine with brain stem aura can affect children and teens but tends to change to other types of migraine with age. It is less common in patients over the age of 50 years. The visual auras are bilateral and include scintillating scotomata, blurring vision, or total blindness. Double vision is not common but may occur if sixth cranial nerve paresis is part of the aura. Sensory symptoms may be bilateral and symmetric but also may alternate from side to side in a hemisensory pattern. These sensory changes can involve the oral region and extend throughout the arms and legs. Motor weakness has been reported in more than 50% of the cases. Changes in level of consciousness are de rigueur. These changes range from a sleep state to syncope and even coma.

The headache itself is bilateral (rarely unilateral) in the frontal or occipital region, is described as throbbing, and is accompanied by photophobia, phonophobia, and nausea and vomiting.

The ICHD-II classification renamed basilar migraine, basilar-type migraine, and included it under rubric of migraine with aura. The ICHD-III beta now classifies this migraine variant as migraine with brain stem aura [3]. Because of the remarkable attending symptoms, this migraine variant was originally thought to be due to a spasm of the basilar artery resulting in ischemia, since many of the accompaniments, such as dizziness, ataxia, or altered states of consciousness, reflected brain stem dysfunction. Bizarre behavior and obscene utterances have been noted as well as slowed EEG recordings. Now, it is thought that the symptoms of this variant of migraine are due to neuronal dysfunction either with or without ischemia.

The aura symptoms include visual, sensory, and/or speech symptoms, and all are fully reversible. There are no motor symptoms associated with this condition. If motor symptoms are observed, the headache should be classified as hemiplegic migraine.

The symptoms include two or more of the following [3]:

1. Dysarthria
2. Vertigo
3. Tinnitus
4. Hypacusis
5. Diplopia
6. Ataxia
7. Decreased level of consciousness

Additionally, the headache should have at least two of the following four characteristics:

1. At least one aura symptom spreads gradually over 5 min, and/or two or more symptoms occur in succession.
2. Each individual aura symptom lasts 5–60 min.
3. At least one aura symptom is unilateral.
4. The aura is accompanied, or followed within 60 min, by headache.

24.2.2.1 Pathophysiology

The pathophysiology of migraine with brain stem aura is still unclear but is considered to be related to neuronal dysfunction with or without vasoconstrictions, e.g., spreading depression in the brain stem, similar to cortical spreading depression associated with migraine with aura.

24.2.2.2 Treatment

Early on, treatment of migraine with brain stem aura was limited to medications that did not cause vasoconstriction due to earlier presumptions that this migraine variant was due to vasoconstriction of the basilar artery. Medications such as triptans, DHE-45, cafergot, isometheptene, methergine, or other vasoconstrictors were avoided. Although this particular issue has been resolved, there is still a lack of research showing that their use is safe with this variation of migraine. Abortive medications such as opioids may be used. Prophylactic medications such as depakote, gabapentin, and topiramate are also useful.

24.2.3 Ophthalmoplegic Migraine

This condition is now termed recurrent painful ophthalmoplegic neuropathy and is no longer classified as a migraine variant.

24.2.4 Hemiplegic Migraine/Familial Hemiplegic Migraine

The description of this migraine disorder is migraine with aura including motor weakness. Familial hemiplegic migraine (FHM) also includes motor weakness, but there must be at least one first- or second-degree relative that has migraine aura including motor weakness. Familial hemiplegic migraine (FHM) is an autosomal dominant genetically heterogeneous form of migraine with aura that is characterized by motor weakness. Researchers have identified four missense mutations in the CACNA1A gene on chromosome 19p. The gene encodes for an alpha 1A subunit of the P/Q type voltage-gated calcium channel [7, 8]. This channel regulates release of specific neurotransmitters such as glutamate. The attacks may represent typical migraine with or without aura and severe attacks with prolonged aura that may last from several days to weeks. Additionally, the patient may experience impaired consciousness ranging from confusion to profound coma. The headache phase of the attack may be absent, precede, or start with the hemiparesis. The hemiparesis may be abrupt and mistaken for a stroke.

The *differential diagnosis* list for hemiplegic migraine includes:

- Focal seizures
- Stroke
- Coagulopathies
- CADASIL
- MELAS

The ICHD-II subdivides hemiplegic migraine into sporadic and familial types. The ICHD-III subclassifies familial hemiplegic migraine into type 1, type 2, type 3, other loci, and sporadic hemiplegic migraine. This headache should be thoroughly investigated including family history by a specialist.

24.2.4.1 Treatment

Typically triptans are best avoided during the aura phase. Flunarizine or topiramate may be the best options for prophylactic treatment.

24.2.5 Retinal Migraine

Retinal migraine is described as repeated attacks of monocular visual disturbance, including scintillations, scotomata, or blindness that are associated with migraine headache. One of every 200 migraineurs has monocular visual symptoms with their headache. The headache is preceded by or accompanies reversible visual impairment or blindness in one eye. The visual impairment will last less than 1 h.

Pathophysiologic studies have demonstrated retinal or optic nerve hypoperfusion from spasm of the central retinal or ophthalmic artery. Burger and associates reported amaurosis fugax episodes due to vasoconstriction during the retinal migraine attacks [9]. Visual symptoms of retinal migraine include unilateral quadratic and altitudinal or total grayout, whiteout, or blackout visual loss. Some patients report a concentric constriction of the monocular visual field proceeding from the periphery to the center. There may be total visual loss or a small part of the visual field preserved. It is presumed that the visual symptoms are due to the retinal or ophthalmic artery. Central retinal artery occlusion and branch retinal artery occlusion can cause infarction of the entire retina or of the affected retinal sector.

The retinal artery usually has two major branches: one covering the upper half and the other the lower half of the retina. An altitudinal scotoma in one eye can result from occlusion of one of the branches. A transient occlusion of the retinal artery whether by vasospasm or by emboli causes amaurosis fugax with a browning or blackout of the vision in one eye for about 10 min. This has been described as being "like a window shade" moving down or up over the eye. Amaurosis fugax may be a warning sign for an impending retinal or cerebral infarct.

The *differential diagnosis* should include:

- Embolic disease
- Ischemic optic atrophy
- Central organic causes
- Retinal spreading depression (part of the spreading depression of migraine)

The examination should include an ophthalmologic examination, CT/MRI, and carotid ultrasound studies.

24.2.6 Progressive Migraine (to Chronic)

Medication overuse has been associated with the development of chronic headache, including migraine. This migrainous headache has been variously called progressive or transformational migraine but is now called chronic migraine in the ICHD-III beta manual. The most common cause of chronic migraine is overuse of symptomatic medications. Chronic migraine is described as a headache occurring on 15 or more days per month for more than 3 months and has the features of migraine headache on at least 8 days per month [2, 3]. The headache can be either tension-type-like or migraine-like and with or without aura. Around 50% of patients with chronic migraine see the headache revert to an episodic headache with disuse of the overused drug. In those patients who are overusing medication and have chronic migraine, they should be given both the diagnosis of chronic migraine and medication overuse headache [3].

Treatment involves withdrawing the offending medication and starting the patient on an appropriate prophylactic medication such as Topamax. Onabotulinum toxin has been approved as a treatment for chronic migraine, and numerous studies have shown it to be very effective in treating the headache [10, 11].

24.2.7 Primary Stabbing Headache (Jabs and Jolts Syndrome)

What had been previously designated as icepick pain, jabs and jolts, or ophthalmodynia periodica is categorized by the ICHD-III beta as *Primary Stabbing Headache*. The pain is described as transient localized stabs of pain in the head, occurring spontaneously and in the absence of organic disease of underlying structures or of the cranial nerves. The diagnostic criteria include sharp or stabbing pain, usually in the V1 distribution of the trigeminal nerve. The stabs last for a few seconds and may recur spontaneously several times per day. The stabs or "jabs and jolts" may move from one area to another on the same side or move to the opposite side. The reason for including this headache in the group of migraine variants is that 40% of migraineurs experience these stabbing pains [12, 13]. They may occur during or between migraine attacks. Jabs or Jolts occurring in the temple, face or external ear may be misdiagnosed as a TMJ disorder or trigeminal neuralgia by an unsuspecting clinician. Although the mechanism is unclear, the condition has been found to respond to indomethacin and possibly other NSAIDs [14].

The *differential diagnosis* should include:

- Myofascial pain
- Epicrania fugax
- Nummular headache
- Occipital neuralgia

Treatment for primary stabbing headache includes indomethacin 25–50 mg three times/day. This has been found to be effective in 65% of patients.

24.2.7.1 Epicrania Fugax

Although not related to migraine, epicrania fugax can be confused with primary stabbing headache that has been associated with migraine. This disorder is characterized by brief paroxysmal stabbing head pains that radiate in a linear or zigzag trajectory across the surface of one hemicranium, although a case series has been reported where the pain crosses to the opposite hemicranium [3, 15]. The recurrent stabbing pains last for 1–10 s. Treatment involves neuromodulators, indomethacin, tricyclic antidepressants, nerve anesthetic blockades, and trochlear steroid injections [16].

The *differential diagnosis* should include:

- Occipital neuralgia
- Primary stabbing headache
- Nummular headache
- Trigeminal neuralgia
- Myofascial pain

24.2.8 Exertional Migraine (Primary Exercise Headache)

Hippocrates may have been the first person to recognize the headache disorder when he wrote, "one should be able to recognize those who have headache from gymnastic exercises, or walking, or running, or any other unseasonable labor, or from immoderate venery." The ICHD-III beta continued to include this headache entity in the fourth category of other primary headaches. The headache is characterized by severe transient headache that occurs after an exertional or straining activity. The diagnostic criteria include a pulsatile headache lasting from 5 min to 48 h that was brought on by or occurred only during or after physical exertion. The first occurrence of this headache should always be followed up with imaging studies to exclude subarachnoid hemorrhage or arterial dissection. It has been reported to occur particularly in hot weather or at high altitude.

The pathophysiology may involve arterial dilatation since the headache develops after exertion and on hot days; however, there is no objective evidence of this. Basoglu and associates, using SPECT (single photon emission computed tomography), noted frontal hypoperfusion in a boy with exertional headache, but the significance of this is uncertain. Paulson has suggested that acute venous distension may be a possible mechanism [17, 18]. Pheochromocytoma has been associated with exertional headache.

Differential diagnosis should include:

- Cardiac ischemia
- Intracranial vascular disorders
- Pheochromocytoma
- Carotid artery stenosis

Treatment should involve undertaking exercise gradually and progressively, since as physical conditioning progresses, the headache occurrences tend to dissipate. Exertional headaches respond to indomethacin in the majority of cases [19, 20].

24.2.9 Vestibular Migraine

This is a migraine-like headache that is associated with vertigo or dizziness. The patient has a past history of migraine fulfilling the migraine criteria with or without aura. The vestibular symptoms are moderate to severe intensity and will last 5 min to 72 h. This disorder may also be associated with transient auditory symptoms and susceptibility to motion sickness. Although vertigo is also reported by more than 60% of patients with migraine with brain stem aura, the ICHD-III requires at least two brain stem symptoms in addition to the visual, sensory, or dysphasic aura symptoms to make the diagnosis of vestibular migraine [3]. Vestibular migraine and Meniere's disease may be an inherited symptom cluster, and migraine headaches, photophobia, and auras are common in Meniere's attacks. Additionally, in the first year of symptom onset, it may be difficult to distinguish the difference between vestibular migraine and Meniere's disease [3, 21].

This headache requires a full neurological assessment because it is important to establish a correct diagnosis. The differential diagnoses include:

- Benign paroxysmal positional vertigo (BPPV)
- Meniere's disease
- Transient ischemic attacks (TIAs)
- Fluid leaks in the inner ear
- Vestibular nerve irritation

Treatment is aimed at preventing the attacks. Typical medications include:

- Beta-blockers
- Calcium channel blockers
- Tricyclic antidepressants
- Gabapentin
- Clonazepam
- Acetazolamide
- Topiramate
- Oxcarbazepine

References

1. Mitrirattanakul S, Merrill RL. Headache impact in patients with orofacial pain. J Am Dent Assoc. 2006;137(9):1267–74.
2. ICHD-II. Classification and diagnostic criteria for headache disorders, cranial neuralgias and facial pain. Headache classification committee of the international headache society. Cephalalgia. 1988;8(Suppl 7):1–96.
3. ICHD. The international classification of headache disorders, 3rd edition (beta version). Cephalalgia. 2013;33(9):629–808.
4. Saper JR, et al., editors. Handbook of headache management – a practical guide to diagnosis and treatment of head, neck and facial pain. 2nd ed. Philadelphia: Lippincott Williams & Wilkins; 1999.
5. Fisher CM. Late-life migraine accompaniments as a cause of unexplained transient ischemic attacks. Can J Neurol Sci. 1980;7(1):9–17.
6. Bickerstaff E. The basilar artery and the migraine-epilepsy syndrome. Proc R Soc Med. 1962;55(Mar):167–9.
7. Mullner C, et al. Familial hemiplegic migraine type 1 mutations K1336E, W1684R, and V1696I alter Cav2.1 Ca2+ channel gating: evidence for beta-subunit isoform-specific effects. J Biol Chem. 2004;279(50):51844–50.
8. van den Maagdenberg AM, et al. A Cacna1a knockin migraine mouse model with increased susceptibility to cortical spreading depression. Neuron. 2004;41(5):701–10.
9. Burger SK, et al. Transient monocular blindness caused by vasospasm. N Engl J Med. 1991;325(12):870–3.
10. Barbanti P, et al. Rationale for use of onabotulinum toxin A (BOTOX) in chronic migraine. Neurol Sci. 2015;36(Suppl 1):29–32.
11. Russo M, et al. The use of onabotulinum toxin A (Botox((R))) in the treatment of chronic migraine at the Parma Headache Centre: a prospective observational study. Neurol Sci. 2016;37(7):1127–31.
12. Raskin NH. Chapter 2 migraine: clinical aspects. In: Raskin NH, editor. Headache. New York: Churchill Livingstone; 1988. p. 35–98.
13. Raskin NH. Chapter 11: facial pain. In: Raskin NH, editor. Headache. New York: Churchill Livingstone; 1988. p. 333–72.
14. Robbins MS, Evans RW. Primary and secondary stabbing headache. Headache. 2015;55(4):565–70.
15. Casas-Limon J, et al. Pain paroxysms with coronal radiation: case series and proposal of a new variant of epicrania fugax. Headache. 2016;56(6):1040–4.
16. Cuadrado ML, Guerrero AL, Pareja JA. Epicrania fugax. Curr Pain Headache Rep. 2016;20(4):21.
17. Basoglu T, et al. Demonstration of frontal hypoperfusion in benign exertaional headache by Technetium-99 m-HMPAO SPECT. J Nucl Med. 1996;37:1172–4.

18. Paulson GW. Weightlifters headache. Headache. 1983;23(4):193–4.
19. Diamond S, Medina JL. Prolonged benign exertional headache: clinical characteristics and response to indomethacin. Adv Neurol. 1982;33:145–9.
20. Mathew NT. Indomethacin responsive headache syndromes. Headache. 1981;21(4):147–50.
21. Radtke A, et al. Vestibular migraine: long-term follow-up of clinical symptoms and vestibulo-cochlear findings. Neurology. 2012;79(15):1607–14.

Part IX

Health Care Approaches in Orofacial and Widespread Pains

Interdisciplinary and Multidisciplinary Approaches to Orofacial Pain Care

25

Shawn McMahon

Pearls of Wisdom

- Biomedical and biopsychosocial models are two approaches to health care that have been proven effective when utilized in the appropriate situation. Health-care providers must understand that chronic pain is a disease of the person and that a traditional biomedical approach cannot adequately address all of the individual pain-related physiological, psychological, and social needs of this patient population.
- Chronic pain patients generally present with complex, multimodal problems that often involve two or more coexisting chronic pain conditions (e.g., chronic headaches, chronic fatigue syndrome, fibromyalgia, inflammatory bowel disease, interstitial cystitis, temporomandibular joint dysfunction, vulvodynia, and gastric reflux disease). They often describe disturbed sleep, increased stress, anxiety, depression, and even anger resulting in a decreased quality of life. With so many overlapping factors, it makes sense that current literature supports a "whole person" approach to chronic pain diagnosis and management.
- Current literature describes various models to address chronic pain using a multimodal approach. Although they differ in areas such as organization, structure, format, and cost, they do have common core features:
  - A biopsychosocial approach to diagnosis and care that not only addresses the associated biology but also the psychological and social aspects of the pain condition

S. McMahon, DDS, MS
Orofacial Pain Clinic, Joint Base San Antonio, San Antonio, TX, USA

Uniformed Services University of the Health Sciences, Bethesda, MD, USA
e-mail: shawnmcmahondds@gmail.com

J.N.A.R. Ferreira et al. (eds.), *Gene Therapy for Radiation-Induced Salivary Hypofunction*, DOI 10.1007/978-3-319-51508-3_25

- Providers from multiple disciplines working in an integrated fashion with shared treatment goals
- Goals: to reduce effects of pain, improve function, and achieve independence from the health-care system

- Multidisciplinary care involves care provided by health-care providers from several disciplines which may, or may not, be coordinated, and treatment may occur with different goals in parallel rather than an integrated approach.
- Interdisciplinary care involves a team of health-care providers from different specialties that play complementary roles that when implemented together enhance patient care.

25.1 Introduction

As evidenced by the topics presented in this clinical guide, orofacial pain disorders comprise a wide range of conditions. Thus, when evaluating an orofacial pain patient, the clinician may face a formidable diagnostic challenge. The differential diagnoses for an orofacial pain complaint may include conditions from a variety of categories: musculoskeletal, inflammatory, infectious, neurovascular, neuropathic, neoplastic, metabolic, endocrine, and autoimmune disorders [1]. Patients with orofacial disorders may present with a complex medical and psychosocial clinical history, which may include acute or chronic symptoms, and present as single or coexisting disorders that may share perplexing interrelationships that involve psychosocial behavioral factors as well as underlying physical pathology.

A successful treatment is frequently compromised by the chronic nature of the disease and by long-standing maladaptive behaviors, attitudes, and lifestyles that may actually perpetuate or result from the illness. Factors such as disability, chemical dependency, inadequate nutrition, sleep disturbances, and countless others are beginning to be studied and understood. Failure to help the patient change these factors often plays a major role in failure to obtain successful long-term management of these disorders.

Traditional medicine often fails to educate and support the patient in making these changes. Even when these problems are identified by the clinician or the patient, the ability to help deal with factors involved is limited by the nature of dental or medical training, the system in which dentistry or medicine is practiced, and the complex nature of each factor. In addition, the traditional approach to treatment employs a biomedical approach (Fig. 25.1), is usually singular in nature, and varies according to the clinicians' favorite theory of etiology (Table 25.1).

When history and examination do not indicate a clearly identifiable etiology for a patient's pain (i.e., trauma, infection, neoplasm, etc.), patient care should be approached with a comprehensive biopsychosocial mind-set to enable the best possible prognosis (Fig. 25.2) (Table 25.2).

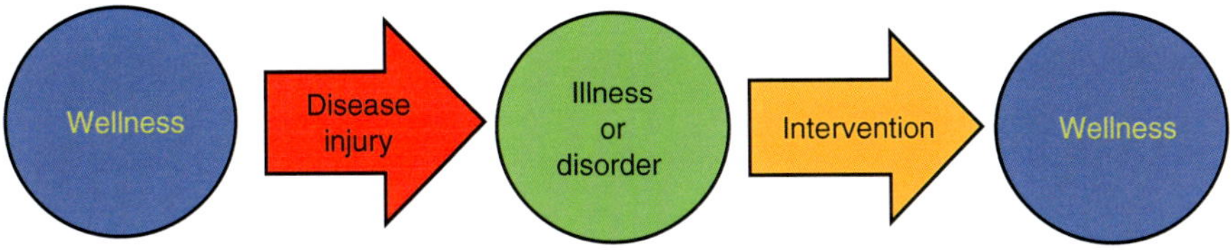

Wellness → Disease injury → Illness or disorder → Intervention → Wellness

Fig. 25.1 The biomedical model is a conceptual model of illness that excludes psychological and social factors and includes only biologic factors in an attempt to understand a person's medical illness or disorder [21]

Table 25.1 Biomedical model

Definition: assumes etiology is disease based and effective treatment is a medical approach
Advantages:
Embraces a simpler or more fundamental level of care
Effective in the management of acute illnesses that have predictable outcomes (i.e., bone fracture)
Suitable for health-care providers focused on similar individual areas of a patient's health
Potentially less expensive
Disadvantages:
Does not account for situations involving persistent pain even after damaged tissue has healed
Focuses on disease mechanisms and does not take the person's thoughts, emotions, or social effects into consideration

Table 25.2 Biopsychosocial model

Definition: combines the physiological, psychological, and social aspects of the pain experience
Advantages:
Comprehensive, often independently unique, care that fits individual physiological, psychological, and social needs and wants
Often utilizes interdisciplinary or multidisciplinary care
Incorporates patient, family, and health-care provider participation to promote patient "ownership" and social support for well-rounded care (i.e., avoiding or reducing patient catastrophizing)
Defines how and why psychological disorders or social factors can sometimes result in physiological problems
Promotes good mental and emotional health in order to maintain a healthy lifestyle – cost-effective
Disadvantages:
Assumes that all pain conditions are biopsychosocial; however, the model is not necessarily applicable to every condition (i.e., acute pain)
Can be confusing and misleading method to use correctly. Requires training beyond the biomedical approach
Could result in delayed care. It can be impractical and time-consuming when trying to analyze and manage a patient's problem
Potentially more expensive

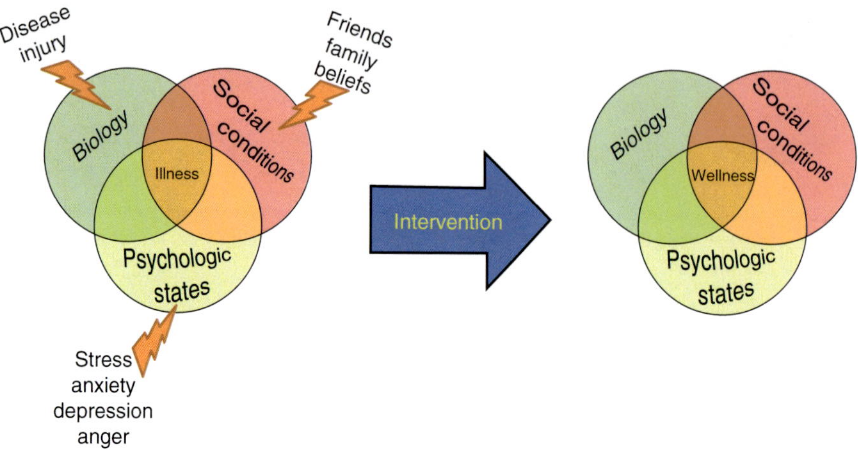

Fig. 25.2 The biopsychosocial model encompasses the complex interactions between biology, psychological states, and social conditions that bring about and/or maintain dysfunction [1]

The past president of the American Society of Physical Medicine and Rehabilitation, William Fowler, states that "Schools continue to emphasize diagnostic skills, quick complete cures, and the patient with acute disease as the teaching model for medical students and house staff…. as a result, clinical management as well as research and teaching regarding chronic disease and rehabilitation tends to take second place and is often done outside the usual academic channels." This may be partially because the practice of health care focuses on evaluation and management of a chronic illness by a single primary practitioner. It is estimated that 30–50% of patient presentations to primary care will not yield a specific diagnosis. Furthermore, when distressed patients continue to shop for care from a multiple providers, they are at increased risk for iatrogenic injury and cost to themselves and the health-care community [2]. It may be unrealistic to expect a single clinician to address the multitude of contributing factors that may be present in a patient with chronic pain.

25.2 Defining Multimodal Approaches to Orofacial Pain Care

There are various ways in which a comprehensive approach may be implemented. Evidence supports both multidisciplinary and interdisciplinary approaches to care. The terms multidisciplinary and interdisciplinary are often used interchangeably; however, there are subtle but important differences.

Multidisciplinary care is defined as care provided by specialists from several disciplines which may, or may not, be coordinated, and treatment may occur with different goals in parallel rather than an integrated approach (Fig. 25.3). In this model each provider has a clearly defined role in the overall care of the patient. They contribute individualized expertise in relative isolation from one another under the overall care manager (generally a physician) [3–5] (Table 25.3).

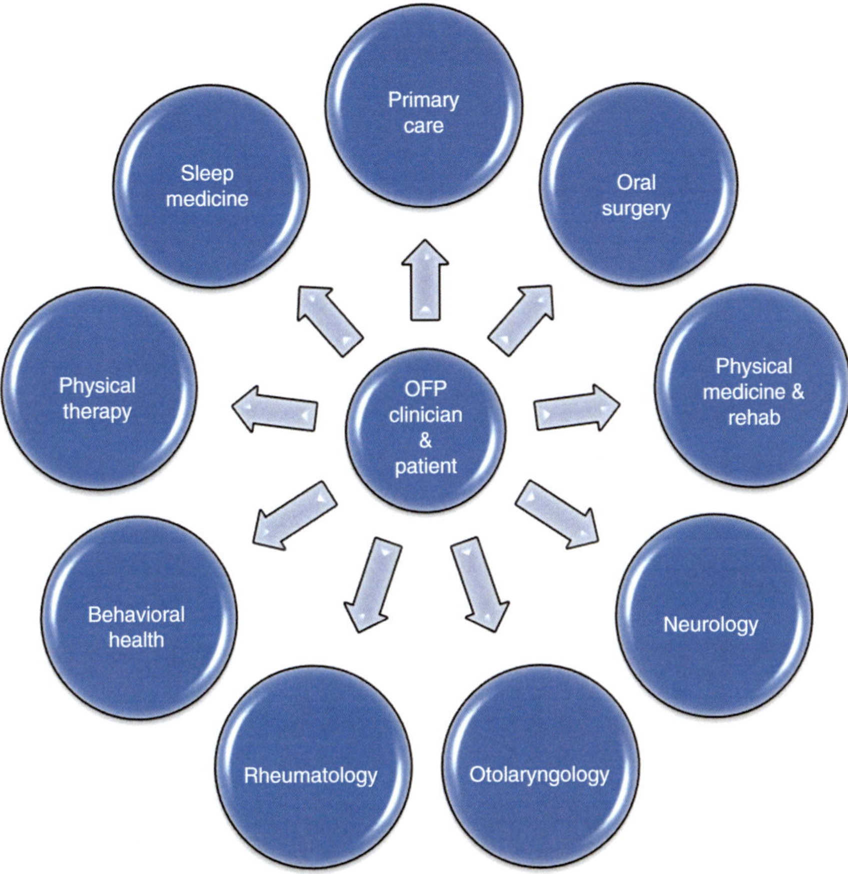

Fig. 25.3 Multidisciplinary orofacial pain care model

Table 25.3 Defining multidisciplinary and interdisciplinary care

Multidisciplinary care
Multiple providers from multiple disciplines
May, or may not, be coordinated between providers
Each provider has a clearly defined role but contributes individualized expertise in relative isolation from one another
Generally care is coordinated by one provider
Interdisciplinary care
Providers from various differing specialties play complementary roles that, when integrated, enhance patient care
Team members share responsibilities, problem solve as one, and share accountability
Planned or recommended treatments, therapeutic interventions, and other activities reflect the team's consensus view rather than the view of any single provider

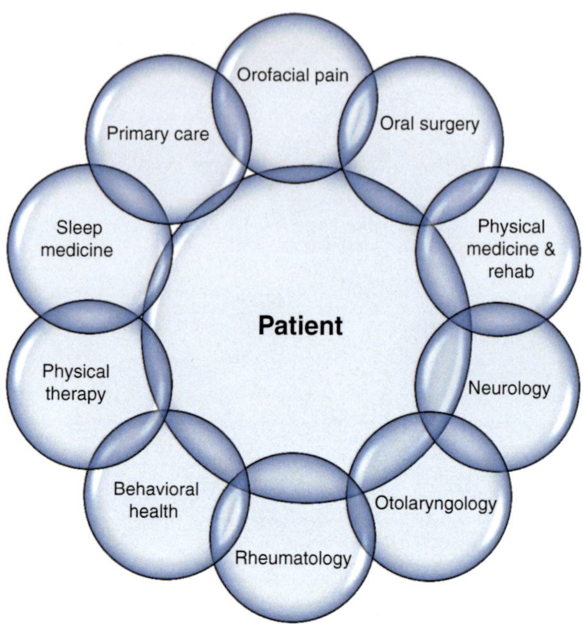

Fig. 25.4 Interdisciplinary orofacial pain care model

Interdisciplinary care, on the other hand, involves providers from various differing specialties that play complementary roles that when implemented together enhance patient care (Fig. 25.4). In an interdisciplinary model, team members have complementary roles and responsibilities, problem solving as one, and sharing accountability for an overlapping continuity of care. Treatment decisions are consensus based, and the process of arriving at a decision is essential to the team's recommendations and treatment implementation. Planned or recommended treatments, therapeutic interventions, and other activities reflect the team's consensus view rather than the view of any single provider [5] (Table 25.3).

Although each clinician may have limited success in managing the "whole" patient alone, the assumption behind a team approach is that it is vital to address different aspects of the problem with different specialists in order to enhance the overall potential for success. Although these programs provide a broader framework for treating the whole complex patient, they have added another dimension to the skills needed by the clinician: those of working as part of a coordinated team. Failure to adequately integrate care may result in poor communication and distrust among team members, fragmented care, and eventually confusion and failure in the clinical management process. Team coordination can be facilitated by a well-defined evaluation and management system that clearly integrates all team members [6].

As previously discussed, the complex neurobiological, behavioral, and psychosocial problems associated with most patients with orofacial disorders can best be managed by an organized multimodal approach that integrates self-care and health care. Patient education, self-responsibility, long-term change, and lasting doctor-patient relationships must be emphasized from initial visit onward.

A prerequisite to implementing a team approach is an inclusive medical model and conceptual framework that places the physical, behavioral, and psychosocial aspects of illness on an equal and integrated basis. Although each clinician understands a different part of the patient's problem, he or she can integrate them with other clinicians' perspectives and see how each part is interrelated in the whole patient. For example, a dentist or physician will evaluate poor postural habits, a psychologist will evaluate emotional problems or social stressors, and together they may address other variables such as sleep disturbance. Each factor will become part of the problem list to be addressed in the treatment plan. In the process, the synergism of each factor in the etiology of the disorder becomes apparent to clinicians (e.g., social stressors lead to depression, depression leads to poor posture and muscle tension, and the poor posture and muscle tension may lead to myalgia or myofascial pain).

Likewise, a reduction in each factor will work synergistically to improve the whole problem. Treatment of only one factor may improve the problem, but relief may be partial or temporary. Application of these concepts requires an interspecialty collaboration of evaluation and management where the providers of health care accept responsibility for addressing the multifaceted problems that exist.

The problem list for a patient with a specific chronic illness includes both a physical diagnosis and a list of contributing factors. This broad understanding of the patient is then used in a long-term management program that both treats the physical diagnosis and helps reduce these contributing factors.

The purpose of treatment includes four goals:

1. Alleviating symptoms
2. Improving functional capacity
3. Reducing negative effects of the illness on the patient's lifestyle
4. Restoring the patients' independence from the health-care system

Treatment of the physical problem includes the accepted dental, medical, physical, or surgical therapy for that diagnosis. Reduction of contributing factors is accomplished through appropriate behavioral or psychological techniques such as education, behavior modification, biofeedback, family therapy, and exercise. Patient education of the pathophysiology of the pain condition can be a key tool in successful treatment and is often overlooked in routine care.

Clinicians must rely on the patient and family self-responsibility for making changes through a home program of self-care, and this begins with having a basic understanding of how the pain condition is affecting them. Improved understanding often equates to improved treatment adherence. Self-care facilitated in a supportive environment in which the patient hears the same message from multiple clinicians and gains the sustained insight, support, and care needed to make the changes that both reduce the pain and improve health, and independent functioning also strengthens the prognosis.

25.3 Implementation of an Interdisciplinary Approach to Orofacial Pain

Patients in both interdisciplinary and multidisciplinary systems may undergo three phases of care: evaluation, management, and follow-up. A breakdown of each phase is listed in Tables 25.4, 25.5, and 25.6:

25.3.1 Evaluation

A patient with a recurring problem presents to the clinic and is examined to determine the physical diagnosis and whether the patient can be helped by the team approach. The clinician explains the diagnosis (if known), what diagnostic tests are necessary, and how the team program can help the patient.

The clinician may explain [6]:

> The symptoms you are experiencing are caused by (physical diagnosis). This diagnosis is characterized by (signs, symptoms, and pathophysiology in lay terms). As you can see, these characteristics fit your situation closely. However, in addition to the diagnosis, there are other factors such as (direct contributing factors) that will lead to (physical diagnosis) and need to be considered. These factors will (put strain on muscles or joints, irritate blood vessels, nerves). We need to do (diagnostic and lab tests or consults) to confirm the diagnosis and other (behavioral, sleep) evaluations to evaluate other contributing factors. The

Table 25.4 Interdisciplinary evaluation

Interdisciplinary evaluation
Initial comprehensive history/examination
Establish an initial diagnosis to determine if a team approach is applicable
Explain the diagnosis, additional tests if necessary, and how the team program can help the patient
Complete informed consent to care if the patient desires treatment
Determine problem severity
Additional diagnostic testing
Special consultations
Thorough health and illness history
Listing of contributing factors
Evaluation by each of the team clinicians to establish a problem list
Chief complaint
Corresponding physical diagnoses
Contributing factors
Treatment planning conference: team members only
Discuss individualized and common findings
Establish a consensus on the diagnosis
Create an integrated, treatment plan designed to treat the diagnosis and reduce contributing factors
Synthesis meeting: team members, patient, and family/significant others to:
Review the diagnosis and contributing factors
Explain the interrelationships of these factors
Assure mutual understanding
Present the individualized treatment plan

Table 25.5 Interdisciplinary management

Primary goals:

1. Reduction of symptoms and their negative effects
2. Return of normal function without need for future health care

Long-term individualized management program (with same team) that integrates:

- Long-term patient education and training with each clinician
  - Review diagnoses and contributing factors
  - Discuss the need to change these factors
  - Educate on how to change
- Short-term medical/dental care and behavioral and physical therapy
  - Physician or dentist
    - Physical diagnoses
    - Short-term care as indicated
    - Monitoring of treatment efficacy
  - Psychologist or behavioral therapist
    - Instruction about contributing factors
    - Diagnosing, managing, or referring for primary psychological disturbances
    - Establishing a program to support the patient and family in making changes
  - Physical therapist
    - Provides support, instruction, and management program (i.e., exercise regimen)
    - May also provide special care modalities (i.e., occupational therapy)

Ensure clear, concise, and ongoing communication (written and verbal) between the various providers and with the patient

Typically involves a sequence of weekly to monthly visits for over 6 months

Table 25.6 Interdisciplinary follow-up

First, a brief follow-up synthesis meeting

- Provide positive reinforcement of progress
- Terminate the program (an option if treatment is complete or as otherwise indicated)
- Provide a "diploma" with goals for maintaining improvement

Second, follow up sessions with one clinician to reinforce changes every 2–3 months

- Changes are considered to be temporary unless they are sustained for over a year
- If a sustained exacerbation of the problem occurs, the clinician and patient determine why and decide if the team should resume efforts

Two common reasons for lack of symptom reduction are:

- Incorrect or incomplete diagnosis
- The presence of a diagnosis with pain that is intractable (i.e., continuous neuralgia)
- Lack of compliance or ability to change a major contributing factor

In these situations, it is important to help prepare the patient for living with the pain, preferably without addictive medications

- Three goals:
  - Reduce effects of pain
  - Improve function
  - Achieve independence from the health-care system
- Provide palliative relief with the use of an individualized home program:
  - Self-care: regular behavioral techniques and home care modalities
  - Pharmacotherapy
  - Complementary and alternative therapies

> treatment program is designed to reduce the (signs and symptoms) by treating the (diagnosis) and reducing these contributing factors. This is done by teaching you to (behavior modification i.e., do exercises, change clenching), doing physical therapy to make muscles and joints more comfortable, and asking you to wear a splint to protect and improve the posture of the muscles and joints (if needed). In addition, we can help you get back to your normal life style by helping to change (indirect contributing factors). Although we can do some things, the majority of work is done by you, at home or work. It is a commitment and it does take time. If you do the things necessary, you should expect to feel much better in as little as 6 months. Although you still may have some pain, you usually will not notice it and if you do, you will learn how to improve it on your own. Does this all makes sense to you? What questions do you have? Do you want to participate in such a program?

If and when the patient desires management, evaluation can begin with diagnostic tests or other consultations to confirm the diagnosis, determine health and illness history, establish a contributing factor list, and utilize indices to measure problem severity. This is followed by an evaluation session with each of team clinicians (dentist and/or physician, psychologist, physical therapist, and other specialty providers as indicated) to assess the characteristics of the problem and establish the patient's unique problem list. The list includes the chief complaint, the corresponding physical diagnoses, and a list of the contributing factors. The evaluation is followed by a synthesis meeting (treatment planning conference), first among the team members, and then with the patient and family or significant others to review diagnosis and contributing factors, explain the interrelationships of the factors, assure mutual understanding, and present an integrated management program designed to treat the diagnosis and reduce the contributing factors (Table 25.7). The purpose of

Table 25.7 Synthesis meetings (interdisciplinary treatment planning conferences) are designed to enhance communication between clinicians, patient, and patient's significant others

Synthesis meeting layout
Clinician synthesis
1. All clinicians included
2. Timing: 5–20 min
3. Establish a problem list and individual patient characteristics
4. Establish specific goals and priorities of treatment, prognosis, and potential problems
5. Determine individual clinician responsibilities in management program
Clinician-patient-family synthesis
1. All clinicians, patient, and significant others, in needed
2. Timing: 15–30 min
3. Dentist or physician reviews diagnoses, characteristics, and causal factors
4. Physical therapist reviews related behavioral and postural contributing factors, how they related to physical diagnoses, and how to change them
5. Psychologist reviews behavioral and psychosocial contributing factors, how they related to physical diagnoses, and how to change them
6. Review goals of improving symptoms by treating diagnoses and reducing contributing factors
7. Each clinician describes his or her role in the overall program
8. Describe prerequisites to beginning program, guidelines of the program, and pragmatic aspects
9. Verify patient understanding and desire to proceed

this meeting is to educate the family and to ensure consistent treatment planning and communication among the clinicians, patient, and family [6].

25.3.2 Management Team

The patient then undergoes a long-term individualized management program (with same team) that integrates long-term patient education and training with short-term traditional medical or dental care. The primary goals of the program include reducing the symptoms and their negative effects while helping the patient return to normal function without need for future health care. The patient first participates in an educational session with each clinician to learn about the diagnoses and contributing factors, why it is necessary to change these factors, and how to do it. The dentist or physician is responsible for establishing the physical diagnoses, providing short-term medical or dental care, and monitoring medication and patient progress. The psychologist or behavioral therapist is responsible for providing instruction about contributing factors, diagnosing, managing, or referring for primary psychological disturbances, and establishing a program to support the patient and family in making changes. The physical therapist is responsible for providing support, instruction, and management program such as an exercise program. Depending on the therapist's background and the patient's needs, this person may also provide special care such as modalities or occupational therapy. Each clinician is also responsible for establishing a trusting, supporting relationship with the patient while reaffirming the self-care philosophy of the program, reinforcing change, and assuring compliance. The patient is viewed as responsible for making the changes. The team meets weekly to review current patient progress and discuss new patients.

25.3.3 Follow-Up

The management program typically involves a sequence of weekly to monthly visits for over 6 months. At the end of the management phase, a brief follow-up synthesis meeting is scheduled with the patient to provide positive reinforcement of progress, terminate the program, and provide a "diploma" with goals for maintaining improvement. This is followed by follow-up sessions with one clinician to reinforce the changes every 2–3 months. The changes are considered to be temporary unless they are sustained for over a year. If a sustained exacerbation of the problem occurs, the clinician and patient determine why and decide if the team should resume efforts. Reasons for failing to achieve the four goals are many and varied. Assuming the correct physical diagnoses, contributing factors, and treatment plan, two common reasons for lack of symptom reduction are (1) the presence of a diagnosis with pain that is intractable, such as continuous neuralgia, and (2) lack of compliance or ability to change a major contributing factor. In these situations, it is important to help prepare the patient for living with the pain, preferably without addictive medications. This can be facilitated by helping the patient achieve the other three goals (reduce effects of pain, improve function, and achieve independence from the health-care system) and provide palliative relief with the use of an individualized home program of self-care, regular behavioral techniques, home care modalities, pharmacotherapy, and complementary and alternative therapies as indicated.

25.3.4 Cost Control Using an Interdisciplinary Team

The interdisciplinary team approach is designed to address cost control factors. It replaces high-cost dentist or physician care by using less costly health-care professionals, other support staff, and surveys to collect and tally repetitious patient information; the dentist or physician is maintained as the health-care team manager. It also focuses on education and self-responsibility in order to reduce care-seeking behavior and dependency and help prevent the development of a perceived need for extensive health care for other problems of living.

One of the major factors that lead a patient with a short-term problem into developing a chronic pain syndrome is the lack of adequate recognition and treatment of the whole problem during the first few months of pain. Thus, in order to prevent development of a chronic pain syndrome, a patient needs to be managed comprehensively from the beginning. Although individual clinicians can do this, the time commitment and training required to provide dental or medical treatment, teach exercises, and address contributing factors by one clinician are often prohibitive, typically less effective, and ultimately frustrating for the solo clinician. However, not all patients with pain require a team approach. Sometimes singular treatments such as splints or biofeedback are effective alone. A decision needs to be made at the initial evaluation on the need for a team or not. Criteria for making this decision include factors such as long duration of pain, overuse of medication, the presence of psychological or sleep disturbance, severity or extent of comorbid chronic pain conditions, potential for secondary gain, gross confusion, and significant parafunctional habits. The use of an interdisciplinary, biopsychosocial-derived patient intake form can readily elicit the degree of complexity of a case at initial evaluation.

Potential barriers to implementing this evaluation and management system in clinical practice may include dentists' or physicians' reluctance or inability to deal with behavioral and psychosocial aspects of illnesses, hesitation to add a team approach to their busy individual practices, or lack of motivation to integrate a self-care philosophy to their concepts of disease management. However, the greatest effort involves the implementation of the system (finding the right clinicians, preparing them for working in a team, rearranging schedules, etc.). Once the system is up and running, however, each clinician enjoys the benefits of collegial support, shared patient care, and team comradery. Each learns from the other clinicians and is therefore better able to recognize contributing factors. This system's simplicity, potential office and patient cost-effectiveness, combined use of traditional dental and medical care, and its easily duplicated information system facilitate its replicability and adaptability. The interdisciplinary team model, in the opinion of many clinicians, researchers, and educators, may be the most effective management option.

25.4 Implementation of an Multidisciplinary Approach to Orofacial Pain

It is important to realize, however, that interdisciplinary management does not necessarily mandate that a patient must be assessed and treated by multiple professionals. There are many situations where it is simply not possible, usually due to a lack of resources, location, or availability, to provide truly integrated interdisciplinary care. In these situations individual provider who possesses a broad array of skills may be in the best position to deliver optimum orofacial pain management. Such skills are based upon an expanded understanding of orofacial pain that appreciates the unique anatomic and physiological complexities of cranial nerve systems and incorporates recent advances in the neurobiology of pain. Contemporary neuroscience validates the need for an interdisciplinary approach toward orofacial disorder practice. It moves the provider beyond a simple biomechanical or inflammatory concept of pain, substantiates the biologic basis for the biopsychosocial model of pain, and provides pathophysiologic links between orofacial pain disorders and common comorbid pain conditions such as irritable bowel or fibromyalgia.

Multidisciplinary orofacial pain management also consists of the three basic phases: evaluation, management, and follow-up.

25.4.1 Evaluation

Similar to the interdisciplinary method, multidisciplinary care begins with a comprehensive patient history conducted by an individual provider. Perhaps the most expeditious way to obtain such a history is via a detailed patient questionnaire. Such an instrument seeks not just information about the chief complaint but also records a complete medical and treatment history, asks about any site of pain anywhere in the body, assesses affect, checks for awareness of muscle parafunction, reviews personal habits and nutrition, seeks insight into vocational and family concerns, inquires about negative life events (i.e., abuse, assault, childhood neglect, etc.), and

Table 25.8 Multidisciplinary evaluation

Patient completes a comprehensive, detailed, patient questionnaire that is reviewed by the patient and provider
Discuss history of the chief complaint
Complete medical and treatment history
Ask about any site of pain anywhere in the body
Review personal habits and nutrition
Check for awareness of muscle parafunction
Assess affect (stress, anxiety, depression, anger, etc.)
Vocational and family concerns
Negative life events (i.e., abuse, assault, childhood neglect, etc.)
Solicit information about sleep
Initial comprehensive examination
Complete oral, head, and neck examination
Distinguish sites from sources of pain
Determine the extent of physical dysfunction
Integrate appropriate imaging, diagnostic testing, and/or laboratory studies
Establish a list of differential diagnoses and contributing factors
Explain the etiology and pathophysiology and thoroughly discuss all treatment options and prognosis
Complete informed consent to care if the patient desires treatment

solicits information about sleep. After a detailed history is obtained, comprehensive head, neck, and oral examinations are completed. These exams should distinguish the sites from sources of pain and the extent of physical dysfunction and should also integrate appropriate imaging and/or laboratory studies. The information collected from each step is the foundation for establishing a list of differential diagnoses and contributing factors [1] (Table 25.8).

25.4.2 Management

In some cases, the provider may have the appropriate training, experience, and resources to handle all of the patient's treatment needs and address the relevant contributory factors. In other instances, the assistance of additional practitioners may be required. Health-care providers often involved with the global management of orofacial pain patients include dentists, oral surgeons, primary care physicians, neurologists, physiatrists, physical therapists, psychiatrists, psychologists, otolaryngologists, and rheumatologists (Table 25.9).

Table 25.9 Management

Management
Primary goals:
Reduction of symptoms and their negative effects
Return of normal function without need for future health care
In some cases, the provider may have the appropriate training, experience, and resources to handle all of the patient's treatment needs and address the relevant contributory factors
Consider the impact of all sources of pain, including those outside the orofacial region
Non-trigeminal sources of nociception may:
Refer pain cephalad
Facilitate cranial nerve-mediated muscle parafunction
Induce co-contraction and disrupt sleep
Reduce masticatory and cervical muscle overuse to decrease fatigue, pain, and joint overloading
Employ behavioral strategies that increase parafunctional awareness and diminish the brain activity that may facilitate inappropriate muscle use [7]
Reduce physiological arousal
Use relaxation techniques, such as diaphragmatic breathing and imagery, to affect brain regions that may adversely influence pain thresholds, muscle activity, or sleep
Recognize the need to address negative affect, stressful personal-family-vocational issues, and the excessive use of stimulants (caffeine, nicotine, etc.)
Enhance sleep
Explore all factors that can delay, disrupt, or lighten sleep
Educate patients about the importance of sleep hygiene measures and cognitive behavioral strategies such as sleep restriction, stimulus control, and relaxation techniques [8]
When prescribing sedative-hypnotic medications, give preference to those that promote the later stages of sleep
In other instances, the assistance of additional practitioners may be required
Health-care providers often involved with the global management of orofacial pain patients include:
Dentist specialists
Primary (or internal) care medicine
Behavioral health
Neurology
Otolaryngology
Rheumatology
Physical medicine and rehabilitation/physiatry
Physical therapy
Sleep medicine
Ensure clear, concise, and ongoing communication (written and verbal) between the various providers and with the patient
Typically involves a sequence of weekly to monthly visits for over 6 months (based on individual treatment needs)

25.4.3 Follow-Up

Essentially the same as with the interdisciplinary plan, however, additional consultation from another provider (as discussed above) may be indicated (Table 25.10).

Table 25.10 Follow-up

First, a brief follow-up(s)
Ensure efficacy of treatment
Establish adherence to the treatment plan
Provide positive reinforcement of progress
Adjust/coordinate care as indicated
Second, follow up sessions to reinforce changes every 3–6 months
Changes are considered to be temporary unless they are sustained for over a year
If a sustained exacerbation of the problem occurs, the clinician and patient determine why and decide if they should resume efforts (or seek additional consultation)
Two common reasons for lack of symptom reduction are:
Incorrect or incomplete diagnosis
The presence of a diagnosis with pain that is intractable (i.e., continuous neuralgia)
Lack of compliance or ability to change a major contributing factor
In these situations, it is important to help prepare the patient for living with the pain, preferably without addictive medications
Three goals:
Reduce effects of pain
Improve function
Achieve independence from the health-care system
Provide palliative relief with the use of an individualized home program:
Self-care
Regular behavioral techniques
Home care modalities
Pharmacotherapy
Complementary and alternative therapies

25.5 Neurobiological Considerations in Orofacial Pain Management

One of the difficulties in dealing with orofacial pain complaints relates to the structural complexity of the trigeminal nerve system. It is incumbent for clinicians to distinguish true sources of pain from trigeminal sites of pain and to discern the locations of all non-trigeminal sources of pain. The trigeminal sensory nuclei receive extensive input from structures within the brain stem and midbrain that process sensory information from tissues outside the face. The trigeminal interpolaris and spinal tract nuclei receive convergent sensory input from the facial, glossopharyngeal, and vagus nerves, as well as the upper cervical nerves (C1–C4) [9]. Convergent nociceptive input from non-trigeminal afferent neurons provides an anatomic explanation as to how disorders in remote regions of the head and neck may refer pain to the face.

Another important consideration in orofacial pain is the capability of non-trigeminal brain centers to induce non-volitional trigeminal motor responses, muscle activity that has been often labeled as "parafunction." Integrative centers within the brain stem, such as the parvocellular reticular formation and paratrigeminal nucleus, receive both noxious and non-noxious visceral, cutaneous, and autonomic input and, via connections with the trigeminal nuclear complex, may produce a masticatory muscle response [10]. Similarly, activity in higher brain centers, such as the limbic system and prefrontal cortex, can engage descending neural circuits also capable of inciting masticatory muscle activity [11]. Concurrent with induced masticatory responses, hypoglossal, spinal accessory, facial, glossopharyngeal, and vagal motor centers may also be activated. Afferent input from tissues controlled by these nerves may contribute to the wide constellation of symptoms seen in widespread pain cases with multiple comorbidities.

Persistent, nonfunctional masticatory muscle activity may have significant biologic and clinical consequences. Even low levels of muscle activity excite metaboreceptors that send impulses to the central nervous system via group III and IV afferents (A delta and C fibers) [12], the same classes of first-order neurons activated by peripheral nociceptors. Metaboreceptor activity of sufficient intensity and duration may be noxious and produce pain. Excessive metaboreceptor activity may lead to central sensitization, facilitate the referred pain phenomenon associated with myofascial pain, and induce masticatory muscle co-contraction. Activation may also contribute to pathologic changes within the temporomandibular joint (TMJ). Prolonged periods of increased intra-articular pressure have been associated with local tissue hypoxia, free radical formation, and oxygen reperfusion injury, all factors thought to play a role in the genesis of TMJ osteoarthritis and disc displacements [13, 14].

Interestingly, the presence of muscle pain may also decrease proprioceptive feedback; thus, a patient may not be fully aware of the extent of their muscle parafunction or overuse [15]. There is an increasing body of evidence that many orofacial pain patients frequently possess other remarkable physical and mental health concerns. Turp and colleagues found that 82% of facial pain patients also had additional pain complaints outside the distribution of the trigeminal system [16]. Based on an anonymous self-report survey, 68% of patients referred to a university orofacial pain center indicated a history of physical or sexual abuse [17].

Recent investigations have shown that patients with temporomandibular disorders often have coexisting conditions including irritable bowel disease, fibromyalgia, migraine, panic disorder, and others [18]. The link between these seemingly disparate disorders is the potential of a shared neuropathophysiology involving alterations in hypothalamic-pituitary-adrenal axis, autonomic nervous system, and limbic system-prefrontal cortex responses [19]. Hyperactivity, hypoactivity, or lack of coordination within or between the aforementioned systems could lead to dysfunctional allostasis, changes in vasomotor responses, modification in respiration, and alterations in sensory processing [20].

In summary, when one considers the negative impact of these comorbid chronic pain conditions, an integrated treatment approach, whether interdisciplinary or multidisciplinary, is vital to the successful management of orofacial pain conditions.

Disclosure Statement by the Author The opinions or assertions contained herein are the private ones of the author(s) and are not to be construed as official or reflecting the view of the DoD or the USUHS. The author does not have any financial interest in the companies whose materials are discussed in this article.

References

1. De Leeuw R, Klasser G. In: de Leeuw R, editor. Orofacial pain guidelines for assessment, diagnosis, and management. Hanover Park: Quintessence Books; 2013.
2. Dworkin S, Massoth D. Temporomandibular disorders and chronic pain: disease or illness? J Prosthet Dent. 1994;72:29–38.
3. Verhoef M, O'Hara D, Findlay B, Boon H. From parallel practice to integrative health care: a conceptual framework. BMC Health Serv Res. 2004;4:15.
4. Price SD, Crawford GB. Team working: palliative care as a model of interdisciplinary practice. MJA. 2003;179(suppl):S32–4.
5. Turk D, Paice J, Cowan P, Stanos S, Jamison R, Covington E, Palermo T, Gordon D, Clark M. Interdisciplinary pain management, American Pain Society - Position Statement (White Paper): American Pain Society, 4700 W. Lake Avenue, Glenview, IL 60025; 2009.
6. Fricton J. Untitled paper on interdisciplinary model of care for chronic pain patients, Minneapolis: unpublished. 2005.
7. Carlson CR. Psychological factors associated with orofacial pains. Dent Clin North Am. 2007;51:145–60.
8. Pace-Schott EF, Stickgold R, Otto MW, Jacobs GD. Cognitive behavior therapy and pharmacotherapy for insomnia. Arch Intern Med. 2004;164:1888–96.
9. Sessle B. Acute and chronic craniofacial pain: brainstem mechanisms of nociceptive transmission and neuroplasticity, and their clinical correlates. Crit Rev Oral Biol Med. 2000;11(1):57–91.
10. Copray JC, Liem RS, Van Willigen JD, Ter Horst GJ. Projections from the rostral parvocellular reticular formation to pontine and medullary nuclei in the rat: involvement in autonomic regulation and orofacial motor control. Neuroscience. 1991;40(3):735.
11. Nieuwenhuys R. The greater limbic system, the emotional motor system and the brain. Prog Brain Res. 1996;107:551–80.
12. Hill JM, Kaufman MP, Adreani CM. Responses of group III and IV muscle afferents to dynamic exercise. J Appl Physiol. 1997;82(6):1811–7.
13. Schmitz JP, Milam SB. Molecular biology of temporomandibular joint disorders: proposed mechanisms of disease. J Oral Maxillofac Surg. 1995;53:1448–54.
14. Nitzan DW. The process of lubrication impairment and its involvement in temporomandibular joint disc displacement: a theoretical concept. J Oral Maxillofac Surg. 2001;59:36–45.
15. della Volpe R, Ginanneschi F, Ulivelli M, Bartalini S, Spidalieri R, Rossi A, Rossi S. Early somatosensory processing during tonic muscle pain in humans: relation to loss of proprioception and motor 'defensive' strategies. Clin Neurophysiol. 2003;114:1351–8.
16. KowalskiO'Leary CJN, O'Leary N, Stohler CS, Turp JC. Pain maps from facial pain patients indicate a broad pain geography. J Dent Res. 1998;77(6):1465–72.
17. Sherman JJ, Cunningham LL, Okeson JP, Reid KI, Carlson CR, Curran SL. Physical and sexual abuse among orofacial pain patients: linkages with pain and psychological distress. J Orofac Pain. 1995;9(4):340–6.
18. Burke MM, Buchwald D, Aaron LA. Overlapping conditions among patients with chronic fatigue syndrome, fibromyalgia and temporomandibular disorder. Arch Intern Med. 2000;160:221–7.
19. Mayer EA. The neurobiology of stress and gastrointestinal disease. Gut. 2000;47:861–9.
20. Schatman M. Psychological assessment of maldynic pain: the need for a phenomenological approach. In: Giordano J, editor. Maldynia: inter-disciplinary perspectives on the illness of chronic pain. New York: CRC Press; 2011. p. 157–82.
21. "MediLexicon", MediLexicon International Ltd. [Online]. [Accessed 01 07 2016].

Transformative Care for Orofacial Disorders

26

James R. Fricton

Pearls of Wisdom

- When implementing transformative care for orofacial disorders, our main goals should go beyond management and include training to reduce risk factors and enhance protective factors and education on prevention toward recurrence or toward a chronic pain state.
- Transformative care involves the following tasks:
  1. *Evaluating* the person with chronic pain as a whole by identifying and understanding both their risk and protective factors.
  2. *Improving* the safety of treatments to minimize the development or progression of orofacial disorders as an adverse event.
  3. *Implementing* a transformative model of healthcare through a team approach
  4. *Continuing* medical and dental education courses that review the fundamentals of this new approach to care. New healthcare routines should include toolkits to implement online self-management training with evidence-based therapies.
  5. *Supporting* resources to help implement transformative care.

J.R. Fricton, DDS, MS
Schools of Dentistry, Medicine and Public Health, University of Minnesota and HealthPartners Institute, Minneapolis, MN, USA
e-mail: frict001@umn.edu

J.N.A.R. Ferreira et al. (eds.), *Orofacial Disorders*,
DOI 10.1007/978-3-319-51508-3_26

Table 26.1 Common orofacial disorders that require special diagnostic and treatment needs with estimated prevalence

Orofacial pain disorders	Estimated prevalence
Temporomandibular disorders	5–7%
Orofacial pain disorders (burning mouth, neuropathic, atypical pain, neurovascular)	2–3%
Headache disorder (tension-type headaches, migraine, mixed, cluster)	20%
Orofacial sleep disorders (e.g., sleep apnea, snoring)	3–4%
Neurosensory and chemosensory disorders (e.g., taste, paresthesias, numbness)	0.1%
Oromotor disorders (e.g., oral habits, occlusal dysesthesias, dystonias, dyskinesias)	4%
Oral lesions (herpes, aphthous, precancer, cancer)	3–5%
Oral mucosal disease (e.g., lichen planus, candida)	1–2%
Dry mouth, salivary disorders, and xerostomia related to caries	2%
Oral systemic disorders (e.g., autoimmune, cancer, heart disease, etc.)	2–3%
Total estimated prevalence in general population	42–50%

26.1 Introduction

Orofacial disorders are among the most common conditions and include headache, temporomandibular pain, orofacial pain, obstructive sleep apnea/snoring, dry mouth, and many other conditions in the mouth, face, head, and neck with a collective prevalence of at least 40% of the population (Table 26.1) [1–5]. Because oral and facial structures have close associations with functions of eating, communication, sight, and hearing as well as form the basis for appearance, self-esteem, and personal expression, persistent pain or disease in this area can deeply affect an individual both psychologically and systemically. A national poll found more adults working full-time miss work from head and face pain than any other site of pain [6]. Unfortunately, access to care for patients with these disorders is often difficult because the limited number of dentists and physicians who specialize in this area and the fact that they care lies between medicine and dentistry. This book presents a brief summary of the treatment needed for each type of orofacial disorders. However, to best care for these disorders, this chapter describes a transformative approach to care that has more success long term by shifting the paradigms of care to be more patient centered with integration of patient training with treatment of the condition.

26.2 The Problem with Orofacial Disorders

With at least 100 million US adults suffering from orofacial disorders, it has also become a primary reason for seeking healthcare. Over half of all healthcare visits are attributed to some type of pain condition, with pain from orofacial disorders including headache, temporomandibular disorder pain, facial pain, and mouth pain being the most common [1–4]. Since most health professionals including physicians and dentists are not trained in orofacial disorders, patients often shop around seeing an array of medical and dental primary care and specialists and can end up on trials of different medications, therapies, surgeries, and other treatments. Yet, a survey of 405 health professionals found that 95% would like to refer these patients to a specialist because of their complex nature [5, 6]. Because the specialties of orofacial pain and oral medicine are just emerging, there are insufficient numbers of specialists in the field to provide adequate access to care for these problems. If pain continues, care may escalate to higher cost, higher-risk passive interventions such as ongoing opioid analgesics, polypharmacy, implantable devices, injections, and surgeries [1–3, 14–19]. If opioid analgesics are used, especially at high doses, there is an increased risk of abuse leading to unintended overdose-related deaths, which now outnumber motor vehicle-related deaths in some states [5–11]. Unfortunately, many people with pain after 1 month still have persistent pain 5 years later despite these extensive interventions [16, 17].

This delayed recovery and progress of pain has less to do with failed treatment than it is due to the presence of multiple risk factors that contribute to persistence of the conditions. Although genetic factors may predispose one to chronic pain, there is also much research which suggests that repetitive strain, depression, poor sleep, stress, maladaptive postures, and ergonomics are among the many contributing factors leading to delayed recovery, failed treatment, and continued pain [12–23]. Despite recognition that many of these factors can be improved with self-management strategies, they are often not addressed in routine care, which can lead to pain persisting for years. Thus, pain becomes a problem when practitioners fail to engage, empower, and educate patients in reducing risk factors and enhancing protective factors to help prevent pain from becoming chronic [20–24]. Prevalence and impact data as well as recommendations from the Institute of Medicine Report and the National Pain Strategy show that more effort is needed in prevention and successful early intervention using a transformative care approach when caring for patients with pain conditions [22, 23]. If health professionals want to improve patient outcomes, they need to consider helping people identify and change the multidimensional risk factors that may contribute to delayed recovery and chronic pain. We can only do this by shifting our care model from a *provider-centric passive care model* to an *active patient-centered transformative care model* that educates, engages, and empowers patients to transform their lives from one of pain and suffering to one of health and well-being.

26.3 Transforming Pain to Health and Well-Being

A new approach that conceptualizes these conditions more broadly with a focus on prevention and early intervention is recommended [32–35]. A *human systems approach* provides a broader understanding of the role of diverse personal risk factors which can delay healing and perpetuate pain and dysfunction through recursive feedback cycles that increase both peripheral and central sensitization [34–39]. A *transformative care model* is the clinical application of a human systems approach;

it integrates risk factor assessments and robust personalized self-management training of patients, integrated with evidence-based treatments [34]. Risk factor assessment identifies both risk and protective factors that tilt the balance between pain and suffering to health and well-being. Self-management programs can then help train patients to reduce the identified risk factors, enhance protective factors, and reverse the perpetuation of chronic pain. This can best be implemented through an *integrative team* approach that supports the patient in implementing lifestyle changes and long-term improvement in preventing chronic pain.

Transformation of our care to a broader conceptual model of care with new clinical paradigms can be challenging even for the most innovative healthcare professional. For this reason, additional training is recommended. One example of a resource for transformative care are toolkits (www.preventingchronicpain.org) intended for health professionals to integrate online self-management training along with evidence-based treatments as part of routine care. In addition, the massive open online course (MOOC) on preventing chronic pain (www.coursera.org/learn/chronic-pain) presents an online continuing education course for health professionals to review the fundamentals of this new approach to care [40, 41]. This chapter briefly discusses this new approach to care.

26.3.1 Human Systems Model

This human systems conceptual model assumes that people are complex, multidimensional, and dynamic and live within an ever-changing social and physical environment. In contrast, the traditional biomedical model is based on a scientific paradigm that is unidimensional, reductionist, and inflexible, based primarily on understanding underlying pathophysiology (Table 26.2). Healthcare professionals often tend to see what they treat and treat what they see. If they see only the pathophysiology, the complex set of risk and protective factors in chronic pain will be missed. As a result, success of treatment can be compromised by limited approaches that only address part of the problem. For example, some systematic reviews of biomedical treatments for chronic pain have found that even with the most efficacious treatments, the improvement occurs only slightly above placebo [28–30].

A broader conceptual basis is required for orofacial disorders, one that includes understanding how different realms of our lives can interact and contribute to chronic pain. Human systems theory (HST) stems from research in general systems theory and originated in ecology out of the need to explain the interrelatedness of organisms in ecosystems [33–40]. A human systems approach integrates concepts—neuroplasticity, mind-body connectedness, positive psychology, cybernetics, chaos theory, social psychology, cognitive behavioral science, and mindfulness—to help explain the delicate balance between health and illness (Table 26.3) [33–40]. While many distinct pathophysiological mechanisms may occur in chronic pain conditions, HST suggests that it is the complex interaction of diverse factors below, which can initiate, perpetuate, or even protect people from the chronic pain progression

Table 26.2 Comparison of the traditional biomedical model and a human systems model

Concept	Biomedical model	Human systems model
Conceptual basis	Reductionist, mechanistic, inflexible	Holistic, fluid, flexible
Application of scientific methods	Relies on objective physical measures, single brief interventions, and randomized controlled trials	Relies on objective and subjective measures, multiple interventions over longer periods, and pragmatic clinical trials
Etiology	Pathophysiologic etiology based on single static etiology (e.g., infectious agent, structural change, cancer)	Multifactorial dynamic etiology of chronic illness (e.g., influence of risk and protective factors on physical tissues)
Problem list	Identify chief complaint and diagnoses in the physical or psychiatric realm	Identify chief complaints, diagnoses, along with contributing factors in each aspect of life—body, mind, spirit, lifestyle, emotions, environment, and society
Treatment strategy	Unidimensional—encourages single sequential treatments	Multidimensional—integrates multiple interventions with self-management of risk and protective factors
Providers	Single clinician providing single intervention that is easy to implement. May lead to fragmented approaches	Interdisciplinary, integrative team of clinicians who address multiple levels of contributing factors. More complex to implement
Reimbursement	Well supported by traditional healthcare delivery system with an economic model that rewards procedures over process	Supported by evolving healthcare delivery system with economic incentives for patient-centered care
Outcomes	Good outcomes with acute conditions; poor outcomes with chronic illness due fragmentation of multiple single treatments	Good outcomes with chronic illness due to use of transformative care model with self-management, biomedical interventions, and a team approach

Table 26.3 Human systems theory provides an inclusive conceptual framework for transformative care and integrates multiple theories

Systems theory and ecology	*See the big picture*	All realms of an ecosystem are interrelated and impact each other
Neuroplasticity and mind-body connections	*The brain can change pain*	We can learn to turn the volume up and down on pain with changes that influence peripheral and central sensitization
Positive psychology	*Positive wins over negative*	Strengthening protective factors, cultivating strengths, and encouraging what is best within a person have more impact than reducing the negative
Cybernetics	*What goes around comes around*	Each element of a system generates a change, which causes positive or negative feedback to the entire system and leads to first-order reactive change, second-order revelation change, or third-order transformative change

(continued)

Table 26.3 (continued)

Chaos theory	*It's the little things every day that matter*	Small differences in initial conditions may yield widely diverging outcomes within dynamic systems like humans. Thus, the influence of multiple small risk and protective factors can play a significant role in shifting the balance between health and illness
Social psychology	*Relationships matter to our health*	Our thoughts, feelings, and behaviors are influenced by the actual, imagined, or implied presence of others
Cognitive behavioral science	*We are what we repeatedly think, do, and feel*	How we think (cognition), how we feel (emotions), and how we act (behavior) all interact and can influence each other
Mindfulness	*Be here now*	By training our minds to be in the present moment and nonjudgmental, our health and well-being are enhanced

Table 26.4 Description of the seven realms (with the acronym BLESS ME) in human systems approach to preventing chronic pain

Realm	Description	Protective factors	Risk factors
Body	Physical and physiologic aspects of the body	Balanced relaxed posture, stretching, strengthening, and conditioning exercise	Genetic risk, comorbid conditions, poor posture, tight weak muscles, hypo- or hypermobile joints, poor conditioning, and injury
Lifestyle	Lifestyles and behaviors that we do regularly	Protective diet, steady pacing, being active, regular sleep, low-risk behaviors, high energy, and compliance with protective actions	Poor diet, sedentary life, prolonged sitting, poor sleep, hurrying/rushed, repetitive strain, high-risk behaviors, chemical use, low energy
Emotions	Positive and negative feelings we experience	Sustained positive emotions, such as joy, excitement, confidence, optimism, happiness, and contentment	Prolonged negative emotional experiences, anger, anxiety, sadness, fear, and depression
Society	Social relationships with the people around us	Positive relationships, social support, helping others, reward for recovery, e.g., family, friends, colleagues, community, society	Poor relationships, conflict, abuse, posttraumatic stress, low social support, isolation, secondary and tertiary gain
Spirit	Higher beliefs and purposes that drive us	Purpose, direction, beliefs, faith, hope, self-compassion, and self-esteem	Stress, burnout, disbelief, cynicism, doubt, helpless, and hopelessness
Mind	Thoughts and attitudes	Whole understanding, resilience, self-efficacy, self-control, accepting responsibility, realistic expectations, and engaging in active coping	Ignorance of problem, low resilience, low self-efficacy/control, refuse responsibility, poor compliance, unrealistic expectations, and passive coping
Environment	Physical environment that surrounds us	Clean, organized, safe environment, and an approach that is protective, cautious, and careful	Living within an unclean, chaotic, and disorganized environment with activities that are negligent, dangerous, risky, and increase risk of injury, accident, and trauma

and peripheral to central sensitization. HST views a person as a whole, with the interrelationship between different realms of their life contributing to this balance (Table 26.4). These realms are not static and independent but rather are dynamic, evolving, and interrelated processes that involve sets of risk and protective factors that can shift the balance between health and illness.

Successful management of orofacial disorders includes preventing the progression from acute pain to chronic or even intractable pain. An illness such as a pain disorder often begins with initiating factors such as an acute physical injury. In most cases, this condition is transient and heals without complication or persistence. However, if a sufficient, even small, number of risk factors are present, it can shift the balance from the healing of acute pain to a delayed recovery and chronic pain. Strengthening protective factors and successful reduction of multiple risk factors in the cycle may have the significant impact in healing the injured tissues. This strategy supports the concepts of multimodal and interdisciplinary team care that amplifies the small effect of interventions by including self-management training to achieve the best possible outcomes. To achieve these outcomes, several new strategies are needed by the healthcare provider including recognizing their role as agent of change, employing an inclusive problem list (see below), determining the complexity of patient, following a decision tree for increasing the potential for successful management, and employing interdisciplinary and integrated treatment protocols to address the whole problem list. When evidence-based biomedical treatments are combined with robust patient training to reduce risk factors and enhance protective factors, the potential of transforming a person's life from one of illness to health and wellness is enhanced. This premise is the basis for a transformative model of pain care.

26.3.2 Transformative Care

The Institute of Medicine's (IOM) monograph, *Relieving Pain in America*, emphasizes the need to *transform* our current passive model of *doctor-centered* care into one that is *patient centered* [1]. The document states, "Healthcare provider organizations should take the lead in developing educational approaches and materials for people with pain and their families that promote and enable self-management." The IOM further states that health professionals' primary role in caring for chronic pain requires guiding, coaching, and assisting patients with day-to-day self-management in addition to evidence-based biomedical treatments [22]. Unfortunately, most health professionals lack the time and training to perform this role and find little support and reimbursement from health plans for doing so. Transformative care is a new care model that integrates robust self-management training with the best and safest evidence-based treatments. Clinical trials of self-management strategies that activate the patient through exercise and cognitive and behavioral changes have equal or better efficacy than passive treatments in preventing or alleviating chronic pain [24–33]. When self-management training supplements treatments, the long-term outcomes can be dramatically improved while also reducing

Table 26.5 Clinical paradigms associated with transformative care and a human systems approach to preventing chronic pain

New paradigm	Statement that shifts to the new paradigm
Understand the whole patient	Identify all diagnoses, risk factors, and protective factors in the seven realms of life (body, mind, spirit, lifestyle, emotion, social, and physical environment) to shift the balance from illness to health
Each patient is complex	Multiple conditions and interrelated contributing factors may initiate, result from, increase risk, or decrease risk of illness. Each needs to be addressed as part of management strategy
Self-responsibility is key to recovery	You have more influence on the problem than any treatment provided. Will you take ownership and control of the condition?
Self-care	You will need to make daily changes in order to improve your condition
Education and training	We will teach you how to make these changes
Long-term change	Change only occurs over time, and it may take months for the changes to have a large impact on reducing pain and symptoms
Strong provider-patient partnerships	We, as health professionals, will support you as you make the changes. We can be an agent to help you change
Personal motivation	Will you be able to make the changes needed?
Social support	You may need help to make these changes
Change process	Change will occur incrementally over time
Fluctuation of progress	Expect ups and downs during the recovery process

the patient's dependency on the healthcare system. Thus, a transformative care model can help transform not only the patient's life but the healthcare system too.

The clinical application of transformative care involves identifying and reducing risk factors for chronic pain while also training the patients in improving protective factors, as illustrated in Table 26.4. Transformative care includes the use of pain risk assessments to identify risk and protective factors as part of a whole person problem list. Personalized care strategies include integrative teams that can be supported by health coaches, social support networks, and consumer-based health information technology for both patient training and documenting outcomes. Since patients often expect to have a passive role in care, these new paradigms need to be conveyed to the patient as part of the evaluation (Table 26.5). Embracing patient-centered healthcare paradigms such as self-responsibility, education, personal motivation, self-efficacy, social support, strong provider-patient relationships, and long-term change will shift the balance of care from one of a passive, dependent patient to an empowered, engaged, and educated patient [22, 23]. Ultimately, this paradigm shift has potential to not only improve the quality of care and enhance pain and functional outcomes but also will significantly reduce healthcare costs. In the process, the Institute for Healthcare Improvement's triple aim of improving population health, enhancing the patient care experience (including quality, access, and reliability), and controlling or reducing cost of care will be achieved [44].

Table 26.6 Health consciousness

Fifth level	*Transformative health consciousness*
	Wellness warriors live each day with maximum implementation of health and wellness actions in all seven realms and actively act as evolutionary co-creators to help others achieve the same
Fourth level	*Enlightened health consciousness*
	Health actives live each day mindful of the knowledge and decisions that determine their own health and well-being in all seven realms and take active steps to maintain it
Third level	*Informed health consciousness*
	Weekend actives are informed of the importance of health and well-being and take some time each week to practice healthy actions in some realms but are not able to maintain this most days or in all realms
Second level	*Illness-centered health consciousness*
	Illness-centered passives react to illnesses and take only limited short-term actions to help recover from the illness but often do not sustain the changes over time
First level	*Medically dependent health consciousness*
	Medically dependent passives are continuously involved in passive treatment with a health professional and take little to no time and effort to take responsibility and actions to help their own health and well-being

A person's level of health and wellness consciousness determines the degree to which they take actions to maintain their optimal health and wellness and determines the amount of healthcare they require. The higher levels of health consciousness requires less healthcare than lower levels

26.3.3 The Healthcare Provider as an Agent of Transformative Change

Health professionals need to recognize their important role of not only providing treatments but also helping the people transform their health consciousness from being illness centered and healthcare dependent to one of maintaining health and well-being on a daily basis (Table 26.6). As part of this, health professionals need to recognize the limits of biomedical treatments such as medication, interventions, and surgery that may in some cases lead to additional problems, like adverse events, addictions, neuropathic pain, fibrosis from repeated surgeries, and secondary gain from care seeking to validate their illnesses. Rebound pain from medications can actually be part of the patient's pattern of problems and generate self-sustaining chronic pain. If clinicians understand their integral role in tipping the balance from illness to health, they can be an agent of transformative change and part of the long-term solution. They can help patients reconstruct their world into one of health and well-being and not illness. Clinicians can facilitate patients achieving the deepest most permanent order of change—a third-order change, defined as the capacity to change their epistemology of health and illness, i.e., how they understand of their own powerful role in developing illness, thereby learning how they can maintain health and well-being for their lifetime. Through this third order of change, patients may see their world differently as enlightened and transformative wellness warriors. To do so, they first must understand each component of the problem by establishing a complete problem list that includes both the physical problem and the contributing factors.

26.3.4 Determine the Complete Problem List

Human systems theory expands the traditional "problem list" of the chief complaint and physical diagnosis to also include the list of contributing factors in each of the seven realms—mind, body, emotions, spirit, lifestyle, social, and physical environment. The physical diagnosis defines the physical problem that is responsible for the chief complaint and associated symptoms, whereas, contributing factors include those factors that initiate, perpetuate, or result from the disorder but in some way complicate the whole problem. Multidimensional assessment will help determine which contributing factors are present. Specific risk factors for chronic pain are included in Table 26.4 and may range from peripheral factors such as repetitive stress-strain and postural habits to central mediating factors such as anxiety and depression, comorbid conditions, somatization, and catastrophizing [44, 45–49]. Protective factors—level of coping, self-efficacy, exercise, and patient beliefs such as perceived control over pain and understanding that pain is a sign of strain or injury—reduce vulnerability to chronic pain [40, 41]. Social support can also affect outcomes.

26.3.5 Matching Complexity of the Patient with the Complexity of Care

The level of care for patients can vary considerably from simple to complex. Patients with complex chronic illness often present with a frustrating medical and dental situation, which may include persistent aggravation of symptoms, multiple clinicians, long-term medications, repeated healthcare visits, and an ongoing dependency on the healthcare system. Thus, successful management is enhanced if the level of complexity is determined and matched to the complexity of the treatment strategy. Singular treatment strategies such as self-management, physical therapy, or medication can be quite successful with patients with few contributing factors but often fail in patients with complex contributing factors, due to the chronic nature of the disease and the long-standing maladaptive behaviors, attitudes, and lifestyles. Thus, it is helpful to follow a decision-making process that can distinguish simple from complex patients and direct the treatment strategy.

Figure 26.1 outlines the decision tree for sequencing evaluation and management for simple and complex cases. Once the complete problem list is developed, it can be used as criteria to distinguish simple and complex patients. Complexity of the patient increases with the presence of multiple diagnoses, persistent pain longer than 6 months, significant emotional problems, frequent use of healthcare services or

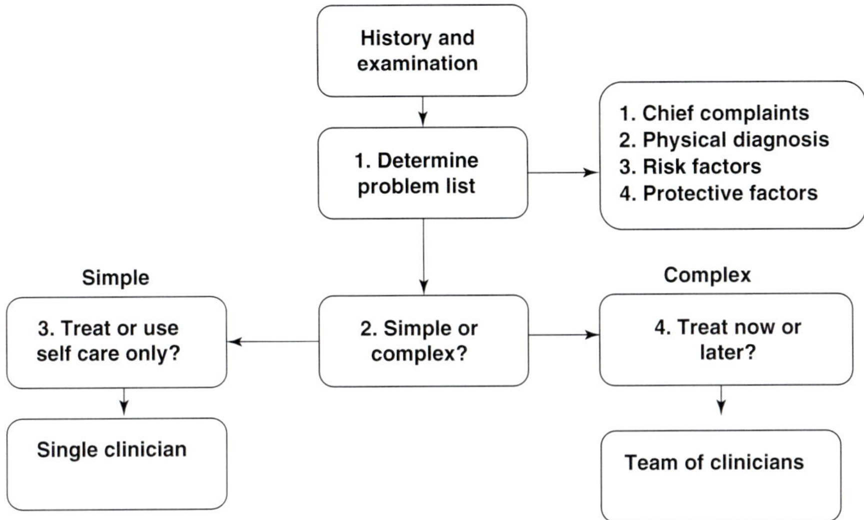

Fig. 26.1 A decision tree for triaging patients and enhancing outcomes and successful care

medication, repetitive muscle strain, and significant lifestyle disturbances. In addition, there are some complex patients who warrant deferral of treatment until more complex problems are addressed. The criteria for not treating until these problems are resolved include primary chemical dependency, primary psychiatric disorder, significant litigation, and a patient unmotivated and/or overwhelmed with other concerns.

26.3.6 Integrative Care

Multimodal treatments within an interdisciplinary integrative care model can best set the stage for a second or third level change in the patient's life by addressing the physical diagnosis and all of its contributing factors. This model includes screening for pain risk assessment; implementing cognitive, emotional, and behavioral change; self-management; patient advocacy; and focus on a patient-centered model. Once complexity is determined, simple chronic illness patients can be successfully treated using a single clinician and treatment to achieve resolution in 2–3 months.

With more complex cases, it is recommended they be managed by an integrative team of clinicians to achieve the best level of improvement in the pain condition typically achieved in 3–6 months. Integrative care is the practical application of this model in clinical practice by combining the practices and care strategies of a team. Different aspects of the problem can be addressed by different health professionals, often including physicians, dentists, health psychologists, and physical therapists, as appropriate, along with pain coaches, in order to enhance the overall potential for success. A pain coach may be an excellent addition to a busy primary care or specialty practice to help guide and support the patient in achieving their goals of reducing pain and its interference in life activities through learning self-management strategies. Teams can be interdisciplinary (one setting) or multidisciplinary (multiple settings). The use of a team helps to understand and manage the whole patient, allows work on multiple aspects of the problem simultaneously, improves patient compliance and outcome, saves time, and is more economical and more enjoyable as the team works together. A consistent philosophy and message to the patient are needed including the importance of self-care, self-responsibility, and education using concepts of the human systems approach and the transformative care model. Success is dependent upon communication and integration among clinicians and proper patient selection.

Conclusion

There are several areas of focus for health professionals in implementing transformative care and managing and preventing chronic pain. These include:

1. *Evaluating* the person with chronic pain as a whole by identifying and understanding both their risk and protective factors. Unaddressed risk factors may lead to treatment failure. Thus, using a broader conceptual basis with a human systems approach and a shift in patient-centered clinical paradigms implicit in the clinician-patient relationship will be the key to success.
2. *Improving* the safety of treatments to minimize the development of orofacial disorders as an adverse event. This is particularly true of adverse events from different types of surgery, dental procedures, chronic opioid use, and side effects related to drug-drug interactions.
3. *Implementing* a transformative model of healthcare through a team approach. A transformative care model includes risk assessment, robust self-management training, and evidenced-based biomedical treatments to improve the outcomes of pain management while reducing the patient's dependency on the healthcare system. Teams of healthcare professionals that may include a patient-centered pain coach will play a growing role in training and supporting patients in self-management, particularly since they are also supported in most health reform efforts.
4. *Continuing* medical and dental education (CE) courses that review the fundamentals of this new approach to care. Make use of the online CE course at www.coursera.org/learn/chronic-pain and the transformative care toolkits to implement online self-management training with evidence-based treatments as part of the new routine of care [40, 41].
5. *Supporting* resources to help implement transformative care. Organizations like the International MYOPAIN Society (www.myopain.org) through their *Campaign for Preventing Chronic Pain and Addiction* (www.preventing-chronicpain.org) [42] have goals to increase research, develop strategies,

expand education of both patients and health professionals on how to prevent chronic pain using online training toolkits to implement a transformative care model, increase advocacy and awareness, and provide media toolkits to health plans, businesses, government agencies, and communities to improve their efforts in preventing chronic pain.

By accomplishing these goals, we will address the Institute for Healthcare Improvement's triple aim of improving the experience of care, enhancing health, and reducing the cost of healthcare for patients with pain conditions [43].

References

1. St Sauver JL, Warner DO, Yawn BP, et al. Why patients visit their doctors: assessing the most prevalent conditions in a defined American population. Mayo Clin Proc. 2013;88(1):56–67.
2. Lipton JA, Ship JA, Larach-Robinson D. Estimated prevalence and distribution of reported orofacial pain in the United States. J Am Dent Assoc. 1993;124(10):115–21.
3. Petti S. Pooled estimate of world leukoplakia prevalence: a systematic review. Oral Oncol. 2003;39:770–80.
4. Lozada-Nur F, Miranda C. Oral lichen planus: pathogenesis and epidemiology. Sem Cutan Med Surg. 1997;16:290–5.
5. Bailey D, Attanasio R, editors. Sleep disorders: dentistry's role. Dent Clin N Am. 2001;45(4):619–30.
6. Taylor H, Curran NM. The Nuprin pain report. New York: Louis Harris and Associates; 1985.
7. Look J, Fricton J. Access to care for patients with orofacial pain: a survey of dentists. JADA, 2017 (in review).
8. Center for Disease Control and Prevention (CDC). Prescription drug overdose in the United States: fact sheet. Available at: www.cdc.gov/homeandrecreationalsafety/overdose/facts.html.
9. Bohnert AS, Valenstein M, Bair MJ, et al. Association between opioid prescribing patterns and opioid overdose-related deaths. JAMA. 2011;305(13):1315–21.
10. Fricton J. The need for preventing chronic pain: the "big elephant in the room" of healthcare. Glob Adv Health Med. 2015;4(1):6–7.
11. Magnusson T, Egermark I, Carlsson GE. A longitudinal epidemiologic study of signs and symptoms of temporomandibular disorders from 15 to 35 years of age. J Orofac Pain. 2000;14(4):310–9.
12. Diatchenko L1, Slade GD, Nackley AG, et al. Genetic basis for individual variations in pain perception and the development of a chronic pain condition. Hum Mol Genet. 2005;14(1):135–43.
13. John MT, Miglioretti DL, LeResche L, Von Korff M, Critchlow CW. Widespread pain as a risk factor for dysfunctional temporomandibular disorder pain. Pain. 2003;102(3):257–63
14. Turk DC, Okifuji A. Psychological factors in chronic pain: evolution and revolution. J Consult Clin Psychol. 2002;70(3):678–90.
15. Turner JA, Holtzman S, Mancl L. Mediators, moderators, and predictors of therapeutic change in cognitive-behavioral therapy for chronic pain. Pain. 2007;127(3):276–86.
16. Gensichen J, von Korff M, Peitz M, et al. Case management for depression by health care assistants in small primary care practices: a cluster randomized trial. Ann Intern Med. 2009;151(6):369–78.
17. Cote P, Cassidy JD, Carroll LJ, et al. The annual incidence and course of neck pain in the general population: a population-based cohort study. Pain. 2004;112:267–73.
18. Aggarwal VR, Macfarlane GJ, Farragher TM, et al. Risk factors for onset of chronic oro-facial pain-results of the North Cheshire oro-facial pain prospective population study. Pain. 2010;149(2):354–9.

19. Coleman EA, Parry C, Chalmers S, et al. The care transitions intervention: results of a randomized controlled trial. Arch Intern Med. 2006;166(7):1822–8.
20. Foster G, Taylor SJ, Eldridge SE, et al. Self-management education programmes by lay leaders for people with chronic conditions. Cochrane Database Syst Rev. 2007;17(4):CD005108.
21. Bair MJ, Matthias MS, Nyland KA, et al. Barriers and facilitators to chronic pain self-management: a qualitative study of primary care patients with comorbid musculoskeletal pain and depression. Pain Med. 2009;10(7):1280–90.
22. Institute of Medicine. Relieving pain in America: a blueprint for transforming prevention, care, education, and research. Washington, DC: National Academies Press; 2011.
23. National Pain Strategy at http://iprcc.nih.gov/docs/DraftHHSNationalPainStrategy.pdf. Accessed on 10 Jan 2016.
24. Macea DD, Gajos K, Daglia Calil YA, et al. The efficacy of web-based cognitive behavioral interventions for chronic pain: a systematic review and meta-analysis. J Pain. 2010; 11(10):917–29.
25. Wantland DJ, Portillo CJ, Holzemer WL, et al. The effectiveness of web-based vs. non-web-based interventions: a meta-analysis of behavioral change outcomes. J Med Internet Res. 2004;6(4):e40.
26. Paul CL, Carey ML, Sanson-Fisher RW, et al. The impact of web-based approaches on psychosocial health in chronic physical and mental health conditions. Health Educ Res. 2013;28(3):450–71.
27. Lau PW, Lau EY, Wong del P, et al. A systematic review of information and communication technology-based interventions for promoting physical activity behavior change in children and adolescents. J Med Internet Res. 2011;13(3):e48.
28. Hayden JA, van Tulder MW, Tomlinson G. Systematic review: strategies for using exercise therapy to improve outcomes in chronic low back pain. Ann Intern Med. 2005;142(9):776–85.
29. Eaton LH, Doorenbos AZ, Schmitz KL, et al. Establishing treatment fidelity in a web-based behavioral intervention study. Nurs Res. 2011;60(6):430–435.4.
30. Kroenke K, Krebs EE, Bair MJ. Pharmacotherapy of chronic pain: a synthesis of recommendations from systematic reviews. Gen Hosp Psychiatry. 2009;31(3):206–19.
31. Devineni T, Blanchard EB. A randomized controlled trial of an internet-based treatment for chronic headache. Behav Res Ther. 2005;43(3):277–92.
32. Lorig KR, Sobel DS, Stewart AL, et al. Evidence suggesting that a chronic disease self-management program can improve health status while reducing hospitalization: a randomized trial. Med Care. 1999;37(1):5–14.
33. Engel GL. The need for a new medical model: a challenge for biomedicine. Science. 1977;196(4286):129–36.
34. Fricton JR, Clavell A, Weisberg M. Transformative care for chronic pain. Pain Week J. 2016;4(3):44–56.
35. Mansour M. Systems theory and human science. Annu Rev Control. 2002;26(1):1–13.
36. Bailey B. Living systems theory and social entropy theory. Syst Res Behav Sci. 2006;22:291–300.
37. Bateson G. Mind and nature: a necessary unity: advances in systems theory, complexity, and the human sciences. New York: Hampton Press; 1979.
38. Rolland JS. Chronic illness and the life cycle: a conceptual framework. Fam Process. 1987;26(2):203–21.
39. Dym B. The cybernetics of physical illness. Fam Process. 1987;26(1):35–48.
40. Fricton J. Preventing chronic pain: a human systems approach. Coursera. University of Minnesota. Available at: www.coursera.org/course/chronicpain.
41. Fricton JR, Anderson K, Clavel A, et al. preventing chronic pain: a human systems approach – results from a massive open online course. Glob Adv Health Med. 2015;4(5):23–32.
42. International Myopain Society. Preventing chronic pain. Available at: preventingchronicpain.org/drupal/pcpnet/about.
43. Institute for Healthcare Improvement. IHI triple aim initiative. Available at: www.ihi.org/offerings/Initiatives/TripleAim.

44. Turner JA, Holtzman S, Mancl L. Mediators, moderators, and predictors of therapeutic change in cognitive-behavioral therapy for chronic pain. Pain. 2007;127(3):276–86.
45. Fillingim RB, Maixner W, Kincaid S, Sigurdsson A, Harris MB. Pain sensitivity in patients with temporomandibular disorders: relationship to clinical and psychosocial factors. Clin J Pain. 1996;12(4):260–9.
46. Gracely RH, Geisser ME, Giesecke T, Grant MA, Petzke F, Williams DA, et al. Pain catastrophizing and neural responses to pain among persons with fibromyalgia. Brain. 2004;127(Pt 4): 835–43.
47. Fricton JR, Nelson A, Monsein M. IMPATH: microcomputer assessment of behavioral and psychosocial factors in craniomandibular disorders. Cranio. 1987;5(4):372–81.
48. Turner JA, Holtzman S, Mancl L. Mediators, moderators, and predictors of therapeutic change in cognitivebehavioral therapy for chronic pain. Pain. 2007;127(3):276–86.
49. Ohrbach R, Fillingim RB, Mulkey F, et al. Clinical findings and pain symptoms as potential risk factors for chronic TMD: descriptive data and empirically identified domains from the OPPERA case-control study. J Pain. 2011 Nov; 12(11 Suppl):T27–45.

Integrative Approaches to Orofacial Pain: Role of Biofeedback and Hypnosis

27

Gabriel Tan, Alan Glaros, Richard Sherman, and Chin Yi Wong

Pearls of Wisdom

- EMG biofeedback procedures in which patients are shown their levels of masticatory muscle tension and taught to recognize and then control tension levels is a highly effective way to treat muscle tension-based orofacial pain.
- Biofeedback-based interventions are at least as effective as traditional dental and medical therapeutic approaches for muscle related pain and may last indefinitely.
- Biofeedback for recognizing and then controlling sustained levels of jaw muscle tension works best when patients learn the skills thoroughly and then continue to practice them.
- Patients will probably benefit most by consulting with well-skilled and appropriately credentialed biofeedback providers [21].
- Hypnosis and hypnotherapy could also contribute to management of the orofacial pain by adding the elements of altering pain perception and experience, and improving motivation to respond to treatment.
- Acquisition and maintenance of a low level generalized relaxation state is counter to the experience of TMD pain.

G. Tan, PhD, ABPP (✉) • C.Y. Wong, BSocSci
Department of Psychology, National University of Singapore, Singapore, Singapore
e-mail: gtan46@gmail.com

A. Glaros, PhD
University of Missouri-Kansas City, Kansas City, MO, USA

R. Sherman, PhD
Psychophysiology Program, Saybrook University, Oakland, CA, USA

J.N.A.R. Ferreira et al. (eds.), *Orofacial Disorders*,
DOI 10.1007/978-3-319-51508-3_27

27.1 Introduction

Temporomandibular (TMD)-related orofacial pain is caused by sustained masticatory muscle tension. While sustained activation of the masticatory muscles accounts for a very large proportion of the variance in pain, other factors, including genetic vulnerabilities, stress, and autonomic dysregulation can also play a role in orofacial pain.

27.2 Rationale for Integrative Approaches to Orofacial Pain

Current scientific knowledge about TMD pain, especially myofascial pain in the orofacial region, has changed dramatically in recent years. At least three mutually complementary approaches to understanding the disorder have emerged. One emphasizes that individuals with particular genetic vulnerabilities are particularly responsive to stress and more likely to develop pain in the future [23]. A second approach addresses autonomic dysregulation that characterizes individuals with masticatory muscle pain and with chronic pain more generally [18]. A third approach focuses specifically on the actions of the masticatory muscles and the impact of sustained tooth contact/low-level activation of the masticatory muscles in TMD pain [10].

Taken as a whole these three approaches suggest that an integrated approach that helps patients manage stress, reduce autonomic dysfunction, and decrease masticatory muscle tension will reduce pain. In the sections that follow, we will review the available evidence that address these three main points, emphasizing so-called complementary and alternative approaches to this problem. Importantly, all the treatment strategies described in this chapter are consistent with the U.S. National Institutes of Health's strong recommendation that providers use conservative, reversible therapies in those with TMD pain and avoid invasive, irreversible treatments.

We will focus primarily on myofascial pain in the orofacial region. There is little evidence that biofeedback and hypnosis have particular benefit treating pain caused by degenerative changes in the hard tissues of the temporomandibular joint (TMJ). Similarly, there is little evidence that dysfunction of the soft tissues in the TMJ (e.g., displacement of the articular disc) can be successfully managed by the techniques described in this chapter. Instead, we will focus on myofascial pain, as defined by the Diagnostic Criteria for Temporomandibular Disorders (DC/TMD) [17], where the available evidence base is quite encouraging.

27.3 Integrative Therapies to Orofacial Pain

27.3.1 Stress Management

Long-term studies convincingly show that individuals with particular variants in the genes that code for catechol-O-methyl-transferase (COMT) are vulnerable to the effects of stress (e.g., [23]). There are also multiple studies showing that cognitive-behavioral therapy (CBT), a well-established system for teaching individuals how to better manage stress and reduce pain, can effectively treat individuals with the myofascial pain of TMD. For example, a review of psychosocial interventions for the Cochran Database of Systematic Reviews [4] found 17 trials eligible for inclusion in the review. These trials showed a reduction in long-term pain intensity and depression. A more fine-grained analysis showed that CBT, either alone or in combination with biofeedback, improved long-term pain intensity, activity interference, and depression.

27.3.2 Control of Autonomic Dysfunction

An individual with TMD pain will, by definition, report discomfort in the muscles of mastication or in the TMJ. However, pain in an individual diagnosed with TMD is frequently accompanied by pain in the neck, shoulders, and upper and lower back. TMD patients also frequently report a variety of headaches. These findings suggest that a common mechanism may underlie the complaints of pain.

One promising strategy has examined autonomic functioning in individuals with masticatory muscle pain (MMP). In one study, 22 individuals with masticatory muscle pain and 23 non-pain control participants took part in three-part study examining physiological activation and emotional reactivity during baseline, stressor, and recovery periods. Physiological activity was assessed with frequency domain heart rate variability (HRV) indices. The results showed that the MMP patients had more physiological activation during the baseline period and significantly more physiological activation during the recovery period compared to the pain-free controls [18]. Similar findings using multiple measures, including computerized pupilometry, confirm the presence of dysregulation in TMD patients [5, 13].

These findings suggest that treatments targeting dysregulation may have a beneficial impact. In one such study, individuals with chronic pain practiced a diaphragmatic breathing techniques designed to influence HRV. Those who practiced the technique the most also were better able to tolerate pain generated by a cold-pressor test [19]. Although these results are quite promising, considerably more research needs to be carried out to evaluate the benefits of treatments that minimize autonomic dysregulation on pain in TMD patients.

27.3.3 Decreasing Masticatory Muscle Tension via Biofeedback

Both experimental and observational studies indicate that masticatory muscle tension is very strongly associated with TMD pain [9], with muscle tension accounting for nearly 70% of the variance in facial pain. Longitudinal multi-level modeling examining the impact of stress, emotional distress, and muscle tension on facial pain points to muscle tension as a causal factor in facial pain, also showing that muscle tension accounts for about 70% of the variance in facial pain, an extraordinarily high value. These findings suggest that control of muscle tension will have a clinically significant benefit in those who suffer from chronic facial pain (e.g., [11]).

Multiple biofeedback modalities can be used to treat TMD-related myofascial tension-related pain. Not surprisingly, the most common modality is EMG biofeedback. EMG biofeedback can be used in various ways to help those with myofascial pain.

When the teeth are separated by 4–6 mm, the activity of the masticatory muscles (i.e., the masseters and temporalis) reaches a baseline minimum. Bringing the teeth in contact increases the activity of these muscles between 2.0 and 3.5 times over the relaxed baseline level. And, increasing the contact pressure between the teeth will increase the activity of the masseters and temporalis muscles even more.

Interestingly, many TMD patients are not aware that their teeth are in contact or that the masticatory muscles are activated. Similarly, TMD patients may not be aware of the length of time that their teeth are in contact during the day (up to 75% of waking hours). The reasons for this lack of knowledge may stem from problems in proprioceptive awareness in those with masticatory muscle pain or from a definitional problem involving the concept of "clenching." Patients with TMD pain may not be as accurate in their reports of internal states as those without pain, especially when stressed. Alternatively, patients may believe that their personal tooth contacts are "normal," but they may not be aware of the amount of time when the teeth are touching (a form of clenching, to be sure) [9]. These findings suggest that increasing awareness of tooth contact and changing patient definitions so that any unnecessary tooth contact becomes defined as clenching can be a reasonable starting strategy for assisting those with TMD pain.

Biofeedback techniques can be used to illustrate the degree of change that occurs in the masticatory muscles when the teeth are in contact or when individuals are clenching. Electrodes can be placed on the surface of the skin above the main body of the masseters and temporalis muscles, and the feedback display can be set to show individuals how much EMG activity changes with even very slight tooth contact. Seeing the impact of tooth contact, in real time, can provide very convincing evidence to those suffering from myofascial pain of the need to control masticatory muscle activity and reduce tooth contact.

Standard EMG biofeedback techniques with the aim of reducing masticatory muscle activity can then be used to help individuals learn the necessary skills. The activity in these muscles is highly dependent on jaw position and tooth contact. If individuals are instructed to allow their teeth to separate, they can quickly learn to reduce the activity of the masticatory muscles and then to learn the subtle signs of increased masticatory muscle activity. Individuals can also be exposed to relevant stressful stimuli and utilize feedback to maintain relaxation in the masticatory muscles. There is considerable evidence showing that EMG biofeedback is an effective treatment for those reporting TMD pain. Used alone, biofeedback improves pain, pain-related disability, and mandibular functioning [8]. Multiple reviews and meta-analyses conclude that EMG biofeedback is an effective treatment for TMD-related pain (e.g., [4, 6]). Furthermore, studies comparing EMG biofeedback-based treatment to traditional dental treatments (i.e., mouth guards or "splints") show that biofeedback is at least as effective as splints and other standard techniques (e.g., [7]). The studies using EMG biofeedback report treatment effectiveness lasting up to 2 years (e.g., [7]), longer than the benefits generated by splints and CBT.

The process of EMG biofeedback training can be summarized as a three-step process involving increasing awareness of muscle tension, calibration, and control. As these examples make clear, these clinical strategies deliberately build in generalization strategies to help patients learn and utilize newly-learned skills in their everyday lives [20].

1. Awareness of masticatory muscle tension
   (a) First in the office while looking at the biofeedback display
   (b) Then in the office without the need of the display
   (c) Then at home
   (d) Then in the stress-producing environment
2. Calibration
   (a) People with chronic masticatory muscle tension cannot tell how tense their painful muscles are as accurately as they can tell how tense non-painful muscles are.
   (b) Biofeedback is used to teach people to accurately calibrate their muscle tension by having them tense to 25%, 75%, or 50% of max (at random), watch the display, attend to the sensations produced, and then tense to the given extent accurately without the display.
3. Control
   (a) Everyone reacts physiologically to stress.
   (b) Nobody can be trained not to react, but people can control the extent and duration of the reaction.
   (c) Patients can learn to avoid keeping muscles tenser than necessary for longer than necessary
      (i) First in the office
      (ii) Then at home
      (iii) Then in the stress-producing environment

As mentioned earlier, individuals with myofascial pain appear to have autonomic dysfunction. In addition to relaxation strategies, individuals may also benefit from biofeedback modalities such as HRV biofeedback or other psychophysiological techniques to reduce the degree of dysfunction in autonomic functioning. Cognitive restructuring can also be used to assist patients in minimizing physiological responses to stress.

27.3.4 Hypnosis and Hypnotherapy

Hypnosis is used to alter pain perception, increase openness to suggestion, alter emotional states (e.g., anxiety), and change behavioral activities/habits (e.g., muscle tension and bracing; body posture) which may be contributing to the experience of pain. With respect to the three elements on targeting TMD pain previously discussed, hypnosis would be most applicable in regulating autonomic dysregulation, reducing masticatory muscles tension, and correcting sustained tooth contact/low-level activation of the masticatory muscles.

A meta-analysis of 18 studies utilizing hypnosis as analgesia across various pain conditions found that 75% of patients experienced substantial pain relief [14]. Reviews of controlled trials [12, 15] have also shown the ability of hypnotic treatments to reduce pain perception in comparison to non-hypnotic interventions.

However, hypnosis for the treatment of orofacial pain specifically has been less common, with most studies focusing on headaches [12]. Recent studies have shown promise in addressing this gap. For TMDs, Simon and Lewis [22] reported significant decreases in pain and increases in daily functioning for recalcitrant patients, with treatment gains maintained at follow-up and decreases in medicine usage. Abrahamsen et al. [2] also found significant reduction in pain intensity for hypnosis, compared to baseline and non-hypnotic relaxation.

Abrahamsen et al. [3] studied oral functions and psychological outcomes for TMD patients, randomized to hypnotic intervention or simple relaxation. Pain scores decreased significantly only in the hypnosis group with a significant increase in usage of 'reinterpreting pain sensations' as a coping strategy. However, both groups experienced significant decreases in painful muscle palpation sites, awakenings, somatisation, obsessive-compulsive symptoms and anxiety. Thus, hypnosis appears to be uniquely effective only in some areas of TMD.

Abrahamsen et al. [1] found similar reductions in pain scores with the treatment of persistent idiopathic orofacial pain (PIOP). Patients more susceptible to hypnosis also experienced a greater decrease in pain. Hypnosis aided in dealing with PIOP, dependent on hypnotic suggestibility. Winocur et al. [25] assigned myofascial pain patients to hypno-relaxation, occlusal appliance or education/advice. The first two conditions were more effective in alleviating sensitivity to palpation, but a significant decrease in pain was seen only in hypno-relaxation.

Although there is a paucity of randomized controlled trials showing the efficacy of hypnosis in the treatment of orofacial pain, the above studies display the potential of this method in alleviating or managing pain disorders. Stam et al. [24] reported that suggestibility scores of facial pain patients predicted decreases in pain experience following treatment. These findings suggest that the efficacy of hypnosis in treatment of orofacial pain disorders is dependent in part on patient characteristics and preference. This could be tested with other alternate treatments, and patients could be pre-assessed to identify a suitable modality in managing their pain conditions. Additionally, as concluded by Pistoia et al. [16], treatment is most effective when a variety of therapies are used, including behavioral and pharmacological interventions. Pain management is most effective when an integrative, multidisciplinary approach is utilized, combining multiple treatment modalities.

References

1. Abrahamsen R, Baad-Hansen L, Svensson P. Hypnosis in the management of persistent idiopathic orofacial pain – clinical and psychosocial findings. Pain. 2008;136(1–2):44–52.
2. Abrahamsen R, Baad-Hansen L, Zachariae R, Svensson P. Effect of hypnosis on pain and blink reflexes in patients with painful temporomandibular disorders. Clin J Pain. 2011;27(4):344–51.
3. Abrahamsen R, Zachariae R, Svensson P. Effect of hypnosis on oral function and psychological factors in temporomandibular disorders patients. J Oral Rehabil. 2009;36(8):556–70.
4. Aggarwal VR, Lovell K, Peters S, Javidi H, Joughin A, Goldthorpe J. Psychosocial interventions for the management of chronic orofacial pain. Cochrane Database Syst Rev. 2015;12:CD008456.
5. Chen H, Nackley A, Miller V, Diatchenko L, Maixner W. Multisystem dysregulation in painful temporomandibular disorders. J Pain. 2013;14(9):983–96.
6. Crider A, Glaros AG, Gevirtz RN. Efficacy of biofeedback-based treatments for temporomandibular disorders. Appl Psychophysiol Biofeedback. 2005;30(4):333–45.
7. Flor H, Birbaumer N. Comparison of the efficacy of electromyographic biofeedback, cognitive-behavioral therapy, and conservative medical interventions in the treatment of chronic musculoskeletal pain. J Consult Clin Psychol. 1993;61(4):653–8.
8. Gardea MA, Gatchel RJ, Mishra KD. Long-term efficacy of biobehavioral treatment of temporomandibular disorders. J Behav Med. 2001;24(4):341–59.
9. Glaros AG. Temporomandibular disorders and facial pain: a psychophysiological perspective. Appl Psychophysiol Biofeedback. 2008;33(3):161–71.
10. Glaros AG, Marszalek JM, Williams KB. Longitudinal multilevel modeling of facial pain, muscle tension, and stress. J Dent Res. 2016;95(4):416–22.
11. Glaros AG, Owais Z, Lausten L. Reduction in parafunctional activity: a potential mechanism for the effectiveness of splint therapy. J Oral Rehabil. 2007;34:97–104.
12. Jensen M, Patterson DR. Hypnotic treatment of chronic pain. J Behav Med. 2006;29(1):95–124.
13. Monaco A, Cattaneo R, Mesin L, Ortu E, Giannoni M, Pietropaoli D. Dysregulation of the descending pain system in temporomandibular disorders revealed by low-frequency sensory transcutaneous electrical nerve stimulation: a pupillometric study. PLoS ONE. 2015;10(4):e0122826.
14. Montgomery GH, Duhamel KN, Redd WH. A meta-analysis of hypnotically induced analgesia: how effective is hypnosis? Int J Clin Exp Hypn. 2000;48(2):138–53.
15. Patterson DR, Jensen MP. Hypnosis and clinical pain. Psychol Bull. 2003;129(4):495–521.
16. Pistoia F, Sacco S, Carolei A. Behavioral therapy for chronic migraine. Curr Pain Headache Rep. 2013;17(1):304.
17. Schiffman E, Ohrbach R, Truelove E, et al. Diagnostic Criteria for Temporomandibular Disorders (DC/TMD) for Clinical and Research Applications: recommendations of the International RDC/TMD Consortium Network* and Orofacial Pain Special Interest Group†. J Oral Facial Pain Headache. 2014;28(1):6–27.
18. Schmidt JE, Carlson CR. A controlled comparison of emotional reactivity and physiological response in masticatory muscle pain patients. J Orofac Pain. 2009;23(3):230–42.
19. Schmidt JE, Joyner MJ, Carlson CR, Hooten WM. Cardiac autonomic function associated with treatment adherence after a brief intervention in patients with chronic pain. Appl Psychophysiol Biofeedback. 2013;38(3):193–201.
20. Sherman RA. Pain assessment and intervention from a psychophysiological perspective. 2nd ed. Colorado: Wheat Ridge; 2012.
21. Sherman RA, Amar-Schwartz P, Andrasik F, Criswell C, Csoka L, Walker L. AAPB standards for performing biofeedback. Colorado: Wheat Ridge; 2013.
22. Simon EP, Lewis DM. Medical hypnosis for temporomandibular disorders: treatment efficacy and medical utilization outcome. Oral Surg Oral Med Oral Pathol Oral Radiol Endod. 2000;90(1):54–63.

23. Slade GD, Sanders AE, Ohrbach R, et al. COMT diplotype amplifies effect of stress on risk of temporomandibular pain. J Dent Res. 2015;94(9):1187–95.
24. Stam HJ, McGrath PA, Brooke RI, Cosier F. Hypnotizability and the treatment of chronic facial pain. Int J Clin Exp Hypn. 1986;34(3):182–91.
25. Winocur E, Gavish A, Emodi-Perlman A, Halachmi M, Eli I. Hypnorelaxation as treatment for myofascial pain disorder: a comparative study. Oral Surg Oral Med Oral Pathol Oral Radiol Endod. 2002;93(4):429–34.

Part X

A Comprehensive Approach to Orofacial Disorders

History Taking and Physical Examination for Orofacial Disorders

28

David Ojeda Díaz and Thomas P. Sollecito

28.1 Introduction

As clinicians our goal is to give our patients an answer to their concerns, a relief to their suffering, and ultimately (when available) a cure to their illness. This will be possible, only if we carefully follow a series of diagnostic steps, where every detail is important. To develop consistency in the diagnosis of orofacial disorders, a concise, thoughtful history and physical examination are essential.

The history and physical examination should be based on the specific complaint, while being mindful of the etiology, epidemiology, and pathophysiology of various possible diagnostic entities. The presenting signs and symptoms, temporal characteristics, modifying factors, onset and course of the disease should be obtained, using the knowledge, skills, and values of the clinician. The history and physical examination is based on the type of orofacial complaint presented by the patient. In this chapter we will discuss a systematic way to conduct a history and physical examination to assess various orofacial disorders and successfully reach a diagnosis.

D.O. Díaz, DDS (✉)
Department of Oral Medicine, Penn School of Dental Medicine, University of Pennsylvania, Philadelphia, PA, USA
e-mail: davidojedadiaz@gmail.com

T.P. Sollecito, DMD, FDS, RCSEd
Department of Oral Medicine, Penn School of Dental Medicine, Oral Medicine Division, Penn Medicine, University of Pennsylvania, Philadelphia, PA, USA

J.N.A.R. Ferreira et al. (eds.), *Orofacial Disorders*,
DOI 10.1007/978-3-319-51508-3_28

28.2 Oral Mucosal Diseases

Mucosal diseases affect an important segment of the population and can be debilitating. The evaluation, diagnosis and treatment of mucosal diseases involving the oral cavity, represent an essential element of the oral medicine discipline. Mucosal diseases of the oral cavity affect the mucosal lining of the mouth, including structures such as the gingiva, buccal mucosa, tongue, floor of the mouth, and hard and soft palate. These conditions can arise from multiple etiologies and can present in various patterns. The identification of specific patterns helps clinicians categorize conditions and aids in arriving an accurate diagnosis.

One difficulty facing clinicians managing a patient with a mucosal disorder, lies in the fact that most oral lesions appear similar clinically. Therefore, it is extremely difficult to diagnose based on the examination only [1]. In order to reach a precise diagnosis, one needs to develop a systematic method of inquiry, leading to a list of diagnostic possibilities. A differential diagnosis list should be created based on the history and physical examination and by drawing on fundamental knowledge and the use of critical thinking to order the possibilities. The next diagnostic step might include laboratory studies, imaging, biopsies, or other methods to narrow the list or to arrive at a final diagnosis.

28.2.1 Medical History

A detailed medical history is at the foundation of an accurate diagnosis. The clinician must conduct an interview, which, through a series of questions, will reveal the medical status of the patient. A skilled clinician should use the data gathered to assess and understand the patient's concern, achieve a diagnosis, and propose a management strategy [2].

The medical history should include identification of the patient along with demographic information, useful for epidemiologic purposes. After the demographic information is recorded, the first step in a medical history is the chief complaint. The chief complaint is (the patients stating in their own words) the reason they are seeing you. The history of present illness (HPI) follows and is a description of the details regarding the present condition and will provide a dimension of the problem. The HPI should include attributes of symptoms describing the chief complaint. The past medical history will gather the general health information of the patient such as previous and current medical conditions, diagnosis, and treatments; it also contains the past surgical history, a medication history, and allergy history. The dental history includes previous dental procedure, treatments, and experiences. A family history is necessary to determine possible genetic implications of diseases and should include pertinent information about the patient's blood relative's health history. A social history includes previous and current employment and use of alcohol, tobacco, and recreational drugs. Finally, a review of systems is a comprehensive review of all of the systems of the body, monitoring for signs and symptoms related to disease. It is extremely important to update the medical status of the patient every office visit, including new medical diagnoses, changes in medications or dosages, and new allergies.

28.2.2 History of the Present Illness (HPI)

It is the section of the medical history where the clinician needs to be inquisitive, because the data will provide invaluable information regarding the current patient's condition. The HPI should be presented in a narrative fashion and chronological order [3], taking into consideration underlying medical conditions, signs and symptoms, onset, severity, triggers, modifying factors, previous medical opinions or diagnoses, past medications used for the condition, and imaging and laboratory studies done previously.

Specially for patients with mucosal disease, four questions of the condition need to be clearly established in order to be able to understand the nature of the problem; these are:

1. Acute vs chronic:
   Ask the patient if the symptoms developed recently or been present for over a month.
2. Single vs multiple:
   Refers to the number of lesions in the oral cavity.
3. Primary vs recurrent:
   Differentiate between a first episode and a repeated episode.
4. Local vs systemic:
   Inquire about oral mucosa involvement solely or manifestations in any other part of the body.

28.2.3 Clinical Examination

In mucosal diseases the clinical examination is limited to inspection and palpation, and the main goal is to differentiate normal from abnormal. The inspection process should begin on the initial sight of the patient. A comprehensive and extended oral cavity examination have should be performed in a systematic manner to minimize oversights. All tissues of the oral cavity and visible oropharynx have to be examined. The findings should be recorded in detail (location, size, shape, color, consistency, base of the lesion, and surface appearance) using proper medical jargon (papule, tumor, nodule, vesicle, pustule, fissure, erosions, ulcer, plaque, macule) (Table 28.1) (Figs. 28.1 and 28.2). Palpation is also fundamental to the exam and will provide more clinical information such as consistency (firm, hard, soft, indurated, fluctuant), temperature, or pulsation. The manipulation of the lesion could also provide valuable information regarding the nature of the mucosal disease (peeling, draining, wipeable, friable). Palpation of the cervical lymph nodes is mandatory and should include pre- and postauricular, anterior cervical, deep cervical, posterior cervical, supraclavicular, submandibular, and submental lymph nodes. Normally, lymph nodes in general should be not palpable. If palpable, a description of the nodes' consistency, mobility, sign, and symptoms is required.

Technology has provided a useful tool in helping assessment in mucosal diseases in the oral cavity. Clinical photography is an easy and economical way to document

Table 28.1 Oral mucosal lesions nomenclature [3]

Lesion	Definition
Papule	Superficial, solid, elevated lesion less than 1 cm in diameter
Pustule	Vesicle filled with purulent fluid
Tumor	Solid elevated lesion greater than 2 cm in diameter
Nodule	Solid, elevated lesion, larger than a papule and smaller than a tumor
Vesicle	Superficial, elevated, well-circumscribed lesion less than 1 cm in diameter
Bullae	Superficial, elevated, well-circumscribed lesion greater than 1 cm in diameter
Erosion	Depressed lesion resulting from loss of epithelium
Ulcer	Depressed lesion resulting from the loss of epithelium and connective tissue
Fissure	Deep linear lesion on the connective tissue
Macule	Circumscribed, non-palpable discoloration less than 1 cm in diameter
Plaque	Solid, flat elevated lesion greater than 1 cm in diameter

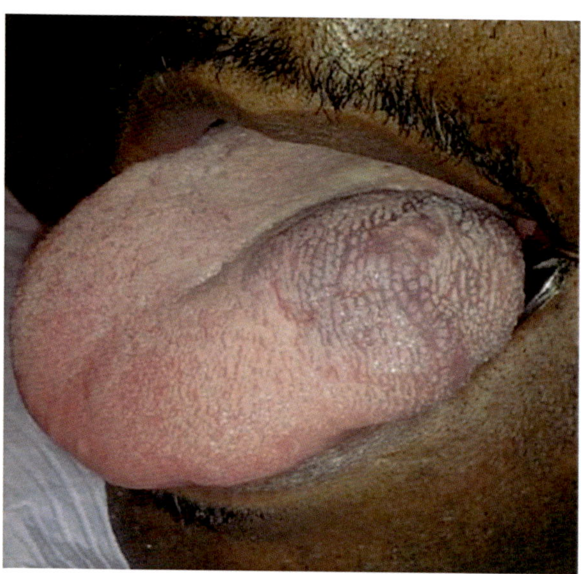

Fig. 28.1 Tumor on the tongue

and monitor oral lesions, due to the availability. Clinical photography allows a closer examination of the surface of the lesion and perhaps allow for the ability to monitor changes in the lesion over time. It could also help educate a patient regarding their condition. Clinical photography must be practiced following the principles of autonomy of the patient, supported by a consent and according to local privacy rules.

28.2.4 Diagnostic Tests

On those occasions where the diagnosis cannot be reached base on the medical history and physical examination, further diagnostic tests are needed. There are innumerable diagnostic techniques available and should be only requested to answer a

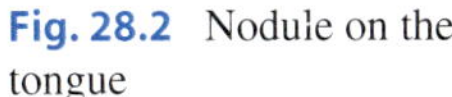
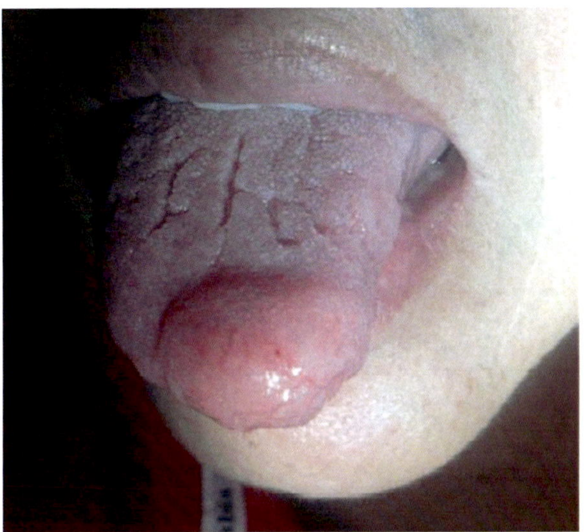

Fig. 28.2 Nodule on the tongue

specific clinical question about the possible diagnosis and not as a routine [4]. The clinician has to be mindful of the limitations, sensitivity, and specificity of each test to interpret the result and accurately reach a diagnosis. Microbiological cultures, Gram smears, and polymerase chain reaction (PCR) are only few examples of methods commonly used in oral medicine (see other chapters for indications).

28.2.5 Adjunctive Techniques for Oral Mucosa Examination

Due to the similar appearance of many mucosal diseases, adjunctive diagnostic techniques have been developed to facilitate the detection of oral premalignant and malignant lesions. These techniques are based on the ability of the tissues to behave under certain stimuli, when metabolic or structural changes are present. Adjunctive techniques have been divided into visual tissue staining, visualization adjuncts, advanced cytopathology [5], and molecular technologies. With different levels of sensitivity and specificity, further study is needed to refine their use in a generalized patient population administered by the general dentist. None of these techniques are substitutes for the surgical biopsy with histological examination, which is the gold standard method to diagnose mucosal diseases.

28.2.6 Serologic Studies

On occasion laboratory tests are required and could be ordered based on the medical history, physical examination and intra oral findings. Laboratory studies are indicated to determine the health status of the patient, to rule out systemic disease and monitor side effects of medications.

Routine blood test such as complete blood count (CBC) with differential and comprehensive metabolic panel (CMP) are tests used to help diagnose a suspected condition, with screening purposes, or to monitor infections, anemia, diabetes, liver and kidney functions which may relate to the oral condition. Other more specific laboratory tests, such as SSA/SSB, antinuclear antibodies (ANA), and rheumatoid factor, could help to diagnose autoimmune disorders. Levels of iron, ferritin, vitamin B12, and folate may provide useful information about possible deficiencies and their impact in oral health and disease.

28.2.7 Surgical Biopsy

Biopsy is a surgical procedure where a sample of tissue is taken for histopathologic evaluation. Two surgical biopsy techniques are described: incisional and excisional. Incisional biopsy is a procedure where a small sample of tissue is taken from the lesion and is indicated in large lesions or when potential malignancy is suspected. Excisional biopsy is a surgical procedure where the entire lesion is removed and is often considered the treatment. It is indicated in benign, smaller lesions. The procedure is usually done in outpatient settings, with local anesthesia and is associated with minimal complications. Routinely the tissue samples are transported and fixed in 10% formalin and sent to the pathology laboratory for hematoxylin and eosin (H&E) staining. In most of the cases after a histological examination under light microscopy, a diagnosis is offered (Fig. 28.3). Other staining techniques are

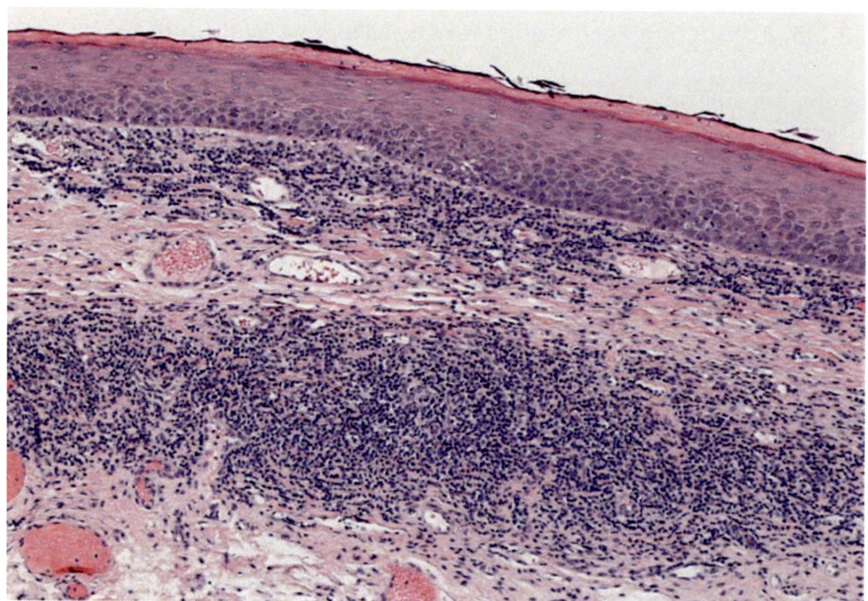

Fig. 28.3 H&E staining of lichenoid mucositis (Courtesy Dr. F. Alawi)

available and are used when the selective staining of cells or cellular components is required. In certain occasions staining for particular infectious agents may also be warranted.

When a diagnosis cannot be achieved through H&E or other staining techniques and autoimmune disease with oral manifestations is suspected, immunofluorescence testing is indicated. Autoimmune diseases are characterized by production of specific autoantibodies; identification of the antibodies and the tissues against they are targeted is important to reach a diagnosis [6].

There are two types of immunofluorescence techniques described: Direct immunofluorescence (DIF) consists in the application of fluorescein-conjugated antihuman Ig antibodies to the patient's tissue specimen containing disease-specific antibodies. If it is positive, a green fluorescence is seen in the patient's tissue specimen when viewed with UV light (Fig. 28.4). Indirect immunofluorescence (IIF) uses the patient's serum with disease-specific antibodies which bind to homologous structures in an animal tissue specimen, and then fluorescein-conjugated antihuman Ig antibodies to animal tissue specimen containing the patient's disease-specific antibodies are applied. If it is positive, the animal's tissue specimen will glow when viewed with UV light [7].

When DIF is planned, Michel's solution (as a conservation and transportation medium) needs to be used in order to preserve immune antigenicity of the tissue sample and ensure an accurate diagnosis. More recently normal saline solution has shown to be also effective, but the tissue sample has to be processed within 24 h [8].

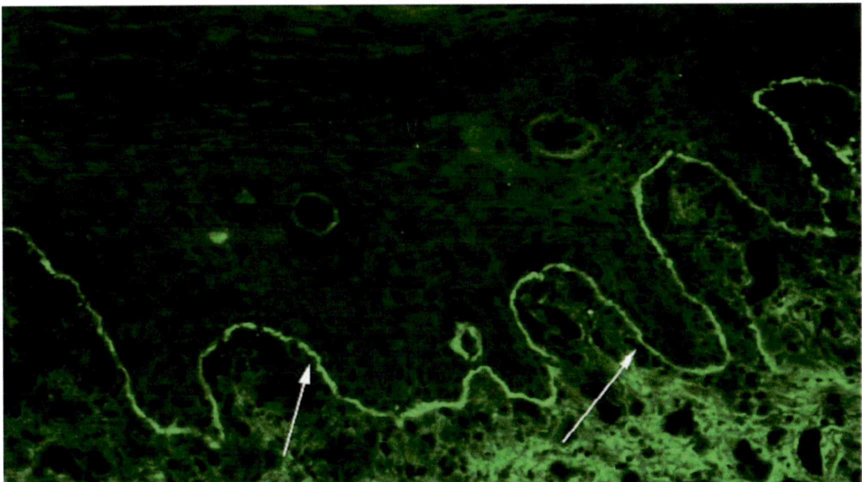

Fig. 28.4 Direct immunofluorescence showing fibrogen (Courtesy Dr. F. Alawi)

28.3 Salivary Gland Disorders

The salivary glands are exocrine glands that play an important role in digestion. They are divided into two groups: the major salivary glands and the minor salivary glands. The major salivary glands (composed of the parotid, submandibular, and sublingual) are distributed in pairs, symmetrically on both sides of the head and neck area. While the minor salivary glands are located throughout the mucosal lining of the oral cavity, both groups are responsible of the production and secretion of saliva, which plays an important role in the homeostasis of the mouth [9].

To effectively assess the salivary glands, it is important to understand their anatomy and the relationship with other important anatomic structures including the facial nerve and the facial artery. One must also understand the possible etiologic factors causing the signs and symptoms of disease such as autoimmune disorders (Sjogren's syndrome), infectious diseases (bacterial or viral parotitis, HIV, etc.), and neoplastic processes. Finally, one must understand the physiology of the glands in mastication and sleeping.

Salivary gland disorders can be suspected subjectively in the setting of symptoms, most commonly oral dryness, and less frequently associated with pain. But salivary gland disorders can also manifest objectively with signs of a swelling, mass in a gland, or objective hypofunction. Patients with salivary gland dysfunctions can develop local and systemic complications, and therefore a careful history and examination will ensure a proper diagnosis.

28.3.1 Medical History

The medical history plays a key role in establishing a differential diagnosis of salivary gland disease, due to the relationship of the salivary gland with systemic disorders. An accurate medical history should establish the complaint and the magnitude of the complaint. When the patient's medical history is consistent with conditions or medications that are known to affect salivary function, the diagnosis is often easily determined. If during the history of present illness or the review of systems, a patient reveals symptoms that are associated with salivary gland dysfunctions, more refined diagnostic methods may be needed to rule out underlying pathology.

Previous and current medications deserve special attention during the medical history, since there are known relationships between certain medications and salivary gland dysfunction. The exact pathophysiologic mechanism involved in medication-induced salivary gland dysfunction is not easily explained, due to the multiple ways this phenomenon could occur. Drugs can interact simultaneously with different nerve inputs at different levels, affecting salivary gland stimulation. Furthermore, polypharmacy could even increase the xerogenic potential of other medications [10]. The most common medications associated with xerostomia are antidepressants, antipsychotics, anticholinergics, antihypertensives, antihistamines, and sedatives [11].

Xerostomia is the most common subjective complaint of salivary gland dysfunction [12]. Although diminished salivary flow is a logical reason to experience dry mouth, studies have shown that xerostomia is not always accompanied by salivary

Table 28.2 Fox questionnaire

Question	Response Yes/No
1. Does the amount of saliva in your mouth seem to be too little and too much, or you do not notice it?	
2. Do you have any difficulty swallowing?	
3. Does your mouth feel dry when eating a meal?	
4. Do you sip liquids to aid in swallowing dry food?	

gland hypofunction. Many methods to identify and categorize patients with dry mouth complaints have been proposed in order to establish if the xerostomia is related to salivary hypofunction. Fox et al. were pioneers developing a system (questionnaire) which predicts salivary gland hypofunction, based on the patient perspective [13] (Table 28.2).

28.3.2 Clinical Examination

Salivary glands are located superficially in the head and neck region which facilitate inspection and palpation during a physical exam. Initial evaluation requires a careful extraoral inspection based on side to side comparison, looking for asymmetry and discoloration. Parotid involvement is perhaps easily recognizable due to the location of the gland and association with preauricular swelling. Submandibular glands may exhibit enlargement anterior and medial to the angle of the mandible while sublingual glands are not possible to inspect extraorally. Usually, bilateral involvement of the salivary glands implies systemic disorders whereas unilateral involvement favor local pathology. Due to the close proximity between the parotid glands and cranial nerve VII (facial nerve), motor function could be tested to rule out neurologic involvement. Intraoral inspection is also important, integrity of the salivary glands and ducts as well as the preservation of their excretory functions should be assessed by palpation.

During extraoral palpation, masses should be assessed, particularly in the context of febrile illness. To maximize the submandibular gland exposure, it is recommended to incline the patient's head forward and slightly flex the neck. Typically, salivary glands palpation is painless or with mild discomfort, and the consistency should be rubbery but not hard. Bidigital palpation (extraoral and intraoral) is recommended looking for possible masses while assessing function. With both hands gloved, one inside the mouth and the other on the face, compression for few seconds should be applied to the major salivary glands, in a milky fashion looking for clear copious saliva.

Minor salivary gland assessment is performed by overall inspection of the oral cavity with special attention on the labial mucosa and the hard and soft palate. Stretching of the upper and lower lip should expose minor salivary glands and reveal a wet nodular surface. In patients with minor salivary gland atrophy as a consequence of salivary gland dysfunction, the result is the tendency for the lower lip to sticking to the teeth.

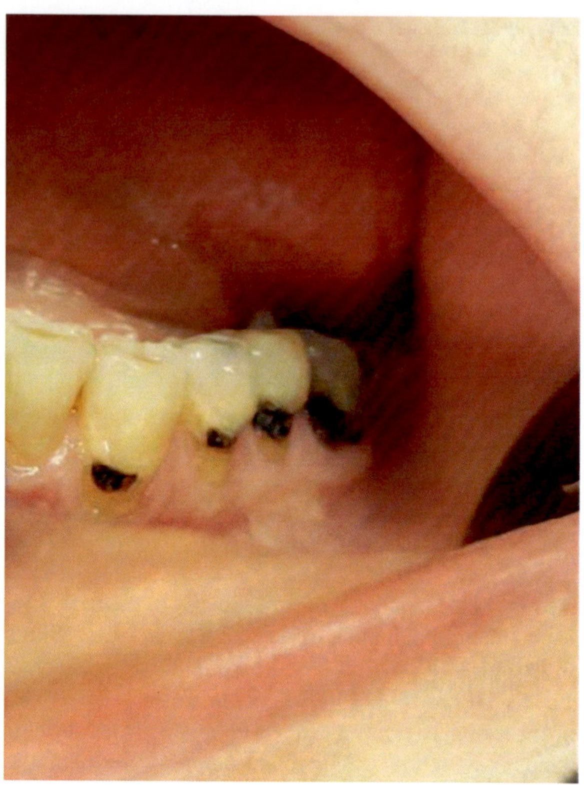

Fig. 28.5 Cervical decay

Salivary gland dysfunction has significant repercussions in the mouth environment. The oral mucosa, lips, and teeth are usually affected. The lips may be dry, cracked, and peeling. The buccal mucosa may look corrugated and shiny to the light while the tongue tends to appears smooth (devoid of papilla) and reddened. Patients are prone to develop cervical and incisal dental decay (Fig. 28.5) due to the accumulation of food debris in areas where usually the saliva would otherwise act as a cleaner. Local complications in patients with hyposalivation are common, including candidiasis involving the tongue and palate. Angular cheilitis of the mouth is quite common as well (Fig. 28.6).

28.3.3 Saliva Collection

In order to objectively determine salivary gland function, salivary flow rates needs to be measured, this is called Sialometry. Different techniques for collection are implemented depending on the aim. For general assessment "whole saliva" (understood as a collection of a mixed sample of oral fluids) is recommended. In contrast, individual major salivary gland function is mostly used for research purposes.

The "spitting method" is the most widely used. It is a simple method to determine unstimulated "whole salivary" flow. The patient should be seated in a vertical

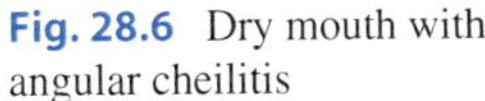
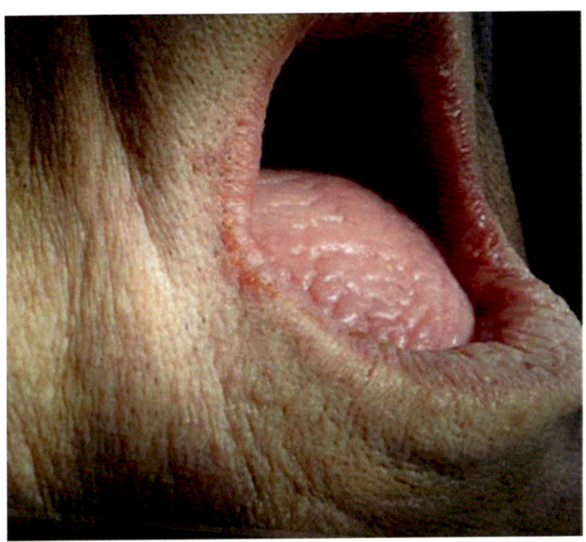

Fig. 28.6 Dry mouth with angular cheilitis

Table 28.3 Saliva flow rates [14]

	Salivary flow (mL/min)
Normal stimulated salivary flow	1.5–2
Normal unstimulated salivary flow	0.3–0.4
Hyposalivation stimulated salivary flow	≤0.5–0.7
Hyposalivation unstimulated salivary flow	≤0.1

position, accumulating the saliva in the mouth for 5–15 min without swallowing. The patient is asked to spit in a pre-weighed tube every 60 s.

Stimulated "whole saliva" can be obtained using a standardized and reproducible method of chewing an unflavored gum or a paraffin wax at a controlled rate (60 times per minute) for 1 min. Stimulating salivary secretion with a 2% citric acid solution by placing on the tongue in intervals of 30 s, while collecting the saliva on a graduated tube for 5 min can also be used. To ensure accurate measures, it is important to abstain the patient from eating, drinking, and smoking or have any oral stimulation for 90 min prior to the collection.

When an individual salivary gland function needs to be measured, more specialized equipment and time is required. For parotid flow measurements, an established suction device called a Carlson-Crittenden collector is used. The collector has to be attached to the Stensen's duct, while an applied suction device extracts saliva through a cannula from the salivary gland. Submandibular and sublingual salivary flow measurements are more difficult due to the location of the excretory ducts. Although many systems have been developed, there is no consensus regarding accuracy, reproducibility, and convenience/easement. One advantage of isolated saliva from a specific salivary gland is that it can be analyzed not only quantitatively but also qualitatively.

General considerations for sialometry recommend to use a standardized and reproducible method (time, position, environment). This will allow accurate, reproducible, and comparative results and allow comparison of various therapies (Table 28.3).

28.3.4 Salivary Gland Imaging

When deciding to proceed with salivary gland imaging, the clinical scenario is one of the most important considerations in choosing the correct technique. Many imaging techniques are available and are useful to determine salivary gland function and anatomic alterations.

28.3.5 Plain Film Radiography

When a salivary stone (sialolith) is considered in the differential diagnosis, a standard dental radiograph may be helpful to define location, size, and number of sialoliths. A mandibular occlusal radiograph will be able to capture the anterior floor of the mouth and rule out a sublingual or submandibular sialolith. If a stone is suspected in the parotid duct, an occlusal film placed in the buccal mucosa on the Stensen's duct opening can be considered. In cases when there is suspicion of a deeper obstruction, a panorex, anterior posterior (AP) or lateral oblique radiograph, may be beneficial. Plain film however is only useful in superficial cases, small or poor calcified stones may not be visible.

28.3.6 Sialography

This technique allows the visualization of the salivary gland duct system on a radiograph, after the administration of a contrast medium throughout the duct. When ductal obstruction (sialolith, tumor, or stricture) is presumed, sialography will allow assessment of the ductal system of the salivary gland. A continuous track is expected to be observed; blockage or dilatation of the contrast are indicative of pathology. Radiographic studies such as panoramic, AP, and lateral oblique are used with this technique. Sialography can be performed both for the parotid and submandibular salivary glands. It is contraindicated in cases of allergy to the contrast dye.

28.3.7 Ultrasound (US)

Due to the superficial location of the salivary glands, ultrasounds may be beneficial. High-frequency sound waves transmitted into the body will result in echo that will be captured to create an image in two perpendicular planes [15]. This image allows a very detailed but superficial study of the salivary glands. Ultrasound study has shown to be very effective differentiating intra-glandular from extra-glandular lesions as well as discriminating solid versus cystic lesions. Sialoliths are also visible and is helpful to determine glandular abscesses. When a malignant neoplasm or vascular lesions are suspected, Doppler ultrasounds can estimate the blood flow through blood vessels utilizing the same principle of high-frequency sound waves. Ultrasounds are a noninvasive and cost-effective procedure. The most significant limitation of ultrasound is the poor ability to evaluate the deep parotid lobe.

28.3.8 Radionuclide Imaging (RI)

RI or scintigraphy is a diagnostic test based on the ability of the radioisotope (technetium) to bind to salivary gland proteins and release to the oral cavity following the normal process of stimulation and excretion of saliva into the oral cavity. After an intravenous administration of the radioisotope, an external detector captures the radiation emitted to create a two-dimensional image. Only the parotid and the submandibular glands can be distinctly visualized [14]. It is considered a dynamic test because it allows for the evaluation of the functional performance of the salivary gland. It is also still considered a noninvasive procedure, since the wash out of the radioisotopes is reached quickly upon salivary gland stimulation.

28.3.9 Computerized Tomography (CT)

CT scan is the result of multiple X-rays taken from different angles and processed in a computer to create cross-sectional dimensional images of the organ to study. The advantage of this technique is in its ability to evaluate both superficial and deep, hard, and soft tissues in a great level of detail. CT is a versatile study; the application of contrast medium will enhance structures for a detailed evaluation of tumors, abscesses, blood vessels, and lymph nodes. This study is indicated to evaluate the deep salivary glands, when there is a concern for neoplastic process or a concern regarding the relationship to vital anatomic structures or when MRI is contraindicated. Some disadvantages include the radiation exposure and the distortion of the image due to dental materials, as well as allergies to contrast dye (iodine, barium).

28.3.10 Magnetic Resonance Imaging (MRI)

MRI uses a strong magnetic field and pulses of radio waves to generate detailed images of organs in different sections/planes. Changes of the pulse sequence (T1 and T2) enhance the structure depending on the nature of the tissue. MRI is highly recommended when neoplastic processes are suspected because of the exceptional capacity to highlight soft tissues with better contrast resolution than any other imaging. However, the ability to identify calcified lesion is not as robust as CT scan. The MRI has become the preferred imaging method for salivary gland masses assessment [16] and preoperative evaluation. MRI is contraindicated in patients with certain implants, claustrophobia, or difficulty keeping in an immobile position.

28.3.11 Positron Emission Tomography (PET)

PET is a functional imaging technique, useful to evaluate the metabolic process of the glands. The system captures gamma rays from a radionuclide after being introduced into the body. It is an accepted method to evaluate for malignancy. The combination of PET and CT has shown to be more accurate in the evaluation of metastasis. Treatment response and long-term surveillance are also common reasons to order a PET scan [17].

28.3.12 Salivary Glands Biopsy

Biopsy is the gold standard method to establish a definitive diagnosis on salivary gland tissue. Minor salivary gland biopsy is included as a major criterion to diagnose Sjogren's syndrome. A routine H&E stain should reveal lymphocytic infiltration into the salivary gland acini [18]. Minor salivary glands can also be used to diagnose amyloidosis, sarcoidosis, and monitoring graft-versus-host diseases [14]. The biopsy is an outpatient surgical procedure. After infiltration of local anesthesia, an incision is made in the inner lower lip mucosa. Blunt dissection should be done to expose the minor salivary glands with removal of five to ten glands. Regarding Sjogren's syndrome diagnosis, major salivary gland biopsies have not shown diagnostic advantage compared with minor salivary glands.

Biopsy of major salivary glands requires significantly more experience. Parotid and submandibular gland biopsies are approach extraorally in contrast with sublingual gland biopsy that is usually done intraorally.

Biopsies of major salivary glands are challenging due to their location and the surgical risk which could compromise vital anatomic structures. When open biopsies cannot be done, fine needle aspiration (FNA) represents an alternative to an open surgical biopsy. The technique is based on the ability to aspirate cellular samples from the gland using a needle, introduced manually into the salivary gland or occasionally with the aid of ultrasound imaging. The sample collected is sent for cytological evaluation.

FNA is widely accepted as a diagnostic tool for head and neck swellings, with high rates of accuracy 73–98% [19]. If the sample is limited or the cytology is report as inconclusive, an open biopsy may be indicated.

FNA has shown to be a reliable method used to differentiate between an inflammatory and a neoplastic process [20]. Fine needle aspiration is a convenient technique that does not require general anesthesia or preoperative testing; it is well tolerated by most patients, while being cost-effective and associated with minimal complications.

28.3.13 Serological Studies

Since salivary gland dysfunction has been associated with autoimmune and systemic conditions, certain laboratory (blood) studies assist in reaching a diagnosis. CMP will allow evaluation of blood glucose levels and help determining if salivary glands enlargement is associated, for example with diabetes mellitus. Other nonspecific blood tests for autoimmune markers, such as antinuclear antibodies (ANA), rheumatoid factor, erythrocyte sedimentation rate, and antibodies directed against

SSA/SSB, are particularly useful to aid in the diagnosis of Sjogren's syndrome. High amylase levels detected in the blood serum could be associated with inflammation in diseases such a viral or bacterial parotitis [21].

28.4 Orofacial Pain Disorders

Orofacial pain is understood as any painful condition involving the head, face, and neck area. The diagnosis and appropriate treatment are complex, because pain can arise from many different structures coexisting in a relatively small anatomic area. The numerous structures and their intricate innervation and functional interaction result in a wide range of diagnostic possibilities, often making interdisciplinary collaboration necessary to achieve a correct diagnosis and treatment [22].

Typically, patients with orofacial pain disorders consult multiple physicians before getting a correct diagnosis and definitive treatment. Clinicians treating patients with orofacial pain can avoid diagnostic errors by developing a careful and systematic method to obtain an accurate and comprehensive history and a thorough head and neck examination.

The differential diagnostic process should include broad various etiologies to pain, including neurologic, vascular, infectious, musculoskeletal entities and the combinations of them. The current definition of pain by the International Association for the Study Pain (IASP) includes the "emotional experience associated," which means that the painful experience is influenced by psychological factors. Okeson outlined a classification system where Axis I comprise the physical factors and the Axis II the psychological factors [23]. Both should be assessed to understand the etiology, the progression, and the prognosis of the condition.

In order to reach a diagnosis, it is important to understand the nature of the problem. Pain is subjective and dynamic and comprises sensations, emotions, and reactions [24], and all of these features require careful evaluation.

28.4.1 Chief Complaint and History of the Present Illness

Orofacial pain patients often present to the office with multiple complaints accompanied by a level of anxiety and frustration. It is favorable to gather all possible information and organize the data in a timeline to have an idea of the progression and severity of the pain. The clinician has to be aware that pain is subjective and is modulated by emotions and can be expressed or interpreted in different ways. For some patients verbal communication of complex symptoms is challenging, Providing examples (burning, stabbing, pressure, etc.) to the patient is often helpful to understand and categorize the complaint.

The clinician should aim to establish the onset of the symptoms, location, quality and quantity of the pain, duration and frequency, relieving and aggravating factors, associated symptoms, and past diagnostic tests.

28.4.2 Location

Starting by determine the location of the pain will help to figure the extension of the pain complaint. It is useful to ask the patients to use their fingers to point the area of pain. Also drawing on a head and neck diagrams can be a convenient method for a better understanding and communication between the patient and the examiner.

Because of the complex interactions between the multiple structures in the head and neck area, do not assume the location of the pain is the source of the pain.

28.4.3 Onset

Determine when the symptoms started and the circumstances that initiated the pain, are helpful as they might provide clues of the possible cause of pain. Local trauma such as car accidents, sport injuries, and/or dental treatment are often clear initiators. Cases with spontaneous onsets deserve a more detailed investigation. It is also essential to listen the patient's understanding of the time when the pain occurs, since it will also offer helpful signs for the diagnosis.

28.4.4 Quality

The characteristics of the pain can offer clues about the etiology. Classically different structures (nerves, muscles, teeth, etc.) express very particular types of pain quality. Even though the description is based on subjective symptoms, if the precise terms are used to describe the pain, different broad categories of disease entities emerge (musculoskeletal, vascular, neurologic, etc.) (Table 28.4).

28.4.5 Quantity or Intensity

The intensity of the pain is important to set as a baseline and to monitor the success or failure of the treatment. The intensity can be recorded verbally (mild, moderate, or severe) or numerically from 0 to 5 or 0–10. The visual analog scale is the most common and validated method used to categorize pain. On a 10 cm vertical line, labeled on one end with "no pain" and on the other end "worst possible pain," the patient is asked to make a mark wherever his/her perception is the level of the pain. Determining the severity of pain may also help to choose the treatment strategy.

Table 28.4 Quality of pain [24]

Pain	Feature
Musculoskeletal	Dull, aching, pressure, depressing, tightness
Vascular	Throbbing, stabbing, pounding, rhythmic
Neurologic	Bright, burning, itchy, electrical, cutting, lancinating, sharp

28.4.6 Timing

Timing includes duration and frequency of the pain episodes, which offers valuable information about the pattern of the pain. These features should be recorded in seconds, minutes, hours, days, or months. The episodes may be described as paroxysmal, episodic, steady, intermittent, or continuous, according to the case.

28.4.7 Modifying Factors

Modifying factors refers to those factors that seem to modulate the pain sensation, either aggravating or alleviating. As the head and neck area is involved in many vital functions (speaking, chewing, swallowing, etc.), some of those processes could aggravate (even trigger) or alleviate the pain. Other ordinary functions, like lying down, yawning, brushing teeth, shaving, and washing the face, could also be a trigger. It is important to inquire about parafunctional habits, either voluntary or involuntary (clenching, grinding, nail and lip biting). High levels of stress and poor sleep quality are often seen and identified as modifying factors. The patient should be advised to avoid known triggers and aggravating factors, while trying to alleviate with different strategies (cryotherapy, moist heat, massages) the pain.

28.4.8 Associated Symptoms

Due to the complex neurologic interaction in the head and neck area, multiple associated symptoms can be present. Autonomic phenomena, such as tearing, redness of eye, nasal congestion, and rhinorrhea, can be associated with myofascial pain and migraines [25]. These findings provide information of sympathetically mediated etiology of the pain. The examiner must to be careful to not confuse the main complaint with the concomitant symptoms.

28.4.9 Past Diagnostic Tests and Medications

By the time a patient consults a specialist, the patient probably has consulted other physicians and has been treated with several therapies and medications. Recording all previous treatments including over-the-counter products or by prescriptions, with their respective outcomes, will optimize patient care.

28.4.10 Cranial Nerve Examination

Cranial nerves provide sensory and motor innervation to head and neck structures. A systematic examination is essential and will facilitate a full assessment of the area. With simple testing a gross cranial nerve examination will bring information regarding the functioning of the 12 cranial nerve pairs, to rule out a central nerve component to

Table 28.5 Cranial nerve function [26]

Cranial nerve	Test
I Olfactory	Sense of smell
II Optic	Visual acuity and visual field
III Oculomotor	Eyeball movements, pupillary reflex, accommodation
IV Trochlear	Down and out movement of the eyes
V Trigeminal	Sensation on the three branches and masticatory muscles function
VI Abducens	Lateral movements of the eye
VII Facial	Movement of facial movements, special sensory taste (anterior 2/3 of the tongue)
VIII Acoustic	Hearing, equilibrium
IX Glossopharyngeal	Elevation of the palate, movement of the pharynx and larynx. Sensation of the palate and the posterior 1/3 of the tongue
X Vagus	Muscles of soft palate, base of the tongue, pharynx, and larynx
XI Accessory	Movement of the sternocleidomastoid and trapezius
XII Hypoglossal	Movement of the tongue

the patient's complaint (Table 28.5). Any deficiency or alteration should be recorded and addressed by referring the patient to the respective specialist (often neurologist).

If the patient is complaining about specific symptoms such as paresthesia and dysesthesia or if during the extra- and intraoral examination they manifest allodynia or hyperalgesia, sensory testing to objectively assess the symptoms should be performed. Light touch, pin prick, two-point discrimination, and thermal discrimination will help to "map out" the area of involvement.

28.4.11 Head and Neck Examination

The head and neck examination uses the basic principles of inspection, palpation, percussion, and auscultation. It is recommended to evaluate the TMJ complex, the masticatory and cervical muscles, the lymph nodes, and the thyroid and salivary glands.

28.4.12 Temporomandibular Joint (TMJ) Evaluation

A comprehensive understanding of the TMJ anatomy and biomechanics is vital to interpret the clinical findings of the TMJ evaluation. TMJ complaints are not limited to pain, but also TMJ sounds and alterations in the range of motion. To fully assess the TMJ, a static and dynamic evaluation has to be performed. With the fingers placed over the TMJ area, light pressure is applied to determine if there is local pain over the preauricular area to establish a diagnosis of capsulitis. The patient is instructed to open and close the jaw slowly a few times for a dynamic evaluation. The fifth digit is also placed into the ear canal while jaw movements are repeated. Pain while performing this test may be a sign of retrodiscitis.

Joint sounds from the TMJ are often signs of biomechanical and/or structural changes, which can also be assessed in a dynamic manner. With the help of a stethoscope placed over the TMJ area, the patient is asked to open and close few times. Distinct clicks are indicative of articular disc displacement. Also crepitus can be present in the TMJ, indicative of osteoarthritic changes of the TMJ. Joint sounds may or may not be accompanied with pain.

Movements of the TMJ are evaluated through the range of motion, in search of restrictions, interferences, or deviations. Alterations of the mandibular movement, either a deviation or deflexion of motion, help in the diagnosis of joint disease.

Maximum opening with and without pain, passive opening, protrusion, and lateral excursions will give information regarding the TMJ complex functioning. For maximum opening measurements, the patient is asked to open as wide as possible without pain (Fig. 28.7). If the patient is reporting pain while opening, he/she should stop and that distance measured. When the maximum opening with or without pain is obviously restricted, attempts to open wider with gentle distraction by the examiner should be performed. This passive opening maneuver results in a sensation of the stop being described as hard or soft.

Protrusion will provide information about condylar translation, and is assessed when the patient is asked to move the mandible forward. For lateral excursive movements, the patient is asked to slightly open the mouth and move as much as they can from side to side (Fig. 28.8). Value in millimeters should be measured and recorded.

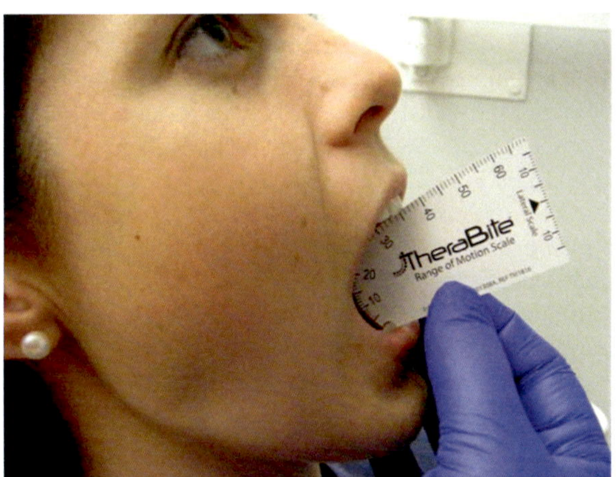

Fig. 28.7 Maximum opening measurement

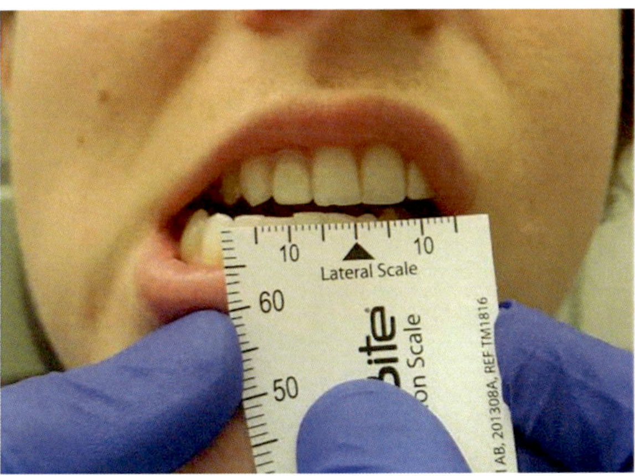

Fig. 28.8 Lateral mandibular excursions

This maneuver will provide information of muscular functionality and TMJ internal disarrangements. Restriction in movement will often indicate a medial or lateral displacement of the articular disc.

28.4.13 Muscle Palpation

Palpation is the best method to directly assess the masticatory muscles, seeking for tenderness or pain. Ultimately trigger points could be also identified. Normally, palpation of the muscles should not provoke tenderness. Muscular palpation often replicates the pain complaint when the muscle is involved. Once the source of pain is identified, the pain severity is recorded. It may be prudent to ask the patient about the use of analgesic prior the consultation, in order to consider its effect on the symptoms during the examination [27].

Through palpation, a muscular pain diagnosis can be easily established. Trigger points, which are hyperirritable foci located within a taut band or fascicle, are tender upon palpation and will reproduce a predictable pattern of referred pain [28]. Despite the lack of consensus for the diagnosis of trigger points, as a general rule, firm and steady pressure for few seconds has to be applied into the muscle in order to be able to replicate the referred pain pattern.

The temporalis and masseter muscles should be assessed extraorally, in addition, the sternocleidomastoid, trapezius and digastric muscles should also be palpated (Figs. 28.9, 28.10, 28.11, and 28.12). Intraorally the masseter origin, temporalis insertion, and medial pterygoid should be palpated (Fig. 28.13). For those masticatory muscles that are impossible to predictably palpate either intraorally or extraorally, such as lateral pterygoids, functional manipulation techniques could be used to assess their role in the symptoms. Protrusive movement, asking the patient to move the mandible forward, will test the lateral pterygoids muscles function as well.

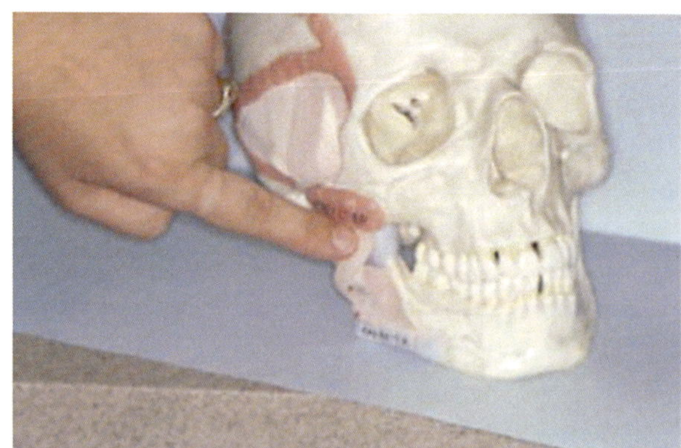

Fig. 28.9 Masseter muscle palpation

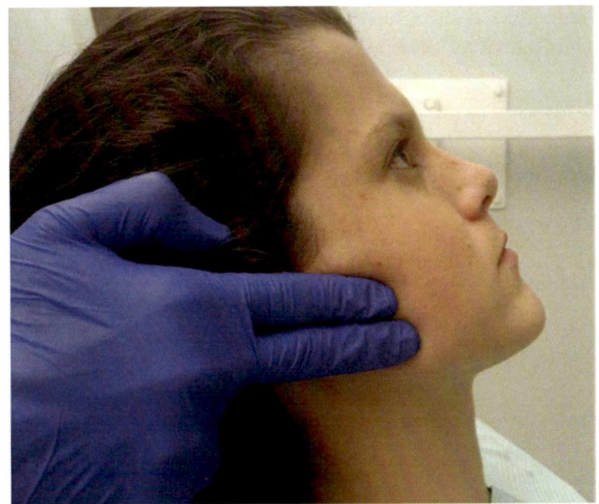

Fig. 28.9 (continued)

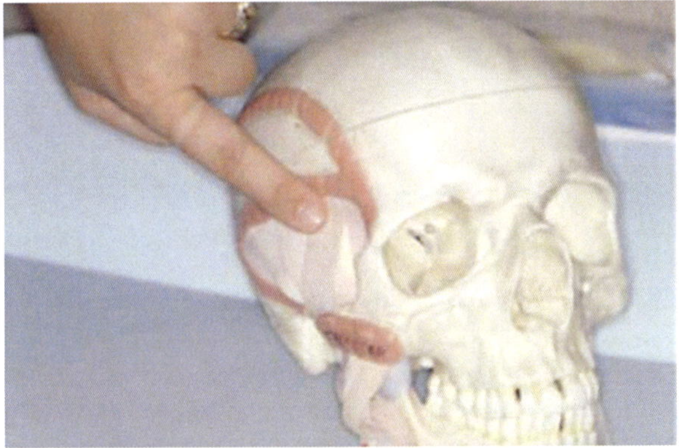

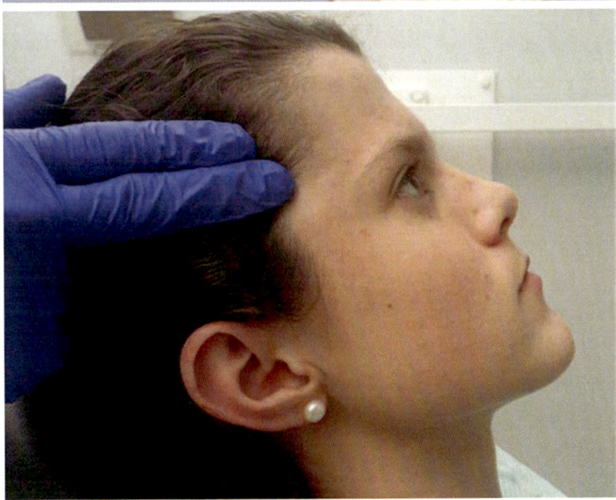

Fig. 28.10 Temporalis muscle palpation

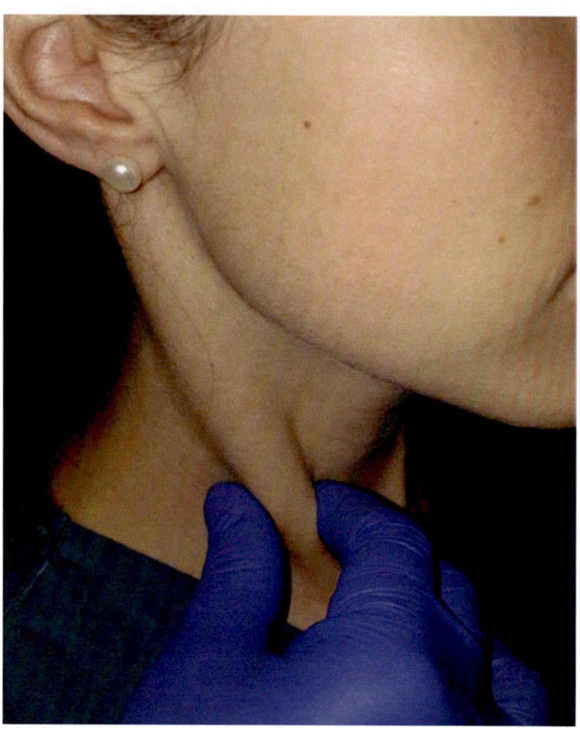

Fig. 28.11 Sternocleidomastoid muscle palpation

28.4.14 Oral Mucosa and Dental Examination

Even when the patient's symptoms do not seem to be odontogenic, an intraoral evaluation should be done. Intraoral findings reveal valuable information especially in regard to patient's parafunctional habits. Crenations on the lateral borders of the tongue and linea alba on the buccal mucosa are common findings in patients with bruxism. Generalized wear facets on the dentition are also commonly found in patients with parafunctional habits.

When the patient's pain complaint mimics dental origin, a dental evaluation should be considered, including radiographs or other imaging techniques, vitality tests, and percussion and periodontal evaluation. Pulpitis, dental fractures, and periapical processes should be also ruled out.

Occlusion should be grossly examined looking for changes. Currently there is no evidence to support the relationship between malocclusion and orofacial pain disorders. Changes in the occlusion can be considered the consequences of temporomandibular disorders rather than the cause [24]. A baseline evaluation allows monitoring the progression of any malocclusion.

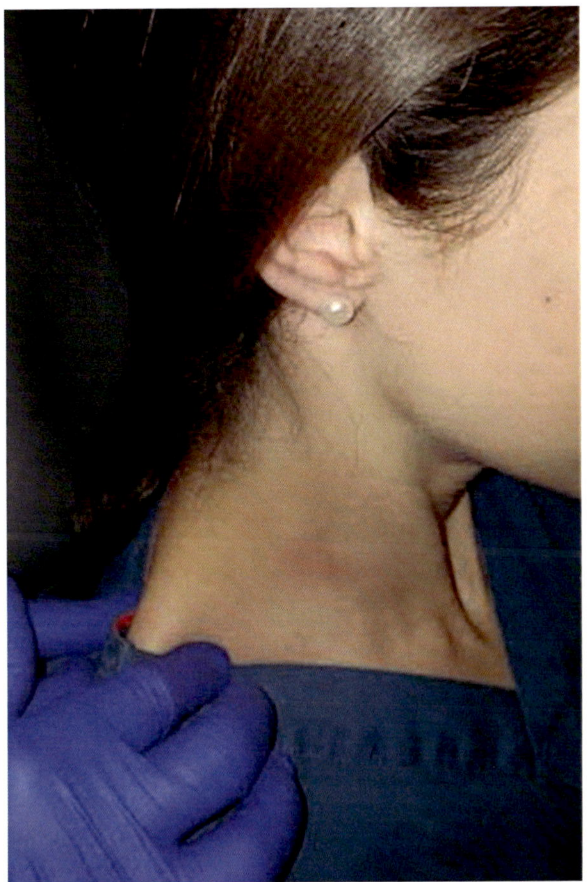

Fig. 28.12 Trapezius muscle palpation

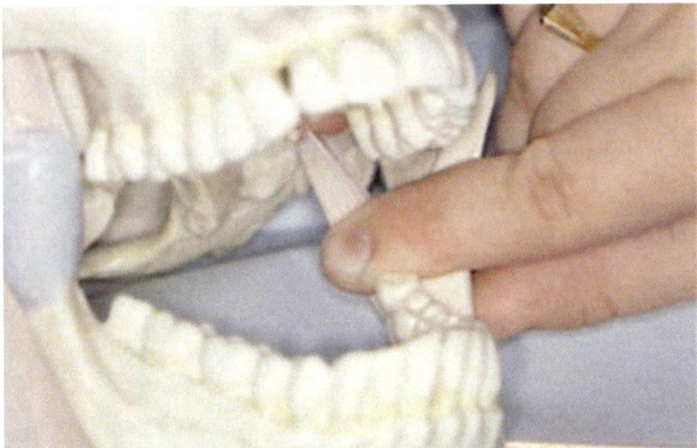

Fig. 28.13 Intraoral medial pterygoid muscle palpation

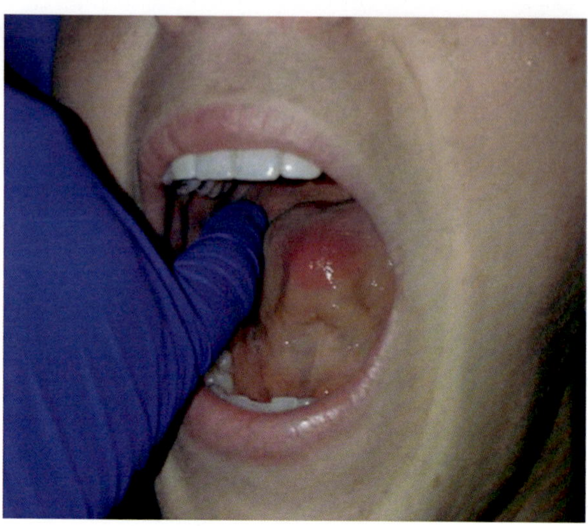

Fig. 28.13 (continued)

28.4.15 Diagnostic Anesthetic Injections

When the source of the pain is difficult to localize, anesthetic injections could be helpful. With a diagnostic block, the clinician might be able to identify the source of the pain and also differentiate a centrally mediated process from a peripheral pain process. There are three types of injections: muscular, nerve, and joint.

Muscular injections with local anesthesia are useful not only to help to determine the source of the pain but also have a therapeutic value, and it may help to educate a patient, regarding the concept of pain referral. Trigger points injections are targeted to an active trigger point. The therapeutic efficacy of trigger point injections is attributed to the mechanical disruption of the trigger point by the needling technique, rather than the anesthesia itself [24].

Nerve blocks are particularly useful to differentiate central sensation of pain from peripheral nerve pain and to identify the pathway that might mediate the peripheral process [24]. In few instances nerve blocks could also have a therapeutic effect. Some of the nerve blocks that are used in orofacial pain disorders are aimed to anesthetize the teeth (anterior, middle, and posterior superior alveolar nerve, inferior alveolar nerve, and mental nerve) and infraorbital nerve.

Joint or intracapsular injections can be of therapeutic value and are indicated when medications have to be released into the TMJ, usually corticosteroids or sodium hyaluronate. For diagnostic purposes a nerve block of the auriculotemporal nerve might help differentiate a joint source of pain from a muscular source [24].

28.4.16 Serologic Studies

Serologic examination is helpful to rule out rheumatologic conditions when there is some suspicion of a connective tissue disease. Rheumatoid factor and antinuclear antibodies (ANA) may provide helpful information when juvenile rheumatoid arthritis or systemic lupus erythematous is suspected. An erythrocyte sedimentation rate (sed rate) and/or C-reactive protein are nonspecific indicators of inflammation and useful to diagnose temporal arteritis in patients complaining about a throbbing aching pain in the temple area. Iron, ferritin, folate, and vitamin B 12 levels can occasionally be useful in patients with burning mouth syndrome, due to the known correlation between deficiencies in them and burning symptoms.

28.4.17 Temporomandibular Joint Imaging

Occasionally imaging is needed to establish an accurate diagnosis. Imaging is indicated in trauma, acute changes in occlusion, limitation of mouth movement, and crepitus and when systemic diseases, swelling, and infections are being considered. Imaging is also important if there is failure to respond conservative treatment [29].

28.4.18 Plain Films

Mainly panoramic radiographs are used as a baseline imaging to rule out an odontogenic source of pain and trauma and to evaluate hard tissue structures of the TMJ. A panorex provides a sectional view of the condyles and may reveal changes in the bone surfaces [30] (Fig. 28.14). An open and closed TMJ series can be done to evaluate the condylar translation and positioning. Other plain radiograph techniques such as transcranial view, transpharyngeal view, and anterior posterior (AP) view are available [24] but rarely necessary today.

28.4.19 Computed Tomography (CT)

CT allows the detailed examination of the bony structures of the TMJ on sagittal, coronal, and axial views. CT is mainly indicated to determine the location and extension of bone alterations: fractures, neoplasm, ankyloses, and degenerative changes [31]. An open and closed sequence can also be performed (Fig. 28.15).

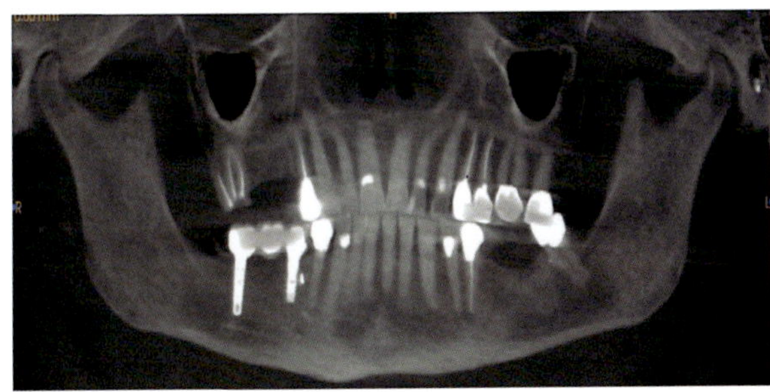

Fig. 28.14 Panoramic reconstruction (Courtesy Dr. M. Mupparapu)

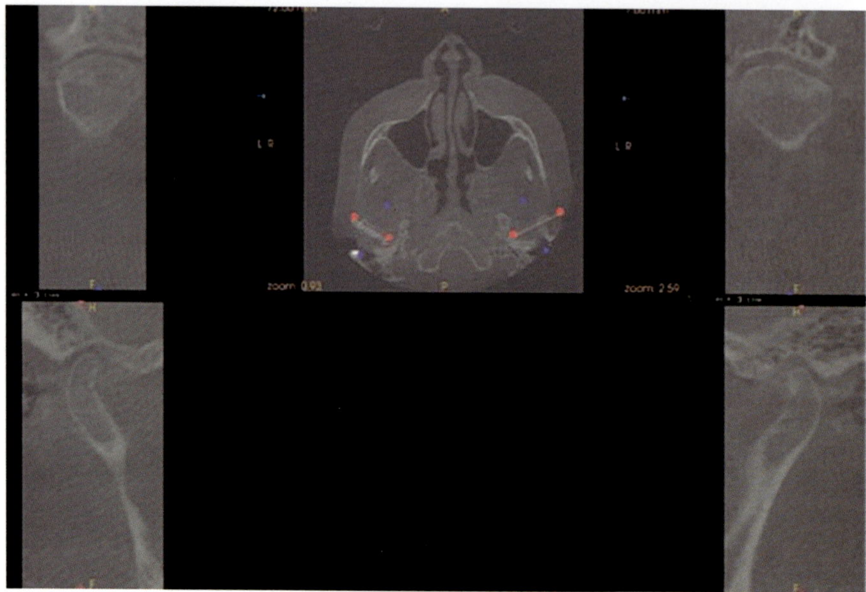

Fig. 28.15 TMJ CBCT showing axial, sagittal, and coronal views (Courtesy Dr. M. Mupparapu)

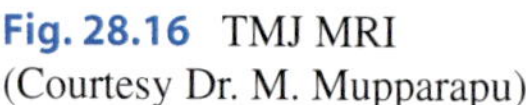

Fig. 28.16 TMJ MRI (Courtesy Dr. M. Mupparapu)

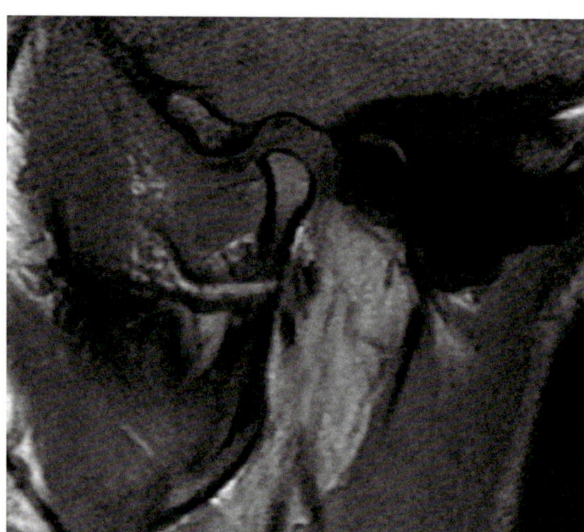

28.4.20 Magnetic Resonance Imaging (MRI)

MRI is a noninvasive (nonionizing radiation) technique based on the ability to capture the signaling from the hydrogen nuclei after a charge in a magnetic field [24]. MRI is used to evaluate the soft tissues of the TMJ, due to the great contrast resolution compared with other imaging techniques [32]. MRI is indicated to assess the position and shape of the articular disc, the presence or absence of fluid within the joint, and bony or synovial changes [30] (Fig. 28.16).

28.4.21 Behavioral and Psychological Assessment

As mentioned before, the pain experience is accompanied by an emotional component that often modulates the pain perception. Pain tends to escalates if it is chronic. When psychological factors (Axis II) predominate over somatic pain factors, therapeutic considerations are required [24]. Due to the known correlation between anxiety, depression, and somatization levels with orofacial pain disorders, the Research Diagnostic Criteria for TMD (RDC/TMD) included a questionnaire to assess the psychologic component [33]. Many other methods to screen or assess the patient psychologically are available and can be used depending on the clinician's experience in interpreting the results.

References

1. Sollecito TP, Stoopler ET. Clinical approaches to oral medicine disorders: part I. Dent Clin N Am. 2014;58:xi–xii.
2. Cole SA, Bird J. The medical interview: the three-function approach. St. Louis: Mosby; 2000.
3. Gomella LG, Haist SA. Clinician's pocket reference. 11th ed. USA: McGraw-Hill, Inc; 2007.
4. Cawson Roderdick A. Odell Edward W. Cawson's essential of oral pathology and oral medicine. 8th ed. Edinbourg, New York: Churchill Livingstone; 2008.
5. Patton LL, Epstein JB, Ross Kerr A. Adjunctive techniques for oral cancer examination and lesions diagnosis. A systematic review of the literature. JADA. 2008;139(7):896–905.
6. Neville BW, Damm DD, Allen CM, Chi AC. Oral and maxillofacial pathology. 4th ed. Canada: Saunders; 2015. p. 690–760.
7. Ettlin DA. Pemphigus. Dent Clin North Am. 2005;49:107–25.
8. Logeina B, Lionel F. Michel's transport medium as an alternative to liquid nitrogen for pcr analysis of skin biopsy specimens. Dermatopathology (Basel). 2014;1:70–4.
9. Christopher F, Bui DT. Anatomy, function and evaluation of the salivary glands. In: Myers EN, editor. Salivary gland disorders. Berlin: Springer; 2007. p. 2–16.
10. Sreebny LM, Schwartz SS. A reference guide to drugs band dry mouth -2nd edition. Gerodontology. 1997;14:33–47.
11. Villa A, Wolff A, et al. World workshop on oral medicine VI: a systematic review of medication-induced salivary gland dysfunction. Oral Dis. 2016;22(5):365–82.
12. Bowers LM, Fox PC, Ship JA. Salivary gland diseases. In: Burket's oral medicine, 13th ed. Connecticut, USA: People's medical publishing house; 2015.
13. Fox PC, Bush KA, Baum BJ. Subjective reports of xerostomia and objective measures of salivary glands performance. J Am Dent Assoc. 1987;115:581–4.
14. Pedersen AM, Bardow A, Jensen SB, Nauntofte B. Saliva and gastrointestinal functions of taste, mastication, swallowing and digestion. Oral Dis. 2002;8(3):117–29.
15. Evirgen Ş, Kamburoğlu K. Review on the applications of ultrasonography in dentomaxillofacial region. World J Radiol. 2016;8(1):50–8.
16. Villa A, Connell CL, Abati S. Diagnosis and management of xerostomia and hyposalivatio. Ther Clin Risk Manag. 2015;11:45–51.
17. Razaf A, Heron DE, et al. Positron emission tomography -computed tomography adds to the management of the salivary glands malignancies. Laryngoscope. 2010;120:734–8.
18. Astorri E, Sutcliffe N, et al. Ultrasound of the salivary gland is a strong predictor of labial gland biopsy histopathology in patients with sicca symptoms. J Oral Path Med. 2015;45:450–4.
19. Shah KSV, Ethunandan M. Tumor seeding after fine-needle aspiration and core biopsy of the head and neck – a systematic review. Br J Oral Maxillofac Surg. 2016;54(3):260–6.

20. Naz S, Khurshid A, et al. Diagnostic role of fine needle aspiration cytology (FNAC) in the evaluation of salivary gland swelling: an institutional experience. BMC Res Notes. 2015;8:101.
21. Nagy A, Barta A, et al. Changes on salivary amylase in serum and parotid gland during pharmacological and physiological stimulation. J Physiol. 2001;95:141–5.
22. De Rossi S. Orofacial pain: a primer. Dent Clin N Am. 2013;57(3):383–92.
23. Okeson J. Bell's oral and maxillofacial pain. 7th ed. US: Quintessence Publishing Co.; 2014.
24. de Leeuw R. Klauusser GD. Orofacial pain. Guidelines for assessment, diagnosis, and management. 5th ed. The American academy of orofacial pain. Chicago, US: Quintessence books; 2013.
25. Geghart GF, Schmidth RF. Encyclopedia of pain. Springer. 2013. p. 239.
26. Ilanit S, Martin G. Clinical assessment of patients with orofacial pain and temporomandibular disorders. Dent Clin N Am. 2013;57:393–404.
27. Romero-reyes M, Uyanik JM. Orofacial pain management: current perspectives. J Pain Res. 2014:99–115.
28. Simon DG. Understanding effective treatments of myofascial trigger points. J Bodyw Mov Ther. 2002;6:81–8.
29. Hunter A, Kalathingal S. Diagnostic imaging for temporomandibular disorders and orofacial pain. Dent Clin N Am. 2013;57(3):405–18.
30. Petersson A. What can you and cannot see in TMJ imaging-an overview related to the CDR/TMD diagnostic system. J Oral Rehabil. 2010;37:609–18.
31. Ferreira LA, Grossman E, Januzzi E, de la Paula MVQ, Carvalho ACP. Diagnosis of temporomandibular joint disorders: indication of imaging exam. Braz J Othorhinolaryngol. 2016;82:341–52.
32. Curry TS, Doedey JE, Murry RC. Christensen's physics of diagnostic radiology. 4th ed. Philadelphia: Lipincott Williams & Wilkins; 1990. p. 432–504.
33. Eric S, Richar O. Executive summary of the diagnostic criteria for temporomandibular disorders for clinical and research applications. J Am Dent Assoc. 2016;147:438–45.

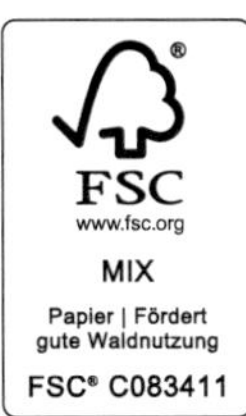

Zeitfracht Medien GmbH
Ferdinand-Jühlke-Straße 7
99095 Erfurt, Deutschland
produktsicherheit@kolibri360.de